Clinical Problems in Medicine and Surgery

P

Commissioning Editor: Laurence Hunter
Development Editor: Sheila Black
Project Manager: Sruthi Viswam
Designer: Charles Gray
Illustration Manager: Gillian Richards

Clinical Problems in Medicine and Surgery

THIRD EDITION

Edited by

Peter G. Devitt MBBS MS FRACS

Professorial Surgical Unit, University of Adelaide and Royal Adelaide Hospital, Adelaide, Australia

Jonathan Mitchell FRCP

Consultant Hepatologist, South West Liver Unit, Plymouth, UK

Christian Hamilton-Craig MBBS PhD BMedSci(Hons) FRACP FSCCT

Consultant Cardiologist, Cardiac Imaging, The Prince Charles Hospital;
Consultant Cardiologist, Heart Care Partners, Mater Private Hospital;
Senior Lecturer in Medicine, University of Queensland, Brisbane, Australia;
Assistant Professor of Radiology, University of Washington, Seattle, USA

Foreword by

Sir John Tooke DM FRCP FMedSci

Vice Provost (Health)
Head of the UCL School of Life & Medical Sciences and
Head of the UCL Medical School
University College London
London, UK

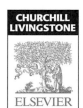

CHURCHILL
LIVINGSTONE

ELSEVIER

Edinburgh   London   New York   Oxford   Philadelphia   St Louis   Sydney   Toronto 2012

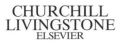

CHURCHILL LIVINGSTONE
ELSEVIER

First Edition 1992
Second Edition 2003
Third Edition 2012
ISBN 978-0-7020-3409-1

British Library Cataloguing in Publication Data
A catalogue record for this book is available from the British Library

Library of Congress Cataloging in Publication Data
A catalog record for this book is available from the Library of Congress

Notices

Knowledge and best practice in this field are constantly changing. As new research and experience broaden our understanding, changes in research methods, professional practices, or medical treatment may become necessary.

Practitioners and researchers must always rely on their own experience and knowledge in evaluating and using any information, methods, compounds, or experiments described herein. In using such information or methods they should be mindful of their own safety and the safety of others, including parties for whom they have a professional responsibility.

With respect to any drug or pharmaceutical products identified, readers are advised to check the most current information provided (i) on procedures featured or (ii) by the manufacturer of each product to be administered, to verify the recommended dose or formula, the method and duration of administration, and contraindications. It is the responsibility of practitioners, relying on their own experience and knowledge of their patients, to make diagnoses, to determine dosages and the best treatment for each individual patient, and to take all appropriate safety precautions.

To the fullest extent of the law, neither the Publisher nor the authors, contributors, or editors, assume any liability for any injury and/or damage to persons or property as a matter of products liability, negligence or otherwise, or from any use or operation of any methods, products, instructions, or ideas contained in the material herein.

ELSEVIER your source for books,
journals and multimedia
in the health sciences
www.elsevierhealth.com

Working together to grow
libraries in developing countries

www.elsevier.com | www.bookaid.org | www.sabre.org

ELSEVIER   BOOK AID International   Sabre Foundation

The publisher's policy is to use paper manufactured from sustainable forests

Printed in China

Contents

THE PROBLEMS

Contents

Contributors

Roger Ackroyd MD FRCS
Consultant Surgeon
Department of Upper GI Surgery
Northern General Hospital
Sheffield, UK

Narin Bak MBBS(Melb) GDE MPH FRACP
Consultant Physician
Infectious Diseases and Internal Medicine
Infectious Diseases Department
The Royal Adelaide Hospital,
Adelaide, SA, Australia

Wendy A. Brown MBBS(Hons) PhD FRACS
FACS
Associate Professor, General and Upper GI
Surgeon
Centre for Obesity Research and Education
Monash University Department of Surgery
The Alfred Hospital
Prahran, VIC, Australia

Philip Clelland MRCP
Specialist Registrar in Gastroenterology
South West Liver Unit, Plymouth, UK

Chris Deans MBChB(Hons) MD(Hons)
FRCS(Gen)
Specialist Registrar
Department of General Surgery
Royal Infirmary of Edinburgh
Edinburgh, UK

Andrew C. DeBeaux MBChB MD FRCS
Consultant General and Upper GI Surgeon
Department of General Surgery
Royal Infirmary of Edinburgh
Edinburgh, UK

Peter G. Devitt MBBS MS FRACS
Professorial Surgical Unit
University of Adelaide and Royal Adelaide
Hospital
Adelaide, Australia

Randall Faull MBBS PhD FRACP FRCP
Professor
Senior Consultant in Nephrology, Royal
Adelaide Hospital;
Dean and Director of the Medical Program,
University of Adelaide
Adelaide, SA, Australia

Robert Fitridge MBBS MS FRACS
Professor of Vascular Surgery
University of Adelaide;
Head of Vascular Unit
The Queen Elizabeth Hospital
Woodville, SA, Australia

Darren Foreman MBBS FRACS
Senior Visiting Urologist
Repatriation General Hospital
Daw Park, SA, Australia

Lucia Gagliardi MBBS FRACP
Consultant Endocrinologist
The Queen Elizabeth Hospital
Woodville, SA, Australia

Mark Gilchrist MB ChB MRCP
Clinical Research Fellow
Diabetes and Vascular Research Centre
Peninsula College of Medicine and Dentistry
University of Exeter
Exeter, UK

John E. Greenwood AM BSc(Hons) MBChB
MD FRCS(Eng) FRCS(Plast) FRACS
Director, Adult Burn Service
Royal Adelaide Hospital;
Director, Skin Engineering Laboratory
Hanson Institute; Associate Professor
Discipline of Surgery, School of Medicine
University of Adelaide,
Adelaide, SA, Australia

Sanghamitra Guha MBBS FRACP
Associate Professor
Director of Diabetes Services
Royal Adelaide Hospital
Adelaide, SA, Australia

Hubertus P.A. Jersmann MBBS MD PhD FRACP
Associate Professor
Respiratory and Sleep Physician
Interventional Pulmonologist
Department of Thoracic Medicine
Royal Adelaide Hospital
Adelaide, SA, Australia

Fiona Kermeen BMBS(Hons) FRACP
Transplant and Thoracic Consultant
Department of Thoracic Medicine
The Prince Charles Hospital
Chermside, QLD, Australia

Sujad Kiani MBChB FRCA
Consultant Intensivist
Department of Critical Care
Royal Derby Hospital
Derby, UK

Michelle Kiley MBBS FRACP
Consultant Neurologist
Director of Epilepsy Services
Department of Neurology
Royal Adelaide Hospital
Adelaide, SA, Australia

Timothy Kleinig MBBS(Hons) BA PhD FRACP
Neurologist
Royal Adelaide and Lyell McEwin Hospitals;
Senior Clinical Lecturer, University of Adelaide
Adelaide, SA, Australia

James Kollias MD FRACS
Consultant Surgeon
Breast and Endocrine Surgical Unit
University of Adelaide and Department
of Surgery
Royal Adelaide Hospital
Adelaide, SA, Australia

Richard J. Krysztopik MD FRCS
Consultant Surgeon
Department of General Surgery
Royal United Hospital
Bath, UK

Jimmy Lam BSc(Med) MBBS(Hons) FRACS(Urol)
Senior Visiting Urologist
Royal Adelaide Hospital
Flinders Medical Centre
Repatriation General Hospital
Adelaide, SA, Australia

Stephen W. Lam MBBS(Hons) FRACP FJFICM
Consultant Intensive Care Physician
Department of Critical Care Medicine
Flinders Medical Centre
Bedford Park, SA, Australia

Jamie Layland MBChB MRCP FRACP
Cardiologist
Department of Cardiology
St Vincent's Hospital
Melbourne, VIC, Australia

Gabriel Lee MBBS(Hons) MS FRACS
Clinical Associate Professor (Neurosurgery)
University of Western Australia;
Department of Neurosurgery
Sir Charles Gairdner Hospital
Nedlands, WA, Australia

Paul C. Leeder MBChB MD FRCS(Gen Surg)
Consultant General, Upper GI and
Laparoscopic Surgeon
Department of Surgery
Royal Derby Hospital
Derby, UK

Robert Ludemann MD PhD
Clinical Assistant Professor
Department of Surgery
Oregon Health and Sciences University
Portland, OR, USA

Naseem Mirbagheri MBBS(Hons) PGDipAnat
Advanced Trainee in General Surgery,
Monash University Department of Surgery
Monash Medical Centre
Clayton, VIC, Australia

Jonathan Mitchell FRCP
Consultant Hepatologist
South West Liver Unit
Plymouth, UK

Charles G. Mullighan MSc MBBS(Hons) MD FRACP FRCPA
Associate Member
Department of Pathology
St Jude Children's Research Hospital
Memphis, TN, USA

Roger J. Pepperell MDBS MGO FRACP FRCOG FRANZCOG FACOGHon
Professor of Obstetrics and Gynaecology
Penang Medical College, Malaysia;
Professor Emeritus
Department of Obstetrics and Gynaecology
University of Melbourne
Melbourne, VIC, Australia

Andrew W. Perry MBBS(Adelaide)
Emergency Medicine Registrar
Lyell McEwin Health Service
Elizabeth Vale, SA, Australia

Matthew Pincus MBBS FRACP
Cardiologist
Cardiology Department
The Prince Charles Hospital
Chermside, QLD, Australia

David Platts MBBS MD FRACP FCSANZ FESC
Staff Specialist Cardiologist
The Prince Charles Hospital;
Senior Lecturer, Department of Medicine
University of Queensland
Brisbane, QLD, Australia

Mohammed M. Rashid MBBS MRCP
Consultant Gastroenterologist and
Hepatologist
Western Sussex NHS Trust
Chichester, UK

Karen E. Rowland MBBS(Adelaide) FRACP
Senior Consultant, Infectious Diseases
Infectious Diseases Unit
Royal Adelaide Hospital
Adelaide, SA, Australia

Jonathan W. Serpell MBBS MD FRACS FACS
Director, General Surgery
Head of Breast, Endocrine and General
Surgery Unit
The Alfred Hospital
Melbourne, VIC, Australia

Cyril Sieberhagen MBChB MRCP(UK)
Hepatology Research Registrar
South West Liver Unit
Plymouth, UK

Sumu Simon MBBS MS
Ophthalmology Registrar
The Department of Ophthalmology
Royal Adelaide Hospital;
South Australian Institute of Ophthalmology
and Visual Sciences;
University of Adelaide
Adelaide, SA, Australia

Stewart Skinner MBBS PhD FRACS
Senior Lecturer and Consultant Surgeon
Monash University Department of Surgery
Alfred Hospital
Prahran, VIC, Australia

Richard A. Stapledon MBBS DipOBS RCOG
MPHC
TB Consultant
Department of Thoracic Medicine
Royal Adelaide Hospital Chest Clinic
Adelaide, SA, Australia

Duncan J. Stewart MD FRCS
Specialist Registrar
Department of Upper GI Surgery
Northern General Hospital
Sheffield, UK

James Sweeney MBBS FRACS
Head, Colorectal Surgical Unit
Flinders Medical Centre
Adelaide, SA, Australia

Sarah K. Thompson MD PhD FRACS
Consultant Surgeon
Department of Upper GI Surgery
Royal Adelaide Hospital
Adelaide, SA, Australia

Anne Tonkin BMBS MEd PhD FRACP
Professor and Director
Medicine Learning and Teaching Unit
Faculty of Health Sciences
University of Adelaide
Adelaide, SA, Australia

David Torpy MBBS PhD FRACP
Associate Professor
Senior Consultant Endocrinologist
Endocrine and Metabolic Unit
Royal Adelaide Hospital
Adelaide, SA, Australia

Usama Warshow MBBS(Lond) MRCP(Lond)
Hepatology Research Registrar
Institute of Biomedical and Clinical Research
Peninsula Medical School
Plymouth, UK

Toby T. Winton-Brown BA BSc MBBS(Hons)
MRCPsych
Clinical Research Fellow
Section of Neuroimaging
Institute of Psychiatry
London, UK

Andrew Zacest MBBS MS FRACS FFPMANZCA
Clinical Associate Professor University of
Adelaide;
Consultant Neurosurgeon
Department of Neurosurgery
Royal Adelaide Hospital
Adelaide, SA, Australia

Foreword

My own medical education began in earnest when I was able to relate the science of medicine to people – the individual cases that make up clinical practice. Their narratives brought medicine alive. As such experience builds, so too does the clinician's awareness of the range of different presentations of even the commonest condition. The third edition of *Clinical Problems in Medicine and Surgery* exploits this 'case-based learning' approach to great effect. A carefully selected array of important clinical problems covering a broad range of medical and surgical conditions provide the substrate for questions that probe the reader's understanding of the underlying pathology and, importantly, link the elements of the clinical reasoning process. The sequential approach adopted resonates with the intrinsic uncertainty of real clinical practice and the requirement to reassess as conditions change. Investigations, including imaging, are clearly presented.

It is increasingly accepted that problem-based learning instills a deeper appreciation of principles. So too does a requirement to reiterate these same principles in a different context – here the Points for Revision sections will prove to be of great value to the student of medical practice.

No compendium of clinical problems can ever be complete. But this is a compelling collection that can contribute much to the acquisition of clinical expertise. Importantly it is a stimulus to a rigorous reasoned approach to diagnosis and management, and the understanding of the scientific basis of medicine upon which sound medical practice depends.

Professor Sir John Tooke

Preface

We are pleased to present the third edition of Clinical Problems in Medicine and Surgery.

First published in 1992, the book has found great popularity with medical students and interns about to experience, or already experiencing, the real world of medical practice. We made a deliberate departure from 'traditional' medical texts in that the original book dealt with the real problems of clinical medicine through scenarios encountered in the emergency department, on the wards and in outpatient clinics: How to manage the comatose patient? How to manage the young man with chest pain? What to do with the rowdy, confused patient on the ward, or the jaundiced patient in the clinic?

Perhaps it was this hands-on, case-based approach which established and maintained its popularity. An often-heard comment has been '*it was the single book that got me through Finals*'. More importantly, however, this book should be recognized as an invaluable guide to the clinical care of patients.

The second edition was Highly Commended by the British Medical Association Book Awards. In this new Third Edition, the basic ethos has remained unchanged, but new cases have been added, the format altered, and the images and web-links updated. The book still relies on real-life medical scenarios to illustrate important everyday principles in clinical medicine, as feedback suggests this is what readers like. The successful format of case presentation, interspersed with questions and answers, and a final synopsis of key material, has therefore been retained.

With the assistance of expert colleagues across three continents, each problem has been revised and updated. For this edition new images reflect the extensive changes in the field of minimally invasive diagnostics. Searching questions have been added to guide the reader towards further self-directed learning.

Despite technological progress, the principles of history-taking and examination remain the cornerstones of sound medical practice. Advanced technology can best be applied if the clinician has taken the appropriate and correct history. Many diseases, however, remain disabling or lethal and in this setting a clinician's empathy with the patient's situation and the ability to counsel the patient appropriately and effectively are of paramount importance. These important aspects of clinical care have been emphasised throughout this edition.

This book does not purport to be an exhaustive text on clinical medicine. Nor is it a replacement for real-life clinical experience and the hands-on teaching of expert clinicians. It is designed rather as a wide-ranging source of information and a practical aid to the management of clinical problems.

Furthermore, we hope to instil in the reader a real sense of excitement and curiosity towards further learning. If this book provides half as much fun and thought-provoking issues for the reader as it has given to us in the writing, then we shall have succeeded in our major aim.

Peter G. Devitt
Jonathan Mitchell
Christian Hamilton-Craig

Adelaide, Plymouth and Brisbane, 2012

Acknowledgements

The visual material in the book has come from many sources and in particular we would like to thank Dr Elizabeth Coates (Fig. 51.2), Dr Angela Barbour (Fig. 5.2), Dr Robert Fitridge (Figs 22.3, 22.4, 23.1–23.4, 24.1–24.3), Dr Jim Kollias (Fig. 5.4), Prof Jeff Maki (Figs 38.3, 38.4, 38.5). The coronary angiograms were provided by Claudio La Posta, Chief Radiographer in the Cardiovascular Investigation Unit at the Royal Adelaide Hospital. The paracetamol nomogram is reproduced by permission of the Clinical Services Unit of the Royal Adelaide Hospital.

The Internet
(or 'Google's good to spot disease')

At the time of the last edition, the Internet had truly come of age and was already established as an almost endless source of medical information. But even then, nobody could have predicted how far it would have evolved by edition three. With one UK tabloid newspaper proclaiming that most diseases could be diagnosed by entering the symptoms into a search engine, could the art of the clinician be waning? And with smartphone apps for clinical scores, cutting-edge evidence-based medicine and entire formularies becoming *de rigueur* for any junior doctor, everybody at every level has the whole world of medicine at their fingertips.

There is no doubt that the Internet and advancing IT systems have revolutionized the way we practise medicine. Few of us can remember having to sift through great envelopes of X-rays in the outpatient department or relying on paper lab reports to work out trends and patterns. How did we cope without e-mail to manage our daily practice and keep up with the ever more complex pathways through which our patients move?

But while we wholeheartedly embrace these technological advances, even with a library of textbooks and journals available at the click of a mouse, the 'art' of medicine remains unchanged: using your knowledge to guide you, while remembering that not all patients or conditions follow 'textbook patterns'; recognizing the sick patient early and knowing when to call for help, realizing that communication is key and remembering that empathy and compassion are at the very heart of everything that we do.

As in the second edition, we have included some weblinks as a guide for each chapter, but remember that addresses change, sites are removed and much of the information on the web is not monitored or peer reviewed. Once again the website of the National Institute of Health in the USA is always a good place to start and the sites of national organizations can usually, but not always, be relied upon for up to date high-quality information.

Meanwhile, in our practice at least, the patients keep coming and there are no plans as yet to replace us with a keyboard and a fast broadband connection.

Normal range of values

Normal values will vary between laboratories. The following ranges are used for the cases described in this book.

HAEMATOLOGY

Haemoglobin	Male:	135–180 g/L
	Female:	115–165 g/L
PCV	Male:	42–52%
	Female:	37–47%
MCV	80–96 fl	
MCH	27–31 pg	
MCHC	300–360 g/L	
Platelets	150–400 x 10^9/L	
Leucocytes	4.0–11.0 x 10^9/L	
Granulocytes	2.0–7.5 x 10^9/L	
Lymphocytes	1.0–4.0 x 10^9/L	
Monocytes	0.2–1.2 x 10^9/L	
ESR	Adult male:	0–10 mm/hr
	Adult female:	0–20 mm/hr
	Elderly:	0–35 mm/hr

CLINICAL CHEMISTRY

Sodium	135–145 mmol/L	
Potassium	3.8–5.2 mmol/L	
Chloride	99–110 mmol/L	
Bicarbonate	22–30 mmol/L	
Anion gap	10–18 mmol/L	
Osmolarity	272–283 mmol/L	
Glucose	3.0–5.4 mmol/L (fasting)	
Urea	3.0–8.0 mmol/L	
Creatinine	0.05–0.12 mmol/L	
Uric acid	Male:	0.25–0.45 mmol/L
	Female:	0.15–0.40 mmol/L
Total calcium	2.20–2.55 mmol/L	

Ionized calcium	1.17–1.27 mmol/L
Phosphate	0.70–1.3 mmol/L
Albumin	36–46 g/L
Globulins	25–36 g/L
Cholesterol	<5.5 mmol/L
Conjugated bilirubin	1–4 µmol/L
Total bilirubin	6–24 µmol/L
GGT	1–55 U/L
Alkaline phosphatase	30–120 U/L
LDH	105–230 U/L
AST	1–45 U/L
ALT	1–45 U/L
Lipase	0–300 U/L
Amylase	30–110 U/L
C-reactive protein	0–5 mg/L

SERUM IRON STUDIES

Ferritin	Male:	20–250 µg/L
	Female:	10–150 µg/L
Iron	Male:	8–35 µmol/L
	Female:	10–35 µmol/L
Transferrin	25–50 µmol/L	
Transferrin saturation	Male:	10–55%
	Female:	10–35%

COAGULATION STUDIES

INR	1.0–1.2
APTT	25–33 seconds
Bleeding time	2–8 minutes

THYROID FUNCTION TESTS

TSH	
euthyroid	0.4–5.5 mU/L
hypothyroid	>4.5 mU/L
hyperthyroid	<0.3 mU/L
Free T4	
euthyroid	16–26 pmol/L
upper borderline	27–30 pmol/L
on adequate T4	15–35 pmol/L
Free T3	
euthyroid	2.1–5.3 pmol/L

| upper borderline | 8.1–10.0 pmol/L |
| hyperthyroid | >10.0 pmol/L |

ARTERIAL BLOOD GAS ANALYSIS (on inspired room air)

pO2	65–83 mm Hg
pCO2	35–45 mm Hg
pH	7.35–7.45
Calculated bicarbonate	22–32 mmol/L

LIPID STUDIES

Total triglyceride	0.3–2.0 mmol/L
Total cholesterol	desirable <5.5 mmol/L
HDL cholesterol	0.9–2.0 mmol/L
LDL cholesterol	desirable <3.7 mmol/L
primary prevention	<3.7 mmol/L
secondary prevention	<2.0 mmol/L
Total cholesterol/	
HDL cholesterol	desirable <3.5

SERUM CARDIAC ENZYMES

Creatine kinase	20–180 U/L
CK–MB isoenzyme	10–4%
Troponin (cTnT)	<0.03 ng/mL

OTHERS

Serum B12	180–1000 ng/L
Serum folate	
(fasting specimen)	2.8–15.0 µg/L

Difficulties with postoperative fluid balance in a 58-year-old man

Richard J. Krysztopik

A 58-year-old man is seen in the emergency department with abdominal pain and vomiting. He has been ill for 36 hours prior to this attendance, with increasingly frequent colicky abdominal pain, distension, and reduced bowel function. In the preceding 24 hours he has not passed any flatus and has vomited four times.

He had a laparotomy for a perforated appendix 5 years ago. Prior to this episode his general health had been good and his past medical history is otherwise unremarkable.

On examination he is in pain, apyrexial, and has a dry, coated tongue with loss of skin turgor. He feels thirsty and has a tachycardia of 115 beats per minute (bpm) and a (lying) blood pressure of 115/75 mmHg. On sitting, his pulse goes up to 135 bpm and his systolic blood pressure drops to 95 mmHg. Examination of his cardiovascular and respiratory systems reveals no significant abnormalities.

He is overweight, with a BMI of 30 kg/m² (height 174 cm, weight 90 kg). His abdomen is distended, with a scar from his previous laparotomy. There are no physical signs of abdominal wall hernia. His abdomen is tense and tender on deep palpation. It is resonant, but not painful to percussion. Bowel sounds are frequent and high pitched.

Q.1 Provide an interpretation of the history and physical findings.

The provisional diagnosis is this patient probably has small bowel obstruction secondary to adhesions.

Q.2 How should this problem be managed?

Blood is collected for haematological and biochemical analysis and an IV cannula placed for fluid replacement. Abdominal and chest radiographs are ordered. A urinary catheter is inserted and 350 mL concentrated urine drains. A NG tube is placed and 800 mL faeculent fluid is drained within the first 2 hours. His blood results are as follows:

Investigation 1.1 Blood results	
Haemoglobin	165 g/L
White cell count	9.6×10^9/L
Platelets	350×10^9/L
Sodium	149 mmol/L
Potassium	3.4 mmol/L
Urea	10.0 mmol/L
Creatinine	0.12 mmol/L
Chloride	112 mmol/L
Bicarbonate	29 mmol/L
Glucose	4.4 mmol/L
Bilirubin	19 µmol/L
Total protein	65 g/L
Globulins	27 g/L
Albumin	38 g/L
ALT	25 U/L
AST	39 U/L
ALP	74 U/L
GGT	17 U/L
LDH	110 U/L
Amylase	65 U/L
Calcium	2.16 mmol/L
Phosphate	1.15 mmol/L
Uric acid	0.21 mmol/L
Cholesterol	3.6 mmol/L

His abdominal X-ray is shown in Figure 1.1.

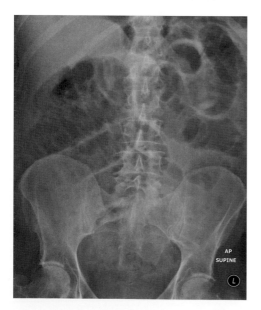

Figure 1.1

Q.3 Comment on the abdominal X-ray, blood results and haemodynamic measurements.

Over the next 12 hours the patient's symptoms fail to improve. His pain becomes more severe, initially more frequent and then constant. He develops increasing abdominal distension and tenderness. He becomes pyrexial.

Conservative management has not been successful and an emergency operation is arranged.

Q.4 What sort of fluid replacement is required before the operation?

At operation there are multiple adhesions involving the small bowel. These are released. A small segment of small bowel is strangulated, necrotic, but not perforated. This is resected and a primary anastomosis formed. A drain is placed.

Q.5 What fluid requirements are likely in the first 24 hours after surgery?

The morning after his operation the patient looks reasonably well and is afebrile. He continues on prophylactic intravenous antibiotics and is on patient-controlled narcotic analgesia. His blood pressure is 130/90 mmHg and his pulse rate is 90 bpm. His fluid balance chart for the 24 hours since admission is as follows:

Investigation 1.2 Fluid balance chart on admission	
Fluid Input	
IV fluids	4200 mL
Fluid Output	
Urine total	400 mL
Urine last 4 hours	22/16/12/0 mL
Nasogastric tube	700 mL
Wound drain	200 mL

With a bolus of 500 mL isotonic saline the urine output is increased to 50 mL over the next hour. A maintenance regimen of 1 L of isotonic saline is ordered, to be followed by 1 L dextrose 5% at 100 mL/hour and a replacement regimen of isotonic saline at 50 mL/hour using an infusion pump.

On review the following morning the patient had been given an additional 500 mL of dextrose 5% overnight when his urine output fell over a 4-hour period to less than 20 mL/hour. He now feels thirsty and there is loss of skin turgor. His abdomen is mildly distended, with absent bowel sounds, but soft and non-tender. His blood pressure is 110/65 mmHg on lying and 90/60 mmHg on sitting. His pulse rate is 100 bpm and he has a dry tongue. His fluid balance chart for the previous 24 hours shows the following:

3

Investigation 1.3 Fluid balance 24 hours later	
Fluid Input	
IV fluids	3700 mL
Fluid Output	
Urine total	800 mL
Urine last 4 hours	15/13/9/8 mL
Nasogastric tube	2800 mL
Wound drain	400 mL

The early morning electrolytes are as follows:

Investigation 1.4 Electrolytes	
Sodium	138 mmol/L
Potassium	2.7 mmol/L
Chloride	102 mmol/L
Bicarbonate	29 mmol/L
Urea	7.0 mmol/L
Creatinine	0.08 mmol/L

Q.6 Comment on this man's fluid balance and electrolytes. What fluids should be given to the patient over the next 24 hours?

Answers

A.1 Colicky abdominal pain, vomiting, abdominal distension and absolute constipation are symptoms and signs suggesting a diagnosis of intestinal obstruction. At initial presentation there is hyperactivity of the bowel leading to colicky pain and tinkling bowel sounds on auscultation. A prolonged period of obstruction can ultimately lead to a paralysis of the bowel with a disappearance of colicky pain and visible peristalsis.

The commonest cause of small bowel obstruction in developed countries is postoperative adhesions (accounting for up to 60% of cases). Abdominal wall hernias account for the majority of the remaining cases of obstruction, with malignancy and inflammatory bowel disease being other causal factors to consider.

Operative procedures most closely associated with subsequent adhesive bowel obstruction are appendicectomy, colorectal surgery and gynaecological operations.

Initially, obstruction of the small bowel leads to proximal dilatation due to accumulation of gastrointestinal secretions and swallowed air. This leads to increased peristaltic and secretory activity in the intestine (both above and below the level of obstruction), which can lead to initially frequent loose stools and flatus. As the degree of obstruction becomes more severe then constipation ensues and dilatation of the proximal small bowel leads to vomiting. The development of fever can occur late and may be associated with bowel ischaemia.

Answers *cont.*

This bowel dilatation is associated with compression of the mucosal lymphatics leading to significant bowel wall oedema. This, combined with increased secretory activity, leads to large third space fluid shifts with loss of electrolytes and proteins into the intestinal lumen.

The pain is often described as 'crampy' and 'intermittent'. This is more prevalent in simple obstruction. Development of more constant pain can be an indication of a more serious complication – suggesting strangulation or ischaemia of the bowel.

Small bowel obstruction can be either partial or complete, simple or strangulated. Uncomplicated obstruction due to adhesions most commonly involves the small bowel. Initially this is best treated conservatively as many episodes will subside spontaneously. Strangulated obstructions are surgical emergencies and if not appropriately treated can lead to vascular compromise – ultimately creating bowel ischaemia and perforation.

A.2 This man is clinically dehydrated and has signs suggesting small bowel obstruction. Initial treatment consists of the following measures:

- Fluid resuscitation – insert an intravenous (IV) cannula and begin resuscitation with 1 litre (L) of isotonic saline over 1 hour. The subsequent rate of administration can be adjusted once laboratory results are back and urine output assessed.
- Administer oxygen by face mask (2–3 L/min).
- Give adequate analgesia (most likely an intravenous opiate).
- Collect blood samples for haematological and biochemical analysis.
- A urinary catheter is often used as an initial measure in the management of fluid balance.

- Arrange for chest and abdominal radiographs.
- Arrange admission and contact a surgeon to give an opinion regarding the management of his likely small bowel obstruction.
- Bowel decompression – initially this can be performed by placement of a nasogastric (NG) tube for suctioning of gastrointestinal contents and to prevent aspiration.

A.3 The supine radiograph shows features of small bowel obstruction. There are distended small bowel loops in the centre of the abdomen with prominent valvulae conniventes. The bowel wall between the loops is thickened and oedematous. No air is seen in the colon or rectum.

However, in up to 30% of cases these radiological features may not be present on a plain abdominal X-ray. In such cases CT scanning can be useful in detecting small bowel obstruction as well as defining the lead point of obstruction and detecting possible aetiological factors or other causes of acute abdominal pain.

The blood results show the following:
- He has a normal white blood cell count.
- The high haemoglobin is probably a reflection of dehydration. This would be supported by an elevated haematocrit or packed cell volume.
- The biochemical values are abnormal with an increased urea, chloride and sodium – all are features of dehydration.

A.4 The key requirement is to correct any pre-existing fluid deficit prior to surgery.

Calculating the exact fluid deficit in patients can be difficult. However, an estimation of the degree of fluid deficit can be made by analysis of clinical signs. A

Answers *cont.*

patient who is thirsty, has dry mucous membranes, loss of skin turgor, tachycardia and postural hypotension is likely to have a loss of 10–15% of total body water. Fluid losses less than 5–10% of body water can be difficult to detect clinically. Once fluid losses exceed 15–20% there is marked circulatory collapse.

The volume of fluid required can be extrapolated from lean body weight. This patient weighs 90 kg but is overweight. His lean (metabolically active) body mass is nearer 70 kg. Fat is a relatively metabolically inert tissue and the percentage of fat relative to lean mass tends to increase with age. Calculations based on body weight alone in obese patients are likely to overestimate fluid needs.

In a 70 kg lean man who has thirst, dry mucous membranes, tachycardia and a slight postural fall in pressure, it is likely that he has a 10% loss of total body water. Body water itself is 60% of body weight and volume deficit is 10%×60% of 70 kg, or 10% of 42 L=4.2 L.

Vomiting or nasogastric aspiration results in loss of electrolyte rich fluid. Similarly, large occult losses occur in intestinal obstruction. Several litres of fluid may be sequestered into the gut contributing to hypovolaemia. These losses are largely isotonic and infusion of isotonic saline would be appropriate with potassium supplementation if serum levels indicate low levels.

Generally, half of this estimated loss is replaced quickly and then the patient re-assessed before replacing the rest, in this case 2 L of isotonic saline over 1 hour.

Resuscitation should be guided by improvement of clinical signs. The most important guide is a resumption of normal urine output (greater than 0.5 mL/kg/h),

stabilization of blood pressure, and reduction of tachycardia.

Careful monitoring of the patient's vital signs during this time is critical, particularly in the elderly or in patients who have associated cardiac disease. In these cases the use of a central venous catheter to measure central venous pressure may be helpful. It may be necessary to nurse the patient in a high dependency unit.

A.5 Fluid requirements in the postoperative period are intended to supply basal maintenance requirements and replace any ongoing losses (e.g. from pre-existing surgical problems, surgical drains, pyrexia).

Normal fluid losses (replaced with maintenance fluids) can be predicted with reasonable accuracy. Under normal circumstances fluid is lost through urinary losses, the gastrointestinal tract and insensible losses.

Fluid losses from the urinary tract are regulated by aldosterone and antidiuretic hormone (ADH). A fall in glomerular perfusion will trigger an increase in aldosterone leading to sodium retention within the kidney. ADH leads to retention of water in the renal tubules. Normal urinary losses are around 1.5–2.0 L/day.

The gastrointestinal tract secretes a large amount of electrolyte rich fluid into the gut. After digestion and absorption the remaining material enters the colon where much of the remaining water is reabsorbed. Approximately 300–400 mL are lost into the faeces each day.

In insensible losses air is humidified as it is inspired into the respiratory system and much of this water is lost with expiration. Fluid is also lost from the skin and these insensible losses can reach levels up to 700 mL per day. However, approximately

Answers *cont.*

300 mL of fluid are produced by endogenous metabolism – leading to a total 'insensible' loss of 400 mL/day. Insensible losses may also be increased by pyrexia or tachypnoea.

Under normal circumstances a 70 kg man needs 2.5–3.0 L of water, 100–150 millimoles (mmol) of sodium and 60–90 mmol of potassium to replace normal losses of water and electrolytes. These maintenance requirements can be met by appropriate intravenous volumes of isotonic (0.9%) saline and 5% dextrose. Isotonic saline contains 154 mmol of sodium ions in 1 L, thus 0.6–1.0 L will provide enough sodium replacement for 24 hours. A further 2.0–2.4 L of 5% dextrose will make up the additional water. An addition of 20 mmol of potassium to each L of fluid will provide sufficient potassium.

When patients undergo surgery this leads to an endocrine response with an increased production of ADH and aldosterone. This in turn leads to renal conservation of sodium and water and by way of exchange, loss of potassium. Potassium is released by damaged tissues during surgery and any reduction in urine output may also lead to impairment of potassium excretion. Usually more potassium is released by tissue damage than is lost in the urine and therefore any potassium supplementation is best guided by serum electrolyte levels in the postoperative period.

Replacement fluid is intended to replace any ongoing losses recorded in a defined period of time. In a previously well patient undergoing emergency surgery this period is usually the previous 24 hours but in seriously ill patients where there have been major fluid shifts or where there are elements of cardiac or renal failure, intravenous fluid adjustment may be required on a more frequent basis. In the

acutely ill general surgical patient fluid replacement is usually on a volume for volume basis with fluid of a similar electrolyte composition to that being lost. Nasogastric losses tend to be lower in sodium but not potassium and are typically replaced with 0.45–0.9% saline with 20 mmol/L of potassium. Gastrointestinal losses (either through a stoma or diarrhoea) have a slightly higher sodium level and similar potassium level – and can be replaced with normal (0.9%) saline with 20 mmol/L of potassium.

Where large volumes of fluid may be required then regular measurement of electrolyte levels is needed to monitor and tailor electrolyte replacement. More importantly, regular clinical examination remains critical in assessing fluid status (blood pressure, pulse rate and urine output).

A.6 The assessment for fluid requirements should begin with a careful clinical examination and a calculation of fluid losses and gains over the previous 24 hours. These show that the patient has lost more fluid than he has received; he is in negative fluid balance and hypokalaemic. He has clinical features of recurrent hypovolaemia, with oliguria, tachycardia, postural hypotension and loss of skin turgor. His mildly distended abdomen suggests likely ileus with ongoing sequestration of fluid into the small bowel.

His fluid requirements include maintenance and replacement fluids, including fluid to restore his existing hypovolaemia and correction of the hypokalaemia. A fluid bolus of up to 2 L of normal saline per hour should be given to restore urine output to at least 50 mL/hour. During this time the patient must be frequently assessed to ensure urine output

Answers *cont.*

returns and avoid heart failure by over-expansion of the intravascular compartment.

Potassium is predominantly an intracellular ion, and provided there is no acid–base disturbance, the serum potassium concentration reflects the total body pool. A serum potassium between 2.5 and 3.0 mmol/L represents a potassium deficit of 200–300 mmoL. The aim should be to replace 25% of this within 6 hours and 50–75% over 24 hours. Using a peripheral line, rates of replacement should not exceed 10 mmol/hour because of the risk of cardiac arrhythmia. With central access, 20 mmol/hour can be replaced without cardiac risk. Rates should never exceed 30 mmol/hour without cardiac monitoring. In this case with a potassium level of 2.7 mmol/L at least 150 mmol of replacement will be required over 24 hours along with ongoing maintenance to compensate for ongoing loss. After the initial replacement, losses may still persist. Further replacement should be guided by repeated serum potassium estimation.

Maintenance fluids are prescribed as already described: 2 L 5% dextrose (with 20 mmol potassium per L). Replacement should be the same in volume and electrolyte content as the losses they replace; particular attention should be paid to increased nasogastric losses, which have been 3.5 L in the previous 24 hours. There is likely to be additional loss from small bowel fluid sequestration secondary to ileus. These losses have been inadequately replaced. In general terms the gastrointestinal losses need to be replaced, litre for litre, with isotonic saline. Sodium (50–100 mmol/L) and chloride (100–140 mmol/L) losses into the stomach and small intestine can be matched reasonably accurately with isotonic saline. Potassium (5–15 mmol/L) must be added to the replacement fluids. In reality, losses of this magnitude in such a complex clinical setting will be replaced on an hour-by-hour basis and serum electrolyte concentrations monitored frequently.

Revision Points

Fluid Balance

Approximately 60% of body weight is made up of water.

In a 70 kg man, this is 42 litres (L):
- Two-thirds (28 L) is intracellular fluid (ICF).
- One-third (14 L) is extracellular fluid (ECF)
  - intravascular (3 L)
  - interstitial (12 L)
  - transcellular (digestive tract, cerebrospinal fluid (CSF), joints, aqueous, etc.) (1 L).

Volume changes may be due to:

- External losses (haemorrhage, vomiting or diarrhoea).
- Internal redistribution of extracellular fluid: for example, sequestration within the gut lumen (so-called 'third-space' loss). This leads to loss of effective ECF into a relatively non-functioning compartment. Only on resolution of the disease is this fluid eventually mobilized back into the effective ECF. Faced with such losses the body's priority is to maintain the intravascular compartment for adequate circulation.

Revision Points *cont.*

Fluid management requires understanding and calculation of three principal factors:

- correction of existing abnormalities
- maintenance of daily requirements
- replacement of ongoing losses.

Some examples of abnormalities include:

- intra-abdominal sepsis (isotonic fluid shifts from ECF to 'third space')
- vomiting or nasogastric tube drainage (electrolyte and water loss)
- dehydration (loss of ICF will lead to compensatory cardiovascular changes).

The aim of perioperative fluid administration is to maintain adequate intravascular volume and thereby optimize oxygen delivery to the tissues. Patients' fluid requirements can rarely be predicted accurately and can change dramatically from hour to hour. Prescribing using a formulaic approach without regular clinical review can lead to excessive fluid administration. Successful fluid management relies on careful anticipation of expected fluid losses and appropriate replacement. Repeated clinical assessment with measurement of pulse, blood pressure and urine output, to determine whether patients are hypovolaemic or overloaded, must be combined with regular measurement of electrolyte concentrations.

Issues to Consider

- How accurately can you clinically assess the extent of dehydration?
- What fluid solutions are available for use in the management of patients with fluid and electrolyte disturbances?
- Consider the differences in these solutions and work out the best combination of fluid and electrolytes for dehydration, paralytic ileus and vomiting caused by gastric outlet obstruction.
- What complications commonly occur as a result of inappropriate fluid prescriptions on surgical wards?
- What do you understand by goal directed fluid therapy?

Further Information

http://archive.student.bmj.com/issues/04/04/education/144.php *A didactic page on fluid balance.*

Shields, C.J., 2008. Towards a new standard of perioperative fluid management. Therapeutics and Clinical Risk Management 4 (2), 569–571. *A useful review of current thinking.*

Grocott, M.P., Mythen, M.G., Gan, T.J., 2005. Perioperative fluid management and clinical outcomes in adults. Anesthesia and Analgesia 100 (4), 1093–1106. *Another review.*

Postoperative fever

Wendy A. Brown

A 25-year-old woman presents back to the emergency department 10 days following an open appendicectomy for perforated appendicitis. She was discharged 5 days ago but she now has swinging fevers, rigors and complains of constant abdominal pain which is worse with movement and coughing. On examination her pulse rate is 100/min, blood pressure 110/80 mmHg, temperature 38.5°C, respiratory 10 breaths/min, and her oxygen saturation is 98% breathing room air. Her wound is red and swollen but there is no discharge. She is tender in the lower abdomen and on rectal examination an area of fullness is noted anterior to the rectum.

Q.1 What is the differential diagnosis?

As part of her initial management the patient will require some investigations and treatment.

Q.2 What investigations are required at this stage – and why?

While the various investigations are arranged, treatment must be started.

Q.3 What treatment is required at this stage?

A CT scan of the abdomen is performed. One slice is shown.

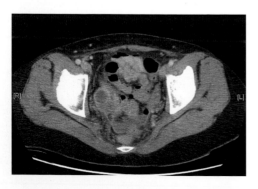

Figure 2.1

Q.4 | What does the image show and what should be done?

Answers

A.1 The most likely diagnosis is a pelvic collection or abscess. Other conditions to consider include a wound infection, urinary or chest infection. A pneumonia is unlikely given this clinical picture.

A.2 Her laboratory studies should include a full blood count (a leucocytosis would support the diagnosis of infection), C-reactive protein (inflammatory response) and electrolytes (dehydration). She is likely to have a septicaemia and blood cultures may help identify the organism(s) and help target antibiotic therapy. A chest X-ray and urinalysis are also required to exclude the respiratory and renal tracts as sources of sepsis. As the most likely source of sepsis is within the abdomino-pelvic cavity some form of imaging is required and a CT scan would be most appropriate.

As the patient is septic she may be coagulopathic and her clotting profile should be established.

A.3 Oral fluids must be withheld in case some procedure or operative intervention is required. Intravenous fluids should be started (see Problem 1) and broad-spectrum antibiotics given on a empirical basis. These should cover Gram-positive cocci and rods and Gram-negative rods and anaerobes. Possible combinations of antibiotics might include ceftriaxone and metronidazole or amoxicillin, gentamicin and metronidazole.

A.4 There are several collections of fluid in the pelvis and specifically in Morrison's pouch. There is also a small collection of fluid in the subcutaneous tissues in the region of the skin incision. The wound needs to be opened. Percutaneous drainage of the pelvic collections needs to be considered. If not feasible, the patient may require open drainage. The antibiotics must be continued and adjusted if need be, depending on the sensitivities of any organisms grown.

Revision Points

Fever is generally defined as a core body temperature of >38°C. It is a relatively common complication following surgery, with the incidence quoted as being 18–70%. When investigating the cause of a postoperative fever, both infective and non-infective causes must be considered. Common causes include the following:
• Pulmonary tract. Fever in the immediate postoperative period is usually secondary to atelectasis. If this is not treated it may progress to pneumonia. Another cause of fever may be aspiration pneumonia.
• Urinary tract (common in patients with indwelling catheters). Generally present on days 3–5 postoperatively.
• Cellulitis in venous access sites, typically occurring days 3–5 postoperatively.
• Surgical wound infections. Generally present 5–7 days postoperatively.
• Intra-abdominal sepsis from abscess is considered after the 5th to 7th postoperative day.

Revision Points *cont.*

• Occasionally the blood may become seeded with bacteria (bacteraemia or septicaemia depending on the clinical presentation). This is usually from contamination of central catheters, particularly in critically ill patients in intensive care units. This may occur at any time, but is more common after day 7 postoperatively.

• Deep venous thrombosis. Typically occurs on day 5–10 postoperatively and is more common in patients who are not mobile.

• Drug fevers are uncommon and are a diagnosis of exclusion.

The time of onset of fever in relation to the surgery can be a useful guide in assessment and determining the underlying cause (Figure 2.2).

When assessing a patient with a postoperative fever it is important to consider the surgery that has been performed, as the risk of complications is directly related to the nature of the surgical procedure and this may guide the investigations. The risk of infection depends on the bacterial load related to the operation (Box 2.1). Similarly, other causes of postoperative fever are more common following certain operations, for example venous thrombo-embolic events are high risks following orthopaedic operations.

When assessing a patient who has a postoperative fever a complete history of symptoms must be taken. These include:

• history and nature of the fever (constant or intermittent)
• associated sweats or rigors
• wound problems (pain, redness, discharge)
• pulmonary problems (cough, dyspnoea, pleuritic pain, haemoptysis, sputum production)
• urinary problems (dysuria, haematuria, discoloration of urine)
• calf pain and tenderness

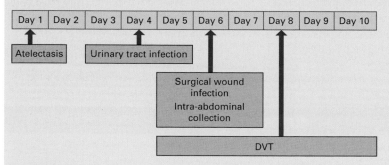

Figure 2.2

Box 2.1 Classification of risk of postoperative infection

• CLEAN operative sites – typically elective procedures (e.g. hernia repair) with 1–2% risk of infection
• CLEAN CONTAMINATED operative sites (e.g. hysterectomy, cholecystectomy) are exposed to some bacteria and risk of infection is 5–15%
• CONTAMINATED operative sites (e.g. colectomy, gastrectomy) are exposed to a significant bacterial load and have a risk of infection of 10–20%
• DIRTY operative sites (e.g. perforated divericulum, pilonidal abcess) have been exposed to a significant bacterial load and the risk of postoperative infection is >50%

Revision Points *cont.*

- cannula site problems (pain, erythema, swelling).

The examination should cover the major sources of postoperative fever listed above and if the patient has had abdominal surgery, a careful rectal examination may be useful to identify a pelvic collection. The standard investigations are those discussed in the case and will often also involve imaging of the operative site, the CT scan being favoured for potential intra-abdominal sepsis. The principles of treatment include tailored antibiotic therapy, drainage of any localized collection and removal of infected foreign materials (e.g. skin sutures, intravenous cannulae or an indwelling urinary catheter). The indications for antibiotics include:

- spreading infection
- septicaemia
- immunocompromise
- presence of a prosthesis such as a heart valve or joint replacement.

Adhering to the principle that prevention is better than cure, all reasonable measures should be taken to reduce the risks of postoperative complications, particularly infection and venous thromboembolism. These include:

- sound aseptic techniques (hand scrubbing, skin preparation)
- appropriate use of prophylactic antibiotics
- good surgical techniques (tissue handling, avoidance of ischaemia, leaving infected wounds open)
- graduated stockings, sequential compression devices and low molecular weight heparin.

Antibiotics should be used on a prophylactic basis for those at increased risk of infection through the type of procedure to be performed (contaminated and dirty procedures – see Box 2.1). Two other groups of patients likely to require prophylactic antibiotics, no matter what the type of procedure, are (i) those who might be immunocompromised (diabetes, steroids, cytotoxic therapy) and (ii) those who have prostheses (e.g. heart valves) in whom any infection could have disastrous consequences. Other patients at increased risk of infection include the obese, those who are malnourished, the anaemic and those who suffer with alcoholism.

In the postoperative period attention must be paid to appropriate analgesia to facilitate early mobilization, deep breathing and coughing and so reduce the chance of chest infection and venous thrombo-embolic problems. Any indwelling device (intravenous cannulae, bladder catheters) should be removed as early as possible.

Issues to Consider

- Would the risk of postoperative infection have been reduced in this case if a laparoscopic procedure had been performed?
- Does bowel preparation prior to elective colonic surgery reduce the risk of infection?

Further Information

Antibiotic Guidelines version 13, 2006. http://www.tg.org.au/

Garibaldi, R.A., Cushing, D., Lerer, T., 1991. Risk factors for postoperative infection. American Journal of Medicine 91 (3B), 158S–163S.

Postoperative hypotension

Paul C. Leeder and Sujad Kiani

You are the resident on call for general surgery and called to the ward to review a 70-year-old man who has become increasingly unwell over the course of the day. The nursing staff are concerned about his deterioration. Five days earlier the patient had undergone an Ivor Lewis oesophagogastrectomy and spent the first 3 days uneventfully on the intensive care unit. He was making satisfactory progress and was transferred to the surgical ward on day 3.

Over the last 12 hours the patient has become more short of breath, his oxygen requirements have gone up and he is now becoming confused and trying to pull his cannulae out. The nurses were concerned that his blood pressure had fallen to 80/50 mmHg.

> **Q.1** What is your differential for the cause of hypotension in this patient?

With the various possibilities in mind, you head towards the ward.

> **Q.2** What sources of information should you seek before you examine the patient?

On arrival at the ward you quickly read the patient's notes to aid your assessment. The man had a 2 month history of dysphagia prior to his diagnosis of oesophageal adenocarcinoma. He was treated with a 6 week course of chemotherapy prior to his surgery. His past medical history included controlled hypertension and reflux, for which he was taking bendroflumethiazide and esomeprazole respectively. He is an ex-smoker with a 40 pack-year history.

He had been making an uneventful recovery from his surgery although his gut has not yet started to function. You note from his charts that a tachycardia has developed over the last 24 hours. Over the last 3 hours his urine output has dropped from over 30 mL/hour to 10 mL/hour. His temperature is 38.4°C. You read the operation record and note that the procedure was uncomplicated and a primary anastomosis was performed. A broad-spectrum antibiotic was given prophylactically and continued for 48 hours.

You attend the patient. He is overweight and you estimate his body mass index (BMI) to be 30. He is slouched in the bed with an oxygen mask on his forehead. He has a triple-lumen central line with a bag of saline attached. An epidural catheter is in situ. His chest drain contains a total of 200 mL of sero-sanguinous material, and there is 300 mL of bile-stained fluid in the nasogastric drainage bag and 400 mL in the urinary catheter bag. All the bags were emptied 12 hours earlier. A feeding jejunostomy is running at 40 mL/hour. Little history is available from the patient because of his confusion.

14

Q.3 What will you look for in your examination?

Before you examine the patient more closely you replace his oxygen mask over his mouth and nose and check that his intravenous fluid is running freely. He is mildly confused and is unable to answer your questions appropriately. His skin is pale and clammy and his pulse is faint but regular at 120/min. You confirm his blood pressure to be 85/65 mmHg. He has a tachypnoea of 28 breaths per minute and oxygen saturations are 87%. He already has peripheral venous access and a triple-lumen central line that was inserted during the operation. Both insertion sites look clean and dry. His JVP is not visible and his tongue is dry. His heart sounds are normal.

His lung examination reveals a dull percussion note and absent breath sounds in the lower third of both lung bases. There are associated crepitations at both mid and basal zones. The upper lung fields are clear. The thoracotomy wound looks clean. The chest drain sites are erythematous but dry (the apical drain was removed 2 days earlier). The drainage bottle contains turbid sero-sanguinous fluid and the fluid level swings with deep respiration.

His abdomen is mildly distended, but soft, with minimal wound tenderness to deep palpation. There are no localizing signs. The abdominal wound looks clean and dry, as are the drain and jejunostomy sites. Bowel sounds are absent.

His urine appears concentrated but clear. He has bilateral lower limb oedema, although his calves are not tender.

Q.4 How would you manage this situation? What would be your initial treatment strategy and what investigations would you perform?

The patient is transferred to the high dependency unit for resuscitation and further management. A bolus of intravenous isotonic saline is given and blood samples collected for laboratory analysis.

The following results become available:

Investigation 3.1 Summary of results

Haemoglobin	105 g/L	White cell count	17.0×10^9/L
Platelets	350×10^9/L	Neutrophils 88%	15.0×10^9/L
PCV	0.39	Lymphocytes 7%	1.2×10^9/L
MCV	86.9 fL	Monocytes 3%	0.5×10^9/L
MCH	29.5 pg	Eosinophils 1%	0.2×10^9/L
MCHC	340 g/L	Basophils 1%	0.2×10^9/L
Sodium	140 mmol/L	Calcium	2.16 mmol/L
Potassium	5.4 mmol/L	Phosphate	1.15 mmol/L
Chloride	106 mmol/L	Total protein	39 g/L
Bicarbonate	18 mmol/L	Albumin	20 g/L
Urea	15.3 mmol/L	Globulins	20 g/L
Creatinine	0.21 mmol/L	Bilirubin	16 µmol/L
Uric acid	0.24 mmol/L	ALT	40 U/L
Glucose	4.4 mmol/L	AST	42 U/L
Cholesterol	3.5 mmol/L	GGT	17 U/L
LDH	151 U/L	ALP	105 U/L

Investigation 3.2 Arterial blood gas analysis on room air	
pO$_2$ 52 mmHg	pCO$_2$ 34 mmHg
pH 7.29	Base excess −9.5

Q.5 What do these results indicate?

Q.6 What do you think is wrong with this patient?

A portable chest X-ray is performed (Figure 3.1).

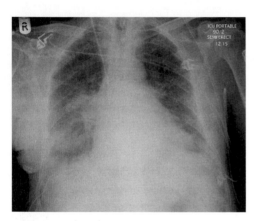

Figure 3.1

Q.7 What does the chest X-ray show?

Q.8 What further investigations will help in the management of this patient and how should treatment proceed?

The patient responds well to your resuscitation measures and his hypotension corrects with intravenous fluid. He is started on broad-spectrum intravenous antibiotics, avoiding aminoglycosides due to concern about nephrotoxicity.

The chest effusions are further visualized with a contrast-enhanced CT scan of the chest and abdomen. One sequence is shown (Figure 3.2).

Figure 3.2

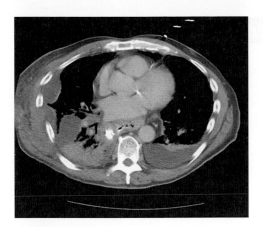

Q.9 What does the CT scan show?

The right-sided pleural collection is drained percutaneously under radiological control. The material is sanguinous and a sample sent for culture grows enterococci, sensitive to the antibiotics you have prescribed. A chest drain is left in the cavity (and removed after a week). His condition rapidly improves over the next 48 hours. An oral contrast study is performed which does not show any evidence of an anastomotic leakage. The postoperative recovery progresses slowly, but without further mishap.

Answers

A.1 The confusion and hypotension suggest this patient is suffering from shock. Shock is defined as inadequate tissue perfusion. The common signs are related to a reduced oxygen delivery to the tissues. There is commonly a loss in effective circulating blood volume. As this occurs, physiological compensatory mechanisms are initiated, with the primary aim of maintaining oxygen delivery to the vital organs, namely the brain, heart and kidneys. As this compensation fails, so the signs of shock develop.

The causes of shock can be classified into those caused by a loss in total blood volume, or where an effective loss occurs due to volume redistribution. Loss of volume can occur with internal or external blood loss, loss in plasma volume secondary to burns, or fluid loss most commonly from the gastrointestinal tract. Volume redistribution can occur secondary to vasodilatation and increased capillary permeability, most frequently seen in sepsis, anaphylaxis or following acute spinal injury.

Cardiogenic shock occurs secondary to a primary pump failure.

There are several potential causes in this case:

1. Hypovolaemia.

This is an important cause of hypotension in the postoperative patient. In this case it could be due to:

Answers *cont.*

- haemorrhage
- gastrointestinal 'third-space' losses (e.g. ileus) with inadequate fluid replacement and subsequent dehydration.

2. Sepsis.

There are many potential sites for infection in the postoperative setting. Look for the presence of a fever that, in the case of an infected collection, may be 'swinging' in nature. This patient had surgery for an oesophageal cancer. There is a significant risk of leak from the gastro-oesophageal anastomosis. Other potential sources of infection are the respiratory tract (retained sputum and inadequate cough reflex), the urinary tract (catheterization) and from intravenous access sites.

3. Low cardiac output.

Cardiogenic shock following an acute myocardial infarct is a common cause for sudden hypotension and requires exclusion. Look for serial ECG changes and a rise in cardiac enzymes, including troponins.

Pulmonary embolus also occurs in the postoperative period and if suspected will need to be excluded with spiral CT. A normal D-dimer blood test has a high specificity for excluding emboli. A high level can occur postoperatively and as such is relatively non-specific – other investigations may be required.

Other cardiac causes include arrhythmias.

4. Anaphylaxis.

Attention must be paid to any medication or blood transfusion that has been commenced over the postoperative period. Penicillin hypersensitivity is common, but be aware that 10% of patients have a cross-sensitivity with cephalosporins.

Anaphylaxis will require emergency treatment with fluid resuscitation, adrenaline (epinephrine) and hydrocortisone.

Signs of shock differ according to the cause and its severity. A previously fit adult can lose 15% of their effective blood volume with minimum, transient effects such as mild tachypnoea. Physiological mechanisms will restore blood volume within 24 hours. This is equivalent to donating blood.

Loss of 30% of blood volume can result in tachycardia and narrowing of pulse pressure (the difference between systolic and diastolic blood pressure). This reduces due to compensatory vasoconstriction producing a rise in diastolic pressure. Urine output may reduce and become more concentrated, due to an increase in ADH (antidiuretic hormone).

Loss of more than 40% of effective blood volume (2000 mL) will normally result in a falling systolic blood pressure and tachycardia, as physiological mechanisms fail to compensate adequately. Patients often become confused owing to reduced cerebral perfusion. Urgent action is required as further loss in circulating volume may be fatal.

You have these thoughts in mind as you head towards the ward.

A.2 Additional information may be available from several sources:

1. As the patient is confused and may not be able to give much history, the nursing staff may be able to provide information on:
   - any symptoms (e.g. chest pain, dyspnoea, chills or rigors)
   - any evidence of blood loss from either the operative site (wound drains) or the digestive tract (bloody return from a nasogastric tube or blood per rectum).

Answers *cont.*

2. The patient record should be studied for information on:
   - the vital signs: recent changes in blood pressure and temperature (the presence of a fever will suggest underlying infection and sepsis)
   - the fluid balance chart: a negative fluid balance and falling weight over the preceding days is in favour of dehydration
   - any medications or blood products the patient has recently received: a recent transfusion or change in antibiotics may point toward anaphylaxis.
3. Ask for the medical records and review the patient's past medical history. Regardless of the cause of the current deterioration, this will be important knowledge in the current management of the patient.

A.3   You must do a speedy, efficient but thorough assessment of the patient looking for clues as to the underlying cause of the shock. In a methodical manner you will:
- adopt an **ABC** (Airway, Breathing, Circulation) approach
- look for evidence of circulatory collapse
- try to identify the underlying cause of the collapse.

Start by taking the pulse and recheck the blood pressure. As you feel the pulse you should check the perfusion of the peripheries by observing the temperature of the hands and feet.

Consider the following:
1. Sepsis.
   Look for evidence of systemic vasodilatation such as warm, flushed peripheries and a hyperdynamic circulation. In other forms of shock, such as volume depletion or haemorrhage, there is peripheral vasoconstriction and the extremities are cool and 'shut down'.
   Look also for sources of infection such as:
   - Thorax: pleural effusion secondary to retained fluid or anastomotic leak. Signs of a respiratory tract infection (pneumonia).
   - Heart: endocarditis.
   - Abdomen: intra-abdominal collection secondary to bleeding or an anastomotic leak or a feeding tube complication. Look for signs of peritonism.
   - Wounds: look for cellulitis, swelling, discharge.
   - Venous access sites: discharge, erythema. How long have the cannulae been in?
   - Drain and jejunostomy sites – any evidence of leakage or infection?
   - Urinary tract: indwelling catheter.
2. Hypovolaemia.
   - Look for evidence of dehydration such as dry mucous membranes, lack of skin turgor.
   - Look at the nature and amount of urine in the urinary drainage bag.
   - Haemorrhage may not be immediately obvious. Examine drains, gastric aspirates and perform a rectal examination if gastrointestinal bleeding is suspected.
3. Cardiogenic.
   - A raised JVP may indicate cardiac failure or pulmonary embolism.
   - Look also for other signs of heart failure such as the presence of pulmonary oedema.
   - Examine the legs for evidence of deep venous thrombosis.
4. Anaphylaxis.
   - Look for a skin rash, angioedema and the presence of wheeze.

19

Answers *cont.*

A.4   The patient requires prompt resuscitation (**A**, **B**, **C**):

- **A + B** – commence high-flow oxygen. A non-rebreathing mask can help to improve high concentration oxygen delivery. Attach a pulse oximeter.
- **C** – ensure there is adequate intravenous access. Look for a wide bore (12 and 14 gauge) peripheral catheter line, which can deliver a higher flow than a central line and is preferred in emergency resuscitation.
- Commence rapid intravenous fluid replacement. Either crystalloid (e.g. isotonic saline) or colloid would be appropriate. Initially, the patient is likely to require a large amount of fluid quickly, e.g. 1000 mL isotonic fluid over 15–30 minutes. Subsequent fluid replacement should be guided by the patient's blood pressure, tachycardia, urine output and central venous pressure. Patients who do not respond quickly to resuscitation or in whom assessing the adequacy of resuscitation is difficult should be transferred to an intensive care unit for closer monitoring.

The type of fluid used for resuscitation is controversial. A common strategy is to aim to replace the type of fluid that has been lost i.e. transfuse blood in haemorrhagic shock, albumin in burns and crystalloid in the presence of gastrointestinal losses.

Most, units have ready access to crystalloid fluid such as Hartmann's solution, or dextrose-saline. Both are isotonic and replace fluid and ions. They are, however, rapidly redistributed, particularly through leaky capillaries, into peripheral tissues. After high volume crystalloid transfusion, patients can become overloaded with fluid, but remain with low blood volume. This situation can ultimately hinder adequate tissue oxygen perfusion. A

potential answer to this dilemma lies in the use of colloid fluids. Common colloids include Gelofusine and dextran. These fluids contain higher molecular weight molecules such as albumin or starch that slow redistribution and are designed to remain within the circulating blood volume. A Cochrane review in 2007 concluded that there was no evidence of improved outcome following resuscitation with colloid in patients with trauma, burns or postoperatively. The authors suggest that as crystalloid was cheaper and more easily available, it should continue to be the fluid of choice for resuscitation of the critically ill patient (Perel and Roberts 2007).

The rate and total volume of fluid infusion should be calculated for each individual and reassessed at regular intervals throughout the resuscitation. A fluid challenge of 1000 mL of crystalloid can be safely administered over a 30 minute period, followed by assessment of response. An improvement in cardiovascular parameters such as blood pressure would point towards hypovolaemic shock. A further drop would suggest inadequate resuscitation. A poor response to a bolus fluid challenge would suggest another cause of shock such as an acute cardiac event. In more complex situations, particularly in the presence of pre-existing cardiac dysfunction, more intensive monitoring may be required with central venous pressure measurement.

A conservative fluid replacement strategy should only rarely be considered in the presence of direct lung trauma or established acute lung injury, without associated hypoperfusion.

- Collect venous blood samples for a complete blood picture and biochemistry, clotting screen, cross-match and blood culture. If central lines are in situ, blood

Answers *cont.*

cultures should be taken through the lines (all ports) and also peripherally. If the lines look infected or are old they should be replaced.

- Perform arterial blood gas analysis looking for evidence of acidosis, hypoxia and high lactate (a measure of poor tissue perfusion).
- If not already in place, insert a urinary catheter to monitor fluid status and renal perfusion. Send a urine specimen for culture.
- Consider a central line if not already inserted and resuscitation is difficult.
- Attach to cardiac monitor. Perform an ECG and arrange a chest X-ray.
- Give a broad-spectrum antibiotic intravenously. The choice of antibiotic should be guided by local protocol and the suspected source of the patient's infection.
- Further specimens should also be sent for infection screen. These may include sputum, and any pus or drain fluid.

A.5 The results suggest the following:
- Dehydration (increased urea and creatinine).
- Infection (leucocytosis due to neutrophilia).
- Renal dysfunction (raised urea and creatinine).
- Metabolic acidosis (negative base excess and reduced pH).
- Hypoxia (reduced pO_2).

The renal dysfunction is probably prerenal in origin, due to hypovolaemia and poor perfusion. The low pH, high base deficit and low bicarbonate level point to a metabolic acidosis, consistent with severe sepsis. Hypoxia could be due to a postoperative basal atelectasis, chest infection or diaphragmatic splinting secondary to surgery.

Low haemoglobin and protein levels are common after major surgery such as oesophagectomy and do not require specific treatment.

A.6 The presence of fever, tachycardia, hypotension, dehydration and confusion indicate this patient most likely has severe sepsis. The development of pyrexia, tachycardia, tachypnoea and abnormal white cell count is defined as *systemic inflammatory response syndrome* or *SIRS*. The criteria for a diagnosis of SIRS are listed in Box 3.1. When SIRS occurs in the presence of infection, this is termed *sepsis*.

In the more advanced cases, there may be evidence of organ dysfunction. Where two or more organ systems are affected this is termed *multiple organ dysfunction syndrome* or *MODS*. Where MODS occurs in the presence of an identified source of infection, this is termed *severe sepsis* or *sepsis syndrome*. Infection and hypotension that fail to respond to initial resuscitation is termed *septic shock*.

Box 3.1 Diagnosis of SIRS

SIRS can be diagnosed when two or more of the following criteria are present:
- Body temperature less than 36°C or greater than 38°C.
- Heart rate greater than 90 beats per minute.
- Tachypnoea (high respiratory rate), with greater than 20 breaths per minute; or an arterial partial pressure of carbon dioxide less than 4.3 kPa (32 mmHg).
- White blood cell count less than 4000 cells/mm^3 (4×10^9 cells/L) or greater than 12 000 cells/mm^3 (12×10^9 cells/L); or the presence of greater than 10% immature neutrophils (band forms) (American College of Chest Physicians 1992).

Answers *cont.*

The body's response to sepsis is mediated through inflammatory cytokines. As well as helping to fight infection, an excessive cytokine response can have a negative effect. Cytokines such as tumour necrosis factor, platelet activating factor and the interleukins can produce peripheral vasodilatation, leaking capillaries and microvascular coagulation. Specific bacterial toxins also have a detrimental effect on myocardial contractility. These actions result in reduced blood pressure, decreased tissue perfusion and reduced oxygen transfer. Excessive clotting within small vessels can lead to a consumptive coagulopathy. Clotting factors are rapidly used up, resulting in excessive bleeding.

Poor oxygen delivery to the tissues leads to anaerobic metabolism and production of lactic acid. A lactic acidosis results from its release back into the circulation. Lung function worsens as fluid leaks into the lungs, reducing oxygen transfer still further. Reduced urine output leads to accumulation of urea and nitrogen into the circulation.

A.7   There is opacification of the right lower zone. The presence of a meniscus and the preservation of the diaphragm and cardiac border suggest that this is a moderate sized pleural effusion. There is associated patchy consolidation. This could be due to a postoperative pneumonia or an underlying anastomotic leak. The mediastinum is widened secondary to the gastric pull up within the chest. There is interstitial shadowing of both lungs consistent with some pulmonary oedema. The basal chest drain and skin staples are visible.

Although an infected pleural effusion and now systemic sepsis is most likely, you still do not know exactly what is happening. The patient could have a nosocomial infection of the bloodstream from infection of his central venous, epidural or urinary catheter. As he is seriously ill, he requires broad-spectrum intravenous antibiotics along with his resuscitation.

A.8   Once the patient has been resuscitated, further imaging studies need to be performed. The preferred investigation is a thoracic and abdominal CT scan with percutaneous drainage of any identified localized collection.

If the patient's condition worsens or there is evidence of peritonitis, surgical intervention may be required. If an anastomosis has leaked, either the anastomosis may need to be refashioned or a proximal (diverting) oesophagostomy may need to be formed. If a leak can be controlled with adequate drainage, a period of conservative treatment often allows a small leak to heal spontaneously.

A failure to respond to initial resuscitation suggests the need for management in an intensive care unit, with facilities for invasive monitoring, vasopressor support and mechanical ventilation.

Definitive treatment of sepsis includes a full screen, looking for common sites of postoperative sepsis. Central to this assessment should be blood cultures prior to any antibiotic therapy and early imaging to identify sites of infection. Infected foreign bodies such as catheters should be removed and infected collections should be drained.

Bacteraemia should be treated with appropriate antibiotics, with close involvement of the microbiologist. Appropriate antibiotic choice should follow local hospital guidelines and will depend on the patient's age, co-morbidity, previous

Answers *cont.*

antibiotic history and length of time in hospital. The length of the course of antibiotic therapy should be guided by clinical response.

An appropriate choice for hospital acquired infection would be an extended spectrum beta-lactam antibiotic such as piperacillin in combination with tazobactam. This combination has activity against Gram-negative, Gram-positive and anaerobic pathogens. Alternative choices include the carbapenems (imipenem or meropenem). Vancomycin is an appropriate choice where resistant infections such as MRSA (methicillin-resistant *Staphylococcus aureus*) or *Clostridium difficile* are suspected.

Whichever antibiotic regimen is used, it must be reviewed on a regular basis and altered according to response and to the results of microbiological (particularly blood) cultures. If there is any suggestion of renal impairment, the use of aminoglycosides should be avoided. However,

aminoglycosides can be used in settings where the risk of uncontrolled sepsis outweighs the risk of renal impairment or failure. In such circumstances, the dose should be adjusted to the calculated glomerular filtration rate (using the Cockroft–Gault nomogram) and the serum concentrations of the drug monitored closely. Caution should also be exercised in the prolonged use of broad-spectrum cephalosporins or quinolones to avoid the risk of developing *Clostridium difficile* colitis.

A.9 The scan shows a view through the lower chest. Contrast has been given to outline the oesophageal remnant and gastric tube within the posterior mediastinum. There is a small left-sided pleural effusion. There is consolidation within the right lower lung with an air bronchogram. Posterolateral to the intrathoracic stomach on the right is a loculated collection of fluid. This is likely to be an infected collection.

Revision Points

Accurate assessment and early treatment of sepsis have been emphasized by the Surviving Sepsis Campaign (Dellinger et al. 2008). Early, goal directed therapy is recommended in the form of 'care bundles'. The immediate 'Resuscitation' care bundle is given within the first 6 hours, followed by the second 'Management' care bundle completed within 24 hours. It is recommended that broad-spectrum antibiotic therapy is commenced within 1 hour of diagnosis of sepsis, with goal directed resuscitation within the first 6 hours of diagnosis. Initial fluid and oxygen resuscitation should aim at maintaining a

central venous pressure of 8–12 mmHg, a mean arterial pressure of 65 mmHg, a urine output of 0.5 mL/kg/hour and a central venous oxygen saturation of over 70%. Noradrenaline (norepinephrine) or dopamine can be used as vasopressors in septic shock as long as adequate fluid resuscitation is ensured (Table 3.1).

Numerous trials have looked at the use of steroids in severe sepsis. A recent trial failed to show any improvement in mortality following administration of hydrocortisone in septic shock. Although shock was seen to reverse more quickly in patients receiving steroids, they were more susceptible to

Table 3.1 Inotropic and vasoactive drugs in shock

Drug	Action	Use
Noradrenaline (norepinephrine)	Alpha agonist Vasopressor	Septic shock, neurogenic shock
Dobutamine	Beta$_1$ agonist Inotropic	Cardiogenic shock, myocardial failure, without hypotension
Dopamine	Beta$_1$ agonist Inotropic and chronotropic	Cardiogenic shock ?Increase renal perfusion in low doses
Dopexamine	Beta$_2$ agonist Inotropic	Septic shock Increase splanchnic perfusion

further infections and sepsis (Sprung et al. 2008).

A key factor in the normal clotting mechanism is activated protein C. Levels of activated protein C are often low in severe sepsis, and its administration is known to have antithrombotic and anti-inflammatory effects. Two multicentre trials looking at the role of activated protein C in the management of severe sepsis have concluded that it may reduce overall mortality, but that it should not be used in patients with a low risk of death because of the associated risk of bleeding complications (Abraham et al. 2005, Bernard et al. 2001).

Other recommended management strategies in sepsis include maintaining a target haemoglobin 70–90 g/L with red cell transfusion, maintaining glycaemic control with infused insulin if required, the use of intermittent haemodialysis in renal failure, thrombosis prophylaxis with low molecular weight heparin and stress ulcer prophylaxis with a proton pump inhibitor.

Shock is defined as inadequate tissue perfusion and its causes are:
• hypovolaemia
• cardiogenic
• sepsis
• anaphylaxis
• neurogenic.

The signs of shock include:
• confusion
• cold, clammy peripheries
• tachycardia and tachypnoea
• oliguria.

A normal systolic blood pressure does not exclude shock. A fit young patient can lose up to 30% blood volume (~1.5 L) before a drop in blood pressure occurs.

Treatment of a patient with shock must include:
• Rapid administration of intravenous fluid with replacement of what has been lost. Aim for 10–20 mL/kg initial bolus.
• High-flow oxygen.
• Identification of the underlying problem (e.g. haemorrhage, anaphylaxis).
• Monitoring of blood pressure, oxygen saturations, urine output and central venous pressure to assess response to resuscitation.
• Consideration of early transfer to intensive care facility.
• Identification and treatment of infection (local and systemic: drainage of collections, antibiotics).
• Removal of infected lines.

Those at high risk of sepsis and septic complications have been defined in Chapter 2 and include the elderly and malnourished, those with diabetes and any immunocompromised patients.

Issues to Consider

- How would your management of this case differ if the CT scan had not yielded an intrathoracic collection?
- What other forms of haemodynamic monitoring are available in the intensive care department?
- What are the limitations of CVP monitoring?

Further Information

Abraham, E., Laterre, P.F., Garg, R., et al., 2005. Drotrecogin alfa [activated] for adults with severe sepsis and a low risk of death. New England Journal of Medicine 353, 1332–1341.

American College of Chest Physicians/Society of Critical Care Medicine, 1992. ACCP/SCCM Consensus Conference Committee. Definitions for sepsis and organ failure and guidelines for the use of innovative therapies in sepsis. Critical Care Medicine 20 (6), 864–874.

Bernard, G.R., Vincent, J.L., Laterre, P.F., et al., 2001. Efficacy and safety of recombinant human activated protein C for severe sepsis. New England Journal of Medicine 344, 699–709.

Dellinger, R.P., Levy, M.M., Carlet, J.M., et al., 2008. Surviving Sepsis Campaign. International guidelines for management of severe sepsis and septic shock 2008. Critical Care Medicine 36, 296–327. [Published correction appears in Critical Care Medicine 2008;36:1394–1396.]

Perel, P., Roberts, I., 2007. Colloids versus crystalloids for fluid resuscitation in critically ill patients. Cochrane Database of Systematic Reviews 2007 Oct 17 (4), CD000567. *Review*.

Sprung, C.L., Annane, D., Keh, D., et al., 2008. Hydrocortisone therapy for patients with septic shock. New England Journal of Medicine 358, 111–124.

Confusion in the postoperative ward

Toby T. Winton-Brown

You are the resident on call covering the night shift and finally about to get some sleep when a concerned nurse pages you requesting a phone order for sedation. A 67-year-old woman has become very agitated 3 days after a left total hip replacement. She has been yelling at the nurses, climbing out of bed and distressing the other patients.

Q.1 What do you tell the nurse over the phone?

This patient evidently has postoperative confusion and needs to be clinically assessed before any psychotropic medication can be given. Over the phone you establish the acuity of the situation – the patient's vital signs are stable and she is not posing immediate danger to herself or others.

On approaching the ward it is obvious which patient is yours from the noise and commotion. She is half out of bed, clawing at her various drains and lines, and is muttering about the nurses stealing her dentures and poisoning her mashed potato.

Q.2 What might possibly have caused postoperative confusion in this patient? What factors put her at risk?

The patient's blood pressure is 140/100 mmHG, pulse 100/min and regular, respiratory rate 30/min. Her temperature is 37.7°C. She is on IV fluids, has an indwelling urinary catheter and the fluids chart records a net deficit of 100 mL over the last 24 hours. The operative report records a routine procedure with no complications.

The nurses confirm an acute increase in her confusion over the last 24 hours, which has seemed to fluctuate and particularly worsened during the evening. There is no known history of prior cognitive or psychiatric problems.

When you attempt to examine the patient she becomes angry. She has trouble understanding your questions and is herself difficult to follow. You inspect the surgical wound, which appears clean and non-infected.

Q.3 How would you describe this woman's clinical state?

Q.4 What investigations will you perform in order to confirm your diagnosis?

Aside from a raised MCV of 104 fL and a GGT of 116 U/L, the results of urinalysis, blood screen and ABGs are normal. The chest X-ray shows a small amount of bibasal atelectasis.

Q.5 What do you think is happening to this patient? What other history would be helpful?

You manage to get the patient's son on the phone, although it is the middle of night. He is surprised to hear his mother is causing a disturbance – she is usually a quiet lady who keeps to herself since her husband died 5 years ago. He tells you his mother does not often use painkillers or sleeping tablets, but she does 'drink quite a bit'. He estimates she drinks around a bottle of wine each evening.

Q.6 How does this information affect your assessment? What other information is useful? What is your management plan?

With appropriate management, and regular monitoring of her condition, the patient's symptoms of delirium due to alcohol withdrawal settle over the next 48 hours.

Q.7 What should be done for this woman before discharge?

After a sensitive chat with you the patient admitted to a habit of drinking that had steadily worsened since her husband's death some years ago. She has begun socializing less and less and now finds her days mostly oriented around her drinking and admitted she feels quite lonely. She accepts your suggestion of a referral for an assessment at the local alcohol outpatient service and she is discharged 10 days after her operation.

Answers

A.1 You need to establish the acuity of the situation, and the degree of risk to the patient and staff. Do you need to call security, or can you handle this yourself?
On attending the ward you will need to:
- Talk to the nurses to establish the time course, fluctuation and severity of the presenting problems, as well as the background level of cognitive functioning.
- Review the case notes to determine previous episodes, preoperative investigations and any co-morbid diagnoses.
- Review the operative record for any intraoperative difficulties.

- Review the observations chart, fluids chart, medication record and recent investigations.
- Seek a collateral history from relatives if available, particularly regarding pre-existing cognitive function and risk factors that may predispose to confusion.
- Talk to and examine the patient.

A.2 Postoperative confusion is common in the elderly and medically unfit, particularly following orthopaedic and cardiac surgery, occurring in up to 65% of cases. Surgical causes include atelectasis, postoperative wound infection or abscess, complications

Answers *cont.*

of anaesthesia and complications specific to the surgery. Postoperative confusion is an instance of delirium, and alongside these factors are the many predisposing and precipitating causes for acute confusion (Table 4.1). Most common are causes of cerebral hypoxia, drugs, infection, pain and iatrogenic factors.

Table 4.1 Predisposing and precipitating factors for delirium

Predisposing Factors	Precipitating Factors
Demographic characteristics	Drugs
• Age of 65 years or older	• Sedative hypnotics
• Male sex	• Narcotics
Cognitive status	• Anticholinergic drugs
• Dementia	• Treatment with multiple drugs
• Cognitive impairment	• Alcohol or drug withdrawal
• History of delirium	Primary neurologic diseases
• Depression	• Stroke, particularly nondominant hemispheric
Functional status	• Intracranial bleeding
• Functional dependence	• Meningitis or encephalitis
• Immobility	Intercurrent illnesses
• Low level of activity	• Infections
• History of falls	• Iatrogenic complications
Sensory impairment	• Severe acute illness
• Visual impairment	• Hypoxia
• Hearing impairment	• Shock
Decreased oral intake	• Fever or hypothermia
• Dehydration	• Anaemia
• Malnutrition	• Dehydration
Drugs	• Poor nutritional status
• Treatment with multiple psychoactive drugs	• Low serum albumin level
• Treatment with many drugs	• Metabolic derangements (e.g. electrolyte, glucose, acid–base)
• Alcohol abuse	Surgery
Coexisting medical conditions	• Orthopaedic surgery
• Severe illness	• Cardiac surgery
• Multiple coexisting conditions	• Prolonged cardiopulmonary bypass
• Chronic renal or hepatic disease	Environmental
• History of stroke	• Admission to an intensive care unit
• Neurologic disease	• Use of physical restraints
• Metabolic derangements	• Use of bladder catheter
• Fracture or trauma	• Use of multiple procedures
• Terminal illness	• Pain
• Infection with human immunodeficiency virus	• Emotional stress
	Prolonged sleep deprivation

Answers *cont.*

A.3 The patient's postoperative confusion is a delirium, variously known as acute confusional state, organic brain syndrome or toxic-metabolic encephalopathy. These are all terms for a clinical syndrome that represents a medical emergency, with significant morbidity and mortality as well as increased length and cost of admission. Delirium should be regarded as a sign of 'brain failure', an important signal of a systemic or cerebral emergency with multiple potential causes, that requires immediate diagnosis and treatment. Clinical features are listed in Box 4.1.

A.4 Based on the wide range of possible underlying abnormalities you consider the following investigations:
- Urinalysis and glucose dipstick at the bedside.
- FBC looking for anaemia and leucocytosis.
- EUC and LFTs for electrolyte imbalance and liver or renal failure.
- Cardiac enzymes for ischaemia.
- Wound, drain, urine and blood cultures for a source of infection.
- Chest X-ray for infection or atelectasis.
- ABGs for acid–base disturbance.

Box 4.1 Clinical features of delirium

Acute onset
- Usually over a period of hours or days. Informant often needed to ascertain the time course of onset.

Fluctuating course
- Symptoms recur and relapse over a 24 hour period with characteristic lucid intervals.

Inattention
- Difficulty focusing, sustaining and shifting attention, manifest in difficulty maintaining conversation or following commands.

Disorganized thinking
- Manifested by disorganized or incoherent speech, rambling irrelevant conversation or an unclear or illogical flow of ideas.

Altered level of consciousness
- Clouding of consciousness, with reduced clarity of awareness of the environment.

Cognitive deficits
- Typically global or multiple deficits in cognition, including disorientation, memory deficits, and language impairment.

Perceptual disturbances
- Delusions or hallucinations in about 30% of patients, particularly visual hallucinations.

Psychomotor disturbances
- Hyperactive, hypoactive and mixed variants. Hypoactive commonly missed.

Altered sleep–wake cycle
- Typically daytime drowsiness, nighttime insomnia, fragmented sleep, or complete sleep-cycle reversal.

Emotional disturbances
- Common – manifested by intermittent and labile symptoms of fear, paranoia, anxiety, depression, irritability, apathy, anger or euphoria.

Answers *cont.*

A.5 There is no obvious postoperative complication or metabolic cause for this patient's delirium.

The isolated mildly raised GGT and macrocytosis raise a possibility of prior alcohol abuse, and the clinical picture would be consistent with a withdrawal state. Drug withdrawal, such as sleeping pills, can cause a similar picture. Collateral history is essential where information from the patient is hard to obtain or unreliable – *now is the time* to call the family, even in the middle of the night. Senior advice should always be sought if it remains unclear what is happening (never be afraid to ask!).

A.6 This extra information is consistent with a diagnosis of alcohol withdrawal. Her alcohol intake is likely to be higher than reported by her son.

Once delirium has occurred, treatment is according to the following principles:
• Treat all evident underlying causes promptly.
• Provide supportive care and prevent complications.
• Manage behavioural symptoms.

In this case, treatment of underlying causes should be directed at optimizing fluid balance and treating alcohol withdrawal. Local hospital protocol should be consulted, involving titrated benzodiazepines and parenteral high-dose thiamine to prevent or treat Wernicke–Korsakoff syndrome. Usually a long-acting benzodiazepine, such as diazepam, is given at an initial dose of 10–20 mg orally, and then symptoms of withdrawal are assessed periodically to determine further dosing.

The key to safe and effective alcohol detoxification is *regular and repeated assessment*, using protocol-based surveillance. Supportive care for delirium should include protecting the airway, maintaining hydration and nutrition, positioning and mobilizing to prevent pressure sores and DVTs and avoiding the use of physical restraints.

Behavioural symptoms of delirium should be treated first with non-pharmacological approaches, creating a calm and orienting environment, with familiar objects and family members, and consistent staff using re-orienting communication. A normal sleep–wake cycle should be encouraged.

Pharmacological treatment should be reserved for when behaviour threatens patient safety or the safety of others. Antipsychotics such as haloperidol and newer agents such as olanzapine and risperidone may be used; however, care should be taken with regard to lowering the seizure threshold, QT prolongation and extrapyramidal effects. As with other medications, the principle of prescribing in the elderly is '*start low, go slow*'.

A.7 The patient should be evaluated for other complications of alcohol abuse (cardiac, hepatic, neuromuscular, respiratory, haematological).

Counselling should address the effects of alcohol abuse on the body, and a formal referral should be made to an appropriate service for further management. An attempt should be made to understand the underlying motivations for continuing to drink. Screening for co-existing mood and anxiety disorders, with their attendant risk of suicide, is a priority. Often there is a family history of alcohol dependence and a vulnerable psychological set that combines with precipitating circumstances leading to dependence. The effectiveness of even very brief interventions in primary care settings to reduce alcohol use has now been established in RCTs, and there are a number of specialized treatments available in secondary settings.

Revision Points

Postoperative Confusion/Delirium

- Occurs in up to 65% of surgical patients. Precipitants may be only minor in the elderly with multiple predisposing factors, which include:
- Age.
- Substance dependence/withdrawal.
- Chronic medical conditions.
- Major surgery, especially orthopaedic and cardiac.
- Malignancy.
- Prior cognitive impairment/dementia.

Cardinal Features

- Acute onset.
- Fluctuating cognitive and perceptual disturbance.
- Altered consciousness.
- Underlying medical cause.

Clinical Management

- Treat underlying cause.
- Provide supportive care and prevent complications.
- Use non-pharmacological measures to treat behavioural symptoms.
- Use psychotropics only when necessary for safety – *'start low and go slow'*.

Alcohol Abuse and Dependence

- Common, often covert – high index of suspicion and collateral history often required.
- Hospitalization leads to acute risk of life-threatening withdrawal syndrome and precipitation of Wernicke–Korsakoff syndrome.
- Long-term abuse leads to multiple complications in most organ systems.
- Often co-morbid with depression and/or anxiety, increases risk of suicide.
- Brief interventions can be effective, longer term specialized team approach in some.

Issues to Consider

- What pharmacological treatments are available for alcoholism?
- How would you distinguish delirium from dementia and depression?
- What other nutritional deficiencies can present as a result of chronic alcoholism?

Further Information

http://emedicine.medscape.com/article/288890-overview *Overview of delirium*.

http://www.health.gov.au/internet/alcohol/publishing.nsf/Content/treat-guide *Guidelines for the treatment of alcohol problems*.

http://www.anesthesia-analgesia.org/content/102/4/1267.full *Postoperative delirium: the importance of pain and pain management*.

Swelling in the neck in a 58-year-old man

Jonathan W. Serpell

A 58-year-old man presents with a 6 month history of a swelling in the neck. This has been getting slowly bigger and is not painful. He has no other symptoms and the history is otherwise unremarkable. The swelling is shown in Figure 5.1. While taking the history you do, however, notice the swelling moves upwards on swallowing.

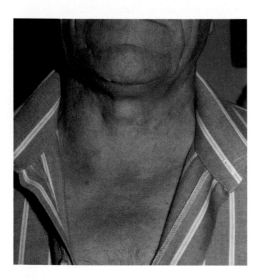

Figure 5.1

Q.1 Describe the abnormality in the photograph.

Q.2 What further information would you like from the history?

Q.3 What are the key features of a problem-oriented examination of a patient with suspected thyroid disease?

Q.4 What are the possible causes of this man's thyroid lump?

Q.5 What investigations would you organize?

Q.6 What does the cytology of the aspirate reveal (Figure 5.2)?

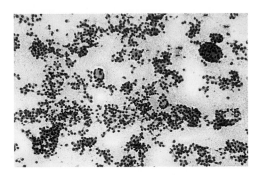

Figure 5.2

Q.7 What does his ultrasound scan show (Figure 5.3)?

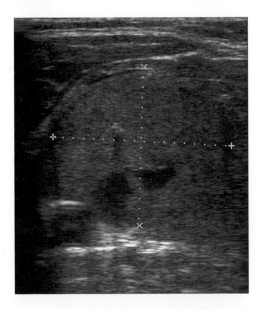

Figure 5.3

Q.8   What would you tell the patient at this stage?

Q.9   What do you tell this patient about the surgery?

The patient undergoes a right thyroid lobectomy and makes an uneventful recovery.

Q.10   What does the specimen (Figure 5.4) show?

Figure 5.4

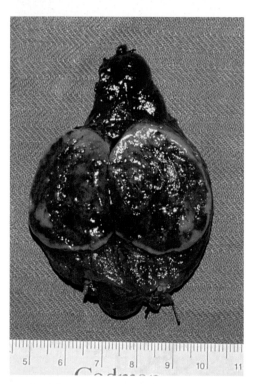

Q.11   What advice will you now give the patient?

Answers

A.1   There is a smooth surfaced swelling at the base of the neck on the right side. You notice that the swelling elevates on swallowing. The swelling is in the anterior triangle of the neck and about 4 cm in maximal diameter. The trachea appears to be displaced to the left. The overlying skin is normal. This may well be a swelling arising in the right lobe of the thyroid gland, as it elevates on swallowing. Thyroid swellings elevate on swallowing because they are enveloped by the pretracheal fascia which attaches the thyroid to the laryngopharynx.

A.2   You will want to know about the following:

- Is there a goitre which has either increased or decreased in size, or perhaps increased in size rapidly, suggesting bleeding or malignancy?
- Are there any symptoms suggestive of local pressure effects on adjacent structures in the neck (local pressure is common and often manifests as the inability to lie flat in bed at night, dysphonia, dysphagia, dyspnoea, noisy breathing)?
- Are there any symptoms suggestive of excessive thyroid hormone production (thyrotoxicosis)? This may occur in cases of toxic adenoma or from a dominant nodule within a multinodular goitre which is toxic. Alternatively the thyroid mass may be incidental to underlying Graves' disease, but the presence of thyrotoxicity may modify the treatment plan.
- Specific enquiry of overactivity will include symptoms related to the metabolic, cardiovascular, neuropsychiatric and ocular manifestations of thyrotoxicosis. These would include increased appetite, weight loss, palpitations, altered bowel habit, temperature sensitivity, tremor, nervousness, muscle weakness, tiredness, low efficiency, anxiety, irritability and excessive sweating.

- An ophthalmic history should make note of any deterioration in vision or any sense of grittiness and diplopia.
- Thyroid nodules may be associated with hypothyroidism in the setting of Hashimoto's thyroiditis. Specific features of hypothyroidism, such as intolerance of cold, constipation, tiredness, poor appetite, weight gain, forgetfulness, dryness of the skin and hair, a general slowing down mentally and physically, menorrhagia, symptoms of carpal tunnel syndrome, and symptoms of anaemia may be present.
- Is there a family history of thyroid cancer (particularly medullary and papillary thyroid cancer)?
- Has there been any previous exposure to ionizing radiation (especially in childhood) to the neck to treat conditions such as acne, tonsillitis, thymic enlargement or excessive facial hair?
- Has the patient lived in an area of endemic goitre or does he have a family history of multinodular goitre.
- Pain in the goitre is uncommon but may suggest haemorrhage into a nodule or subacute thyroiditis or rarely malignancy.

A.3

- The patient is examined with adequate exposure, free of clothing in the region of the neck, and in the sitting position.
- Inspection and palpation are undertaken from the front, laterally and behind the patient.
- Previous thyroidectomy and other neck scars are noted.
- Does the swelling pulsate, and if so is there also a thrill and a bruit?
- Is any venous distension present?

Answers *cont.*

- Is Pemberton's sign positive?
- Does the swelling elevate on swallowing?
- Is the goitre diffuse, i.e. does it affect the whole gland, or is there an apparently solitary nodule within an otherwise normal thyroid gland?
- The specific features of the thyroid mass are noted and should include site, shape, surface, consistency and tenderness.
- Is the cervical trachea palpable and if so is it in the midline or deviated?
- Does the goitre extend retrosternally on the right and/or left sides?
- Is there any regional lymphadenopathy in the anterior or posterior triangles of the neck?
- Are there signs of hyper- or hypothyroidism?
- An assessment of the patient's swallowing, cough and phonation is made.

A.4   The differential diagnosis of this thyroid mass – in order of most to least common – is:

- Dominant nodule in a multinodular goitre (colloid, hyperplastic or adenomatous nodule).
- True solitary nodule:
  - cystic degeneration of a colloid nodule
  - follicular adenoma
  - thyroid carcinoma
  - focal area of nodularity within Hashimoto's thyroiditis.

Even when it is thought that the nodule is a true solitary nodule, further investigation will show that 50% of cases are in fact dominant nodules within a multinodular goitre. Around 8% of the population will have a palpable goitre, and of those subjected to ultrasound of the thyroid, by the age of 50, 50% of the population will have demonstrable ultrasound identified thyroid nodules. Of all these thyroid nodules, only 5% will be malignant. Overall, thyroid cancer is rare, representing only 1% of all malignancies.

A.5

- Thyroid function tests – T4 and TSH. If TSH is suppressed this may indicate thyrotoxicosis due to Graves' disease, toxic adenoma or toxic multinodular goitre.
- Thyroid antibodies – thyroid peroxidase antibodies, anti-thyroglobulin antibodies.
- Calcium, and parathyroid hormone (PTH) as a baseline.
- TSH receptor antibodies will distinguish Graves' disease from toxic adenoma or toxic multinodular goitre.
- Nuclear scanning of a thyroid nodule has a limited role except in the circumstances of thyrotoxicity where it is important to demonstrate that the thyroid gland itself is diffusely hot as in Graves' disease or that there is a dominant nodule within the multinodular goitre or a toxic adenoma which is hot. Nuclear scanning is no longer routinely used to demonstrate whether or not a thyroid nodule is cold.
- Ultrasound of the neck, including the thyroid nodule, the thyroid and cervical lymph nodes:
  - features suggesting malignancy on ultrasound include an irregular margin, micro-calcification or coarse calcification, a predominantly solid as opposed to cystic nodule, and vascularity within the nodule as opposed to peripheral vascularity which is a feature of benign nodules
  - the shape, size and composition and vascularity of the swelling are noted
  - definition of the remainder of the thyroid gland and whether other nodules are present
  - cervical lymph nodes.

Answers *cont.*

- A fine needle aspirate for cytology of the thyroid mass. Cytology obtained by fine needle aspiration (FNA) is the most specific, sensitive and cost-effective of all thyroid investigations. Fine needle cytology has a low false negative rate of 5% and its accuracy increases when samples are taken under ultrasound guidance compared to freehand. The aim of cytology is not necessarily to provide a specific diagnosis of an individual thyroid mass but rather categorize a mass into a diagnostic group, which in turn will dictate subsequent management, either observation or surgery. Accordingly a synoptic method of reporting cytology is utilized.

- Firstly the sample may be non-diagnostic in between 5% and 10% of cases and this will mandate repeating the cytological aspirate.

- Benign thyroid nodules will tend to show a large amount of colloid with a small number of bland follicular cells and these nodules are likely to be benign and can be observed.

- If the thyroid lump is predominantly a cystic structure, this can be aspirated to dryness at the time of obtaining cytology, thus eliminating the lump and providing immediate reassurance to the patient. Of all such cysts, 50% will not re-accumulate and the aspiration will have been definitive treatment.

- Where cytology demonstrates malignant cells (e.g. papillary or medullary carcinoma) or the cytology is suspicious for malignancy, this will indicate the need for thyroidectomy.

- For cases of cellular follicular lesions which are indeterminate, the cytology is unable to distinguish between a well-differentiated tumour such as a follicular adenoma or follicular carcinoma or a benign lesion such as a hyperplastic or adenomatous thyroid nodule. These indeterminate lesions on cytology will therefore require a diagnostic hemithyroidectomy to establish the histological diagnosis. Of these, between 10% and 20% will be malignant.

A.6 The cytological aspirate shows sheets of follicular cells with minimal colloid. There are many clusters of bland epithelial cells which form well-defined circular follicular structures in the centre and to the right of the picture. This is a typical microfollicular pattern. There is, however, no clear evidence of malignancy. When follicular structures are identified on a fine needle aspirate of a thyroid nodule, the differential diagnosis includes a hyperplastic (adenomatous or colloid nodule) follicular adenoma, or follicular carcinoma. A reliable distinction between these is not possible on cytological appearances from an FNA because the distinction between follicular adenoma and follicular carcinoma can only be made histologically by demonstrating invasion of the capsule of the tumour or by vascular invasion.

A.7 The ultrasound scan shows a well-circumscribed, solitary, solid lump in the lower pole of the right lobe of the thyroid gland. The remainder of the thyroid gland appears to be normal. This solid mass lesion, in the context of an otherwise normal thyroid gland, is therefore likely to be a tumour, but still most likely benign.

A.8 You should tell the patient that he has a growth in the thyroid gland. The gland appears to be functioning normally but the lump is solid and solitary and might be a cancer, although you favour a benign

Answers *cont.*

or innocent growth (80–90%). The only way you will be able to tell exactly what the lump is will be to perform an operation and remove the lump. This will involve removal of the right half of his thyroid gland. The pathologist will then assess the excised lump and provide a definitive diagnosis. This process will take at least 48 hours following surgery. Once a definitive diagnosis is reached, you will be able to discuss further treatment with the patient should it be required. At this stage it is probably unnecessary to have a detailed discussion on thyroid malignancy, since the lump is most likely benign.

A.9   A detailed process of consent is essential. The operation and the anaesthetic, the likely inpatient stay and the postoperative recovery phase should all be discussed in detail.

- The details of hemithyroidectomy will include a discussion of the incision in the lower part of the neck which will be expected to heal with a good cosmetic result.
- The right half of the thyroid gland is removed but the left side will not be touched. In 90% of cases one side alone will be sufficient to produce adequate thyroid hormone. In the remaining 10% of patients, the remaining half of the thyroid is not adequate to produce thyroid hormone and therefore these patients will need to go on to thyroid hormone replacement.
- The risks associated with hemithyroidectomy include:
  - those associated with anaesthesia
  - those related to any operation, such as wound infection and bleeding
  - those specific to thyroid surgery.
- The specific risks associated with thyroid surgery include:

- bleeding into the neck (about 1 in 100 cases)
- voice changes (fewer than 1 in 10 cases). These may be due to laryngeal trauma during intubation; recurrent laryngeal nerve injury, temporary in about 5%, permanent in less than 1% and trauma to the external branch of the superior laryngeal nerve
- hypocalcemia is rare after hemithyroidectomy because there are usually two normally functioning glands on each side of the neck.

A.10   The right lobe of thyroid has been opened longitudinally, there is an encapsulated tumour 4 cm in diameter which occupies most of the lobe. The tumour is pinkish red and vascular with areas of haemorrhage. Gross examination does not show any evidence of capsular invasion. Histologically the lesion is shown to be composed of follicular cells and there is invasion through the capsule of the nodule. There is no evidence of invasion in the blood vessels. It was concluded the lesion was an invasive follicular carcinoma.

A.11   You will need to explain to the patient that an invasive follicular carcinoma has been found in the excised half of the thyroid. As a consequence further surgery, treatment and long-term follow-up are required. It is important to emphasize at the start that these tumours have an excellent prognosis (85% 10 year survival).

You therefore recommend to the patient the following measures:

- That the remaining half of the thyroid gland is removed (completion thyroidectomy) to facilitate further treatment and follow-up.
- That further treatment with radio iodine ablation, which is given orally, but

Answers *cont.*

requires an inpatient stay, will ablate any residual thyroid tissue in the neck.

- He will be on lifelong thyroxine (most differentiated thyroid cancers are TSH dependent and the thyroxine will suppress the secretion of TSH and therefore reduce the incidence of recurrence).

- A staging CT scan of the neck and chest will be undertaken as a baseline for metastatic disease, after the patient has had radioiodine.
- Long-term follow-up will be with serum thyroglobulin, neck ultrasound and radioiodine scanning.

Revision Points

Management of the Lump in the Thyroid

Aims

To establish if the lump is solitary and if the lump is malignant.

Process

- Define the anatomy and morphology of the gland (history, clinical examination, and ultrasound).
- Measure thyroid function (T4 and TSH).
- Establish a cytological diagnosis which in turn will dictate subsequent management by fine needle aspiration cytology (FNAC has 95% accuracy).
- Exclude other pathology when indicated (e.g. thyroid peroxidase and anti-thyroglobulin antibodies for Hashimoto's thyroiditis).

Follicular Carcinoma of the Thyroid

- Incidence – less than 1 in 1000.
- Population – less than 10% of all primary thyroid neoplasms.
- Peak age incidence – 40–50 years.

Risk Factors Include

- Endemic goitre.
- Radiation exposure.
- Autoimmune thyroiditis.

Presentation

- Lump in the thyroid.
- Effect of a metastatic deposit, e.g. a pathological fracture in the bone or pulmonary metastases.

Diagnosis

- A follicular and indeterminate cytological aspirate on FNAC.
- Diagnostic hemithyroidectomy to confirm the diagnosis.

Treatment

- Total thyroidectomy, ablation of any remaining thyroid tissue with radioactive iodine, suppressive thyroxine.

Follow-up

- Serum thyroglobulin, clinical ultrasound of the neck, radioiodine scanning.
- Lifelong follow-up required.

Issues to Consider

- How would your management differ if the FNAC reported a papillary carcinoma?
- What other thyroid malignancies exist and how are they treated?

- Why is there such a high incidence of thyroid cancer near to the Chernobyl nuclear plant?
- What is the risk of diagnostic imaging (particular CT scanning) to the development of radiation-related malignancies?

Further Information

www.british-thyroid-association.org *The website of the British Thyroid Association, with a number of useful links.*

www.endocrinesurgeons.org.au *The website of Australian Endocrine Surgeons.*

www.aace.com *The website of the American Association of Clinical Endocrinologists, with clinical guidelines for the management of thyroid carcinoma.*

www.thyroidmanager.org *A site covering all aspects of thyroid disease.*

Yeung, M.J., Serpell, J.W., 2008. Management of the solitary thyroid nodule. The Oncologist 13, 105–122.

A 42-year-old woman with hypertension

Lucia Gagliardi

You are a medical resident in a major teaching hospital. A 42-year-old woman is referred to your outpatient clinic for assessment and management of hypertension. The referral letter states that she was diagnosed with hypertension 8 years ago. She remains hypertensive (blood pressure 150/90 mmHg to 180/100 mmHg when checked by her general practitioner) despite treatment with three agents (irbesartan, indapamide and amlodipine). She was diagnosed with 'anxiety' several years ago, for which she has been taking diazepam. She has had no other major illnesses. There is no family history of hypertension.

Q.1 What are the possible aetiologies of hypertension in this patient?

Q.2 What questions will you ask her and what will you look for on physical examination?

She was diagnosed with hypertension 8 years ago and this has never been well controlled. She has been on the current treatment regimen for the last 3 years and is compliant. She self-monitors her blood pressure at home and obtains readings between 140/90 mmHg and 200/100 mmHg. She has no explanation for this variation.

She was diagnosed with 'anxiety' around the same time the diagnosis of hypertension was made. This diagnosis was based on intermittent episodes of palpitations, shortness of breath, sweating, associated with a feeling of 'impending doom'. She has had no headaches. She has been diagnosed and managed by her local general practitioner.

In the last 2 years she has experienced central weight gain (10 kg), which has occurred despite diet and exercise. She has never had depression and has not had any problems with concentration. She has not experienced increased facial hair or acne. Her muscle strength has always been good. She slipped and fell 2 months ago and sustained a fractured radius. Her periods are regular. She has two children – aged 15 and 10. Both pregnancies were uncomplicated. She is not on the oral contraceptive and does not take any other medications. She drinks 1–2 standard drinks per week and is a non-smoker. Her mother had diabetes; her father is alive and well. There is no other family history of hypertension or endocrine or renal disease.

On examination she appears slightly anxious, and is tremulous. She is overweight, but there are no clinical features of Cushing's. Her blood pressure is 170/90 mmHg lying and 160/85 mmHg standing. Her pulse is 110 bpm and regular. She has a forceful, non-displaced apex beat; examination of the cardiovascular system is otherwise unremarkable. There are no abdominal masses or striae visible or bruits audible. She is able to stand from a squat without difficulty. On fundoscopy there is silver wiring.

Q.3   What investigations will you perform?

The following results are available.

Investigation 6.1 Summary of results	
Fasting glucose (3.8–5.5 mmol/L)	10
Urea (2.7–8.0 mmol/L)	7.3
Creatinine (50–120 µmol/L)	68
eGFR (mL/min/1.73 m²)	>60
Ionized calcium (1.1–1.25 mmol/L)	1.31
Total calcium (2.10–2.55 mmol/L)	2.75
Phosphate (0.65–1.45 mmol/L)	1.27
Plasma metanephrine	18 100 pmol/L (<500 pmol/L)
Plasma normetanephrine	9260 pmol/L (<900 pmol/L)

Q.4   Please discuss the results. What is the diagnosis? What will be your next step(s)?

Some imaging studies are arranged and a CT scan of the abdomen performed. A representative slice is shown (Figure 6.1).

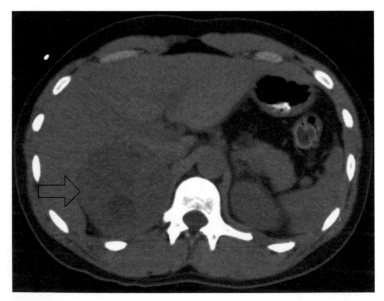

Figure 6.1

Q.5 What does the scan show?

She is tolerating phenoxybenzamine well, but has been tachycardic (heart rate 110–120 bpm for the last 2 days).

Q.6 What should be done next?

She undergoes a laparoscopic adrenalectomy and the large adrenal tumour is removed intact. As soon as the adrenal vein is ligated the blood pressure falls and the anaesthetist is able to reduce the alpha blockade. The opened surgical specimen is shown (Figure 6.2).

All medications are stopped immediately postoperatively.

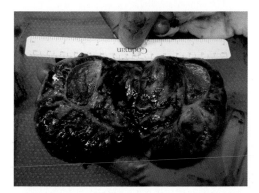

Figure 6.2

Q.7 What postoperative complications should she be observed for?

Over the next week her blood pressure without medication varies between 100/70 and 125/80 mmHg. The histopathology is consistent with a phaeochromocytoma.

Q.8 What follow-up is necessary for this patient?

Answers

A.1 In this patient, secondary hypertension should be suspected because she has refractory/resistant hypertension – remaining hypertensive despite three antihypertensive drugs – and has no family history of hypertension. The possible causes of secondary hypertension in this patient include:

- Endocrine (phaeochromocytoma, Cushing's syndrome, Conn's syndrome).
- Renal (renovascular disease, primary renal disease).
- Other (coarctation of the aorta, oral contraceptive pill).

She must be investigated for a secondary cause of hypertension.

A.2 The following components of the history should be clarified:

- Hypertension – previous treatment; compliance with medications.
- Diagnosis of 'anxiety' – how diagnosis made – including whether psychiatric or psychological evaluation was performed; description of symptoms (chest pain, shortness of breath, increased respiratory rate, sweating, symptoms persistent or episodic, precipitating factors).

Specific enquiry should be made regarding:

- Symptoms of phaeochromocytoma (see Table 6.1).
- Symptoms of Cushing's syndrome (see Table 6.2).
- Symptoms of Conn's syndrome (see Box 6.1).
- Previous renal disease – infections, haematuria, renal calculi.
- Full drug, alcohol and smoking history.
- Family history – hypertension, renal or endocrine diseases.

The physical examination should include inspection both for signs of a secondary cause of hypertension and for complications of longstanding hypertension.

- General inspection – Cushingoid features (see Table 6.2); tremor (phaeochromocytoma).
- Examination of the cardiovascular system:
  - blood pressure – lying and standing
  - pulses – radial pulse rate (tachycardia with phaeochromocytoma); radiofemoral delay (coarctation of the aorta); peripheral pulses
  - praecordium – apex beat – quality and location (forceful – left ventricular

Table 6.1 Phaeochromocytoma – catecholamine excess

Symptoms	Signs
'Classic triad' – episodic headache, sweating, tachycardia (palpitations)	Hypertension (essential or paroxysmal)
	Diaphoresis
	Tremor
	Tachycardia

Box 6.1 Conn's syndrome – primary aldosteronism

Symptoms and Signs

The classic presentation of Conn's syndrome is hypertension and hypokalaemia. Severe hypokalaemia (serum potassium <2.5 mmol/L) may result in muscle weakness.

Answers *cont.*

Table 6.2 Cushing's syndrome – hypercortisolism

Symptoms	Signs
Central (centripetal) obesity (abdominal weight gain, sparing of arms and legs)	Truncal obesity, thin arms and legs ('lemon on a toothpick')
	Moon face, buffalo hump (dorsocervical fat pad); temporal and supraclavicular fossae fullness
Easy bruising	Ecchymoses
Poor or delayed wound healing	Non-healing wounds
Thinning of skin	Atrophic, fragile skin; skin tears
Acne	Facial plethora; broad reddish-purple abdominal striae; acne
Skin infections	
	Fungal infections – nails, skin
Increased facial hair, thinned scalp hair	Hypertension
Oligomenorrhoea, amenorrhoea	Increased facial hair; thinned scalp hair
Muscle weakness – difficulty climbing stairs, combing hair	Proximal muscle wasting and weakness – unable to stand from a squat
Osteoporosis – minimal trauma fractures	
Glucose intolerance – polyuria, polydipsia	
Psychological changes – labile mood, depression, anxiety, psychosis, memory impairment, difficulty concentrating	

hypertrophy; displaced – left ventricular enlargement)
- signs of left ventricular failure which may occur with longstanding hypertension – elevated jugular venous pulse, pulmonary crepitations
- fundal examination – hypertensive changes – silver wiring, AV nipping, haemorrhages/exudates, papilloedema.
- Abdominal examination – Cushing's – striae, bruising; abdominal masses; renal artery stenosis – abdominal bruit.
- Examination of proximal muscle bulk and strength – stand from a squat; strength of shoulder abduction.

A.3 She needs to be investigated for endocrine causes of hypertension – phaeochromocytoma, Cushing's and Conn's syndrome.
   Investigations:
- Phaeochromocytoma – plasma or urine metanephrines or catecholamines.

- Cushing's syndrome – urinary free cortisol or dexamethasone suppression test.
- Conn's syndrome – direct renin concentration, plasma aldosterone and serum K.
- Simple screening tests for renal disease (EUC and urinalysis) and a baseline ECG are also appropriate.

A.4 The elevated plasma metanephrine levels are diagnostic of phaeochromocytoma. Further biochemical testing (e.g. clonidine suppression testing) is not required. Elevated blood glucose may occur in phaeochromocytoma – a result of insulin resistance produced by the elevated catecholamines. This often resolves after treatment of the phaeochromocytoma. The elevated plasma calcium may be seen in phaeochromocytoma due to catecholamine-induced volume contraction/dehydration or to primary hyperparathyroidism – which may be

Answers *cont.*

sporadic (although unusual in this age group) or associated with the phaeochromocytoma as part of a multiple endocrine neoplasia syndrome.

The priority of management of this patient is treatment of the phaeochromocytoma.

With appropriate endocrine consultation the principles of management are:

- Blood pressure and heart rate self-monitoring twice daily.
- Initiation of alpha-blockade to control blood pressure (phenoxybenzamine is most commonly used, although prazocin is a suitable alternative). Alpha-blockade results in vasodilatation. The dose of phenoxybenzamine should be gradually titrated up according to blood pressure (aims of treatment should be individualized – but in this patient a seated blood pressure of 120/80 mmHg is a reasonable goal, provided that this does not induce postural hypotension). In view of the potential orthostatic hypotension, she should be advised to liberalize her salt intake 2–3 days after commencing phenoxybenzamine (to expand circulating blood volume).
- The physiological response to vasodilatation (and therefore to alpha-blockade) is tachycardia (pulse rate >100 bpm). On development of a tachycardia, beta-blockade should be initiated. Beta-blockade should never be started first because blockade of vasodilatory peripheral beta-receptors with unopposed alpha-adrenergic stimulation can lead to a further increase in blood pressure, and could even precipitate a hypertensive crisis.
- Localization of the phaeochromocytoma – she should be referred for a non-contrast (ionic contrast can precipitate a hypertensive crisis) CT scan of the adrenal glands.

A.5 The scan shows a well-circumscribed heterogeneous mass behind the liver in the region of the right adrenal gland. The lesion is 10 cm diameter.

A.6 She is consistently tachycardic so a beta-blocker should be introduced (e.g. metoprolol). The definitive management of this patient is adrenalectomy and she should be referred to an experienced adrenal surgeon and anaesthetist.

A.7 Postoperative hypotension may occur which can be managed with fluid loading. Hypoglycaemia may sometimes occur because of the loss of catecholamine-induced suppression of insulin secretion. Other complications include the surgically related problems of atelectasis, infection and deep vein thrombosis.

A.8 Serum metanephrines should be checked to determine whether she has been cured. There is a risk of recurrence – which is highest in younger patients, those with extra-adrenal or familial disease, or bilateral and/or large tumours. Recommendations are increasingly being made that patients with phaeochromocytoma should undergo long-term surveillance (10 years in sporadic phaeochromocytoma and indefinitely in familial disease) (Lenders et al. 2005). This patient will also need a fasting blood glucose and serum calcium levels checked, as both were elevated preoperatively. If she remains hypercalcaemic then she will need investigation for primary hyperparathyroidism. If a repeat fasting blood glucose level is elevated, then this is diagnostic of diabetes mellitus.

Revision Points

Phaeochromocytomas are catecholamine-producing neuroendocrine tumours arising from chromaffin cells of the adrenal medulla (80–85%) or extra-adrenal paraganglia (10–15%; paraganglioma). Phaeochromocytomas are rare, accounting for 0.1–0.6% of all hypertension. Approximately 25% are diagnosed during the investigation of the 'adrenal incidentaloma' (an adrenal tumour >1 cm in diameter discovered incidentally by radiological investigations performed for another purpose).

Although phaeochromocytomas are usually sporadic, they may occur as a component of a familial syndrome (neurofibromatosis 1 (NF1), von Hippel–Lindau (VHL), multiple endocrine neoplasia 2 (MEN2), succinate dehydrogenase (SDH) syndromes). Features suggestive of familial disease include young age at diagnosis (age <30), bilateral phaeochromocytomas, family history, associated manifestations of NF1, VHL, MEN2, SDH.

The clinical presentation of phaeochromocytoma is variable. The classic presentation is with episodic headache, sweating and tachycardia. Hypertension may be sustained or paroxysmal. Other symptoms include: palpitations, dyspnoea, anxiety, pallor, orthostatic hypotension, weight loss, polyuria, polydipsia. The initial presentation of a phaeochromocytoma may be with an adrenal incidentaloma – such patients are frequently normotensive and asymptomatic – because the phaeochromocytoma is either non-secretory or secreting only low levels of catecholamines.

Measurements of either plasma-free or 24-hour urine metanephrines are increasingly thought to be among the most sensitive of tests for the diagnosis of phaeochromocytoma. Metanephrines are formed as a result of catecholamine metabolism (most of which occurs within the tumour) – and hence increased sensitivity of metanephrine testing is due to the continuous production of these metabolites. Conversely, the production of catecholamines from phaeochromocytomas is highly variable.

Interpretation of investigations can be made difficult because of medications which alter metanephrine or catecholamine levels (e.g. tricyclic antidepressants, phenoxybenzamine, stimulants – caffeine, nicotine, amphetamines). Where possible medications should be stopped prior to repeat testing.

In the clonidine suppression test clonidine is administered to suppress catecholamine release; plasma catecholamines or metanephrines are measured. This should be able to distinguish increased catecholamine levels due to a phaeochromocytoma from increased levels due to sympathetic activation.

Once a biochemical diagnosis is made, imaging (CT abdomen and pelvis) is needed to localize the tumour. If the imaging is negative then there are two possibilities: (a) the diagnosis of phaeochromocytoma is incorrect or (b) the tumour is extra-adrenal (paraganglioma). Nuclear imaging using a tracer compound, MIBG, can help localize the tumour. MIBG is a compound resembling noradrenaline and is taken up by adrenergic tissue. MIBG scanning can also be useful in detecting metastatic disease.

Once the diagnosis has been established and the tumour localized there are several steps in management:

• Control hypertension using alpha- (always first) and beta-blockade (also controls tachycardia).

Revision Points *cont.*

- Coordinated care with a surgical and anaesthetics team experienced in the surgical and anaesthetic management of phaeochromocytoma.
- Assessment for cure.
- Postoperative surveillance for recurrence – there is no consensus on how this is best done, and to an extent this depends on the type of phaeochromocytoma. For example, in sporadic solitary phaeochromocytoma, annual clinical (blood pressure) and biochemical

screening for a few years may suffice, as a proportion of patients with phaeochromocytoma also have essential hypertension. One group has suggested annual follow-up for 10 years for sporadic phaeochromocytoma. All patients with paraganglioma, bilateral or familial phaeochromocytoma should be followed up indefinitely.

- Families with familial phaeochromocytoma should be referred to a clinician/geneticist for screening and follow-up.

Issues to Consider

- What advice should you give to a patient with an incidental finding of an adrenal adenoma?
- What are the risks of non-operative management of a phaeochromocytoma in a patient with easily controlled hypertension?

Further Information

Alderazi, Y., Yeh, M.W., Robinson, B.G., et al., 2005. Phaeochromocytoma: current concepts.

Medical Journal of Australia 183, 201–204. Available online at: http://www.mja.com.au/public/issues/183_04_150805/ald10166_fm.html

Lenders, J.W.M., Eisenhofer, G., Mannelli, M., 2005. Phaeochromocytoma. Lancet 366, 665–675.

A young woman with abnormal vaginal bleeding

Roger J. Pepperell

A 32-year-old woman attends a general practice because she has had some irregular vaginal bleeding for the last 8 days. Her last normal menstrual period occurred 6 weeks ago. Her usual cycle length is between 4 and 6 weeks. She has been trying to conceive for the last 3 years, but has not managed to do so.

Q.1 What further information would you like from the history and why?

In this case the bleeding was only a little heavier than a normal period, there had been no abdominal or pelvic pain, there were no symptoms consistent with early pregnancy. The last PAP smear was done 12 months ago and all previous PAP smears have been normal.

Q.2 What physical findings would assist in making a correct diagnosis?

Physical examination of the patient is unremarkable. In particular, abdominal and pelvic examination is normal. The vagina and cervix appear healthy.

Q.3 What investigations should you perform to define the likely cause of the bleeding?

The results of the tests you arranged were as follows:

Investigation 7.1 Summary of results

Haemoglobin	42 g/L
White cell count	8.5×10^9/L
Platelets	160×10^9/L
Urinary pregnancy test	positive
Serum beta hCG	1200 U/L
Cervical PAP smear	no abnormal cells detected; endocervical cells identified
Cervical swab	no evidence of chlamydial infection

Q.4   Interpret these results. What information do they provide? What further investigations may help formulate a diagnosis?

In this instance the pregnancy test was positive, and the complete blood picture, the cervical swab and PAP smear were normal.

On the basis of the positive pregnancy test a pelvic ultrasound examination is arranged (Figure 7.1).

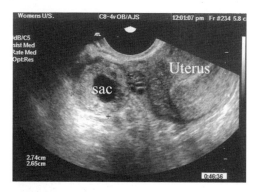

Figure 7.1

Q.5   What does the ultrasound show and what are you going to do now?

Answers

A.1   Further questioning needs to evaluate the extent of the bleeding as compared with a normal period, whether the bleeding occurred after sexual activity, whether there has been any associated pain, whether symptoms of ovulation are usually experienced and whether they were evident during the most recent cycle, and whether there are any symptoms seen consistent with early pregnancy such as more breast enlargement and tenderness than normal, or nausea, or vomiting. When she had her last PAP smear would also be worth defining to evaluate whether the bleeding was likely to be due to a cervical problem.

When taking a history from a woman with abnormal vaginal bleeding the following possible causes need to be considered:

- Is she pregnant and does she have a pregnancy complication? In someone with cycles of variable length, pregnancy is possible so symptoms of pregnancy need to be sought. In someone who has had difficulty conceiving, when a pregnancy is achieved the chance of it being in an ectopic position is increased. You need to ask whether her last menstrual period was of normal volume and duration as it is not uncommon for a 'period' to occur in someone who has conceived although the amount of bleeding at the time of the 'period' is usually less than normally occurs. If she is pregnant the current 8 days of bleeding could be an indication of the pregnancy being in the Fallopian tube, and not the uterus (an ectopic pregnancy), or that one

Answers *cont.*

of the various forms of abortion are occurring (threatened, incomplete, complete or missed abortion).

- If she is not pregnant, the most likely causes are a problem at the level of the cervix, or a disturbance of her oestrogen and/or progesterone levels resulting in irregular shedding of her endometrium (DUB = dysfunctional uterine bleeding).
- Is the bleeding from her cervix? For example, a cervical polyp or carcinoma? Check when her last PAP smear was done, whether PAP smears have ever been abnormal, whether there have been previous episodes of abnormal bleeding and whether she has ever had bleeding after sexual activity. Recurrent bleeding, and especially postcoital bleeding, often has a cervical origin.
- Does she have DUB? This would be suggested by the previous menstrual cycles being irregular, or where the definite symptoms associated with ovulatory menstrual cycles (midcycle mucus change, premenstrual bloating of the abdomen, premenstrual dysmenorrhoea) are absent.
- Abnormal bleeding in a woman with uterine fibroids is generally heavy bleeding at the time of the period. Bleeding between the periods is only likely if one of the fibroids is in the submucosal position and is being extruded.

A.2 The clinical examination is often of limited value in making the correct diagnosis in patients with abnormal vaginal bleeding. Even if this patient was pregnant the uterus is not going to be significantly enlarged. If a cervical cancer was present or a uterine fibroid was being extruded, this should be able to be seen unless it is entirely within the cervical canal. If the bleeding is due to DUB, no abnormality will

be able to be detected on clinical examination. In the absence of pain, even if the bleeding was associated with an ectopic pregnancy, it is likely that the pelvic examination findings will be normal. If pain was present it is more likely that there will be bleeding into the pelvic peritoneal cavity, under which circumstances it is likely that there will be adnexal tenderness, cervical excitation and a 'boggy' feeling in the pouch of Douglas.

A.3 The investigations required are:
- Complete blood picture, to particularly check the haemoglobin level and the white cell count.
- Pregnancy test, to diagnose or rule out pregnancy.
- Cervical swabs, to exclude chlamydia, although this is unlikely.
- PAP smear, to probably exclude cervical cancer.

A.4 She is pregnant; however, the site of this, and whether it is progressing satisfactorily, are not known. The cause of the bleeding has therefore not been defined.

A vaginal ultrasound examination is required to site the pregnancy and to determine if it is progressing normally. Ideally this should not be performed until the quantitative beta-hCG level is assessed and shown to be at least 1000 IU/L, because even a normal intrauterine gestation sac will not be visible at lower hCG levels. If the hCG level is greater than 1000 IU/L and a gestation sac cannot be seen in the uterus, it is highly likely the diagnosis is an ectopic pregnancy. Sometimes the actual sac containing the fetus can be seen outside the uterus, or a mass of clot and the pregnancy can be seen in one adnexum. The other possible

Answers *cont.*

diagnosis if a gestation sac cannot be found under those circumstances is that the whole pregnancy was intrauterine but has been lost (complete abortion).

If the vaginal ultrasound shows the sac is in the uterus, the type of 'abortion' then needs to be defined by the ultrasound examination. Types include:

- Threatened abortion with generally a good prognosis: normal sac size, normal fetal size, fetal heart tones present, gestation and estimated due date (EDD) defined.
- Threatened abortion with increased risk of fetal loss: all the above plus a large amount of intrauterine blood clot, or fetal heart rate less than 100 bpm.
- Inevitable abortion: a very small sac, a normal-sized sac with a very small fetus or a sac with no evidence of a fetus (blighted ovum).
- Incomplete abortion: only placental tissue within the uterus.
- Missed abortion: the gestation sac contains the fetus, but the fetus is dead, i.e. no fetal heart tones are present.

A.5 The ultrasound shows an empty uterus, so the diagnosis is either an ectopic pregnancy or complete abortion, providing the beta-hCG level is greater than 1000 IU/L. The hCG level must therefore be checked.

If it is >1000 IU/L, the diagnosis is probably an ectopic pregnancy and laparoscopic assessment to confirm this diagnosis is usually recommended. The other option would be to reassess the beta-hCG level in 2 and 4 days time, as:

- If a complete abortion was the diagnosis the levels should be falling progressively.
- If the levels were increasing progressively and doubling every second day, a normal intrauterine pregnancy missed on the previous ultrasound examination would need to be considered.
- If the levels were constant, not falling significantly nor doubling every second day, an ectopic pregnancy would be likely.

There are a number of therapeutic options once the diagnosis of ectopic pregnancy has been defined and preferably proven by laparoscopy. The most appropriate option would be the administration of a single dose of intramuscular methotrexate (1 mg/kg) along with folinic acid rescue to destroy the ectopic pregnancy. This is associated with a better chance of tubal patency than when any of the surgical options are employed. It is appropriate treatment, if there is no or minimal intraperitoneal bleeding, especially if the beta hCG level is less than 4000 IU/L, the pregnancy sac size is small or not identified, and no fetal heart tones are detected in the ectopic pregnancy itself if it can be seen. Tubal rupture with resulting intraperitoneal bleeding can occur after methotrexate therapy, but is unusual.

Other options include:

- Salpingostomy performed as an open operative procedure or performed laparoscopically.
- Partial salpingectomy performed as an open procedure or laparoscopically (usually the ovary is not removed at the time of removal of the Fallopian tube).

Revision Points

Ectopic Pregnancy

Incidence
- 1:200 pregnancies.

Risk Factors
- Pelvic inflammatory disease.
- Previous IUD use.
- Previous infertility.
- Pregnancy achieved using IVF or GIFT (gamete intrafallopian transfer).

Clinical Features
- Lower abdominal pain (75%).
- Abnormal vaginal bleeding (75%).
- Usually amenorrhoea (75%).

Management
- Confirm diagnosis:
  - pregnancy test, quantitative beta-hCG pattern
  - pelvic ultrasound
  - sometimes laparoscopy.
- If patient's condition is stable, administer methotrexate.
- In a haemodynamically unstable patient or hCG levels >5000 IU/L: use surgical intervention.

Issues to Consider
- What types of imaging can be used safely in pregnancy?
- What advice would you give to this woman with regard to her further chances of successful pregnancy?

Further Information

www.advancedfertility.com/ectopfot.htm
Laparoscopic images of ectopic pregnancy.

www.emedicine.com/EMERG/topic478.htm
An article from the eMedicine series on ectopic pregnancy.

A scrotal swelling in a 27-year-old man

Jimmy Lam

A 27-year-old man presents to his general practitioner with a 12 month history of a swelling in the left side of his scrotum. This has been causing significant discomfort particularly when walking. During the same time period he has lost 50 kg.

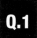

Q.1 What is the most important diagnosis to exclude and what other information should be sought from his history?

The patient is mildly autistic, unemployed, and is looked after by his older brother. He has hypothyroidism and attention deficit hyperactivity disorder. There is no history of any previous testicular or scrotal problems such as maldescent or trauma. There is no apparent history of any infections.

Q.2 What are the key features of the physical examination?

On examination of the scrotum and contents there is a 10 cm irregular firm mass replacing the left testis. This is not tender and not tethered to the scrotal skin. The right testis is normal to palpation. On abdominal examination there is an ill-defined fullness palpable just above the umbilicus to the left of the midline. There was no obvious gynaecomastia or supraclavicular lymph node enlargement.

Q.3 What further investigations are required and why?

You arrange an urgent ultrasound of the abdomen and testis as well as baseline bloods investigations and testicular tumour markers. In addition, and because of the abdominal findings, you arrange a CT of the chest and abdomen (Figures 8.1, 8.2). The haematological and biochemical values are within normal limits. The tumour marker and imaging studies are shown.

Investigation 8.1 Summary results		
LDH	922 IU/L	(50–280)
AFP	3 µg/L	(<11)
HCG	7 IU/L	(<5)

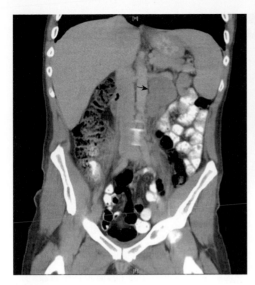

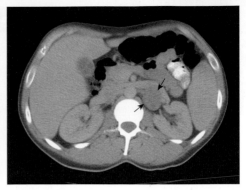

Figure 8.2

Figure 8.1

Q.4 Interpret the laboratory results and imaging studies.

You appreciate that the patient almost certainly has metastatic testicular cancer and this is most likely to be a seminoma. There is no role for a trans-scrotal needle biopsy of the testicular mass and this can potentially result in tumour seeding and scrotal violation as the testis and scrotum lymphatics drain to different sites.

The patient subsequently undergoes a left radical inguinal orchidectomy and the diagnosis of seminoma confirmed.

Q.5 Describe the further management required for this patient.

Answers

A.1 The patient may well have a hydrocele with an underlying testicular malignancy. About 10% of patients with a testicular tumour have a previous history of cryptorchidism. Other conditions to consider include various inflammatory processes producing an epididymitis and/or an orchitis. Any history of pain, acute swelling, urethral discharge or infection might suggest exposure to a sexually transmitted disease or urinary tract infection.

A.2 In any man presenting with a scrotal swelling, it is important to elicit the anatomical characteristics of the swelling in order to define the structures from which the swelling has arisen. Conditions within the scrotum to consider include:

55

Answers *cont.*

- Inguinoscrotal hernia (inability to get above the swelling).
- Hydrocele (testis cannot be palpated as a distinct entity).
- Epididymal cyst (swelling attached to the testis).
- Testicular neoplasm (distinct testicular enlargement).

If a testicular tumour is suspected, a complete physical examination is performed looking for possible metastatic disease. Evidence of any supraclavicular lymphadenopathy, pleural effusion, hepatosplenomegaly or abdominal lymphadenopathy should be sought.

A.3   Baseline investigations to include the following:

- Full blood count (anaemia from chronic disease), serum electrolytes (possible renal impairment), liver function tests (liver metastases).
- Chest X-ray (pulmonary metastases).
- Scrotal imaging with ultrasound to define the testicular mass and to examine the contralateral testis.

Testicular tumour markers are prognostic factors and also contribute to diagnosis and staging. The follow markers are routinely performed:

- Alpha fetoprotein (AFP) (originates from yolk sac cells and may be produced by pure embryonal carcinoma, teratoma, yolk sac tumour or mixed tumours).
- Human chorionic gonadotropin (hCG) (produced by trophoblastic tissue and seen in all patients with choriocarcinoma and 40–60% of embryonal carcinoma and 5–10% of patients with pure seminomas).

- Lactic acid dehydrogenase (LDH) is a less specific marker and its level is usually proportional to tumour volume and may be elevated in 80% of patients with advanced testicular cancer.

A.4   There is elevation of two of the tumour markers and a heterogenous mass occupying most of the left testis. The CT scan shows a large nodal mass in the left para-aortic region. The clinical, biochemical and radiological picture would fit for a stage II seminoma of the testis.

A.5   This patient has stage IIC seminoma (pT2N3M0S2). He will require chemotherapy and a typical regimen would be three cycles of combined cisplatin, etoposide and bleomycin.

With such advanced disease there is a high likelihood of recurrence and he will require regular follow-up. Initially this will be 3 monthly physical examination, tumour markers and CXR and 6 monthly CTs for 2 years, then 6 monthly physical examination, tumour markers and CXR and annual CTs for 3 years, then annual physical examination, tumour markers and CXR thereafter.

Sperm abnormalities are common in patients with testicular tumours and treatment with chemotherapy and radiotherapy can further impair fertility. Therefore patients in the reproductive age group should be offered fertility assessment, semen analysis and cryopreservation. Cryopreservation should be performed prior to chemotherapy treatment.

Revision Points

Testicular cancer more commonly affects young men and prognosis following treatment is excellent. The incidence is estimated at 6–7 per 100,000 Australian Men. Testicular cancer affects young men more commonly with about half of the new diagnoses made in men under the age of 33. There are three peak incidences: late adolescence to early adulthood (20–40 years), late adulthood (60 years and older) and infancy (under 10 years). Testicular cancer is more common in whites than blacks with the incidence of testicular cancer lowest in developing countries, particularly across Africa and Asia.

There has been an increasing incidence of testicular cancer reported in many Western countries but at the same time mortality has also declined substantially, due probably to improvements in chemotherapy. The mortality rate has decreased from 50% in the 1970s to less than 5% in 1997.

Pathology

- 90–95% of testicular tumours are germ cell tumours.
- These are further subdivided into different histologic subtypes:
  - seminoma 30–60%
  - pure embryonal carcinoma 3–4%
  - teratoma 5–10%
  - choriocarcinoma 1%
  - mixed 60%.

Risk Factors

- Cryptorchidism increases the risk by 3–14 times. 10% of testicular cancer has a preceding history of cryptorchidism.
- 2–3 % are bilateral.
- History of exogenous oestrogen exposure.

Presentation

- Testicular nodule or painless swelling of testis (the commonest presentation).
- Acute testicular pain (10–20% of presentations).
- Metastases (10%) e.g. neck mass, back pain, respiratory symptoms.
- Gynaecomastia 5%.

Examination

- Scrotal examination.
- Evidence of metastatic disease.

Investigation

- Scrotal ultrasound.
- Testicular tumour markers.
- Full blood count, serum biochemistry.
- Chest X-ray.
- CT abdomen/pelvis.

Staging

Staging is based on the American Joint Committee on Cancer (AJCC) staging for germ cell tumours, the TNMS staging system.

Treatment

Principles of treatment of germ cell tumours are best approached with multimodal therapy supervised by a multidisciplinary team. Treatment of the primary tumour is via radical inguinal orchidectomy which provides local control as well as histological diagnosis and local staging information. Further treatment with adjuvant chemotherapy (single agent carboplatin or cisplatin-based chemotherapy) or radiotherapy (para-aortic nodes or retroperitoneal) is based on disease factors (such as stage of disease and prognostic factors) and patient factors (likely compliance with follow-up and patient preference based on side-effect profile).

Revision Points *cont.*

Prognosis

The outlook for men diagnosed with testicular cancer has dramatically improved due to advances in chemotherapy and the 5-year relative survival is at least 92.8% for all age groups under 60 years.

Testicular cancer accounted for 0.1% of all cancer-related deaths and in 2004 there were 675 cases nationally with 14 deaths related to testicular cancer. In Western communities the lifetime risk of developing testicular cancer by age 75 is about 1 in 200.

Issues to Consider

- How would the management have differed if the tumour had been a teratoma?
- Why is maldescent a risk factor for testicular cancer?
- Are there other reasons apart for advances in chemotherapy that could explain the improved prognosis in these patients?

Further Information

www.cancer.org.au *The website of the Cancer Council Australia.*

www.andrologyaustralia.org *The website of Andrology Australia.*

www.uroweb.org *The website of the European Association of Urology.*

www.auanet.org *The website of the American Urological Association.*

A 63-year-old woman with a screen-detected abnormality

James Kollias

A 63-year-old woman underwent a screening mammogram which demonstrated an abnormal opacity in the left breast. There is no previous history of breast problems. Her sister was diagnosed with breast cancer at the age of 64 years 2 years previously.

Current medications include combined oestrogen and progesterone hormone replacement therapy (HRT) that she has been taking for 12 years. Menarche was at the age of 10. She is married with two adult children aged 34 and 32 years.

Q.1 What risk factors place this patient at increased breast cancer risk?

The mammogram is reviewed (Figure 9.1).

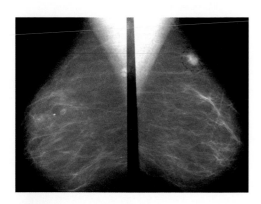

Figure 9.1

Q.2 What abnormal features would you look for? What are the abnormal features in the image?

Q.3 What should be done next?

An ultrasound examination is performed and shows a hypoechoic lesion with irregular margins, distorting and invading the surrounding breast tissue.

A fine needle aspiration (FNA) is arranged. In the outpatient clinic and with ultrasound guidance a 23 gauge needle is passed several times through the lesion. The aspirate is spread on a microscope slide and examined immediately. Benign cells with atypia are seen, but there is no evidence of malignancy.

Q.4   What should be the next step in management?

A core biopsy is arranged. This procedure requires the use of an automated biopsy gun and 12–18 G biopsy needle. The biopsy is performed under local anaesthesia using ultrasound guidance. A core of architecturally intact breast tissue is removed and invasive ductal carcinoma of intermediate nuclear grade is confirmed.

Q.5   What will you tell the patient at this stage?

In this particular case, staging investigations (liver function tests, CT scan chest and abdomen, whole body bone scan) did not reveal any evidence of metastatic disease.

Q.6   What treatment options for the breast cancer are available? What factors influence which are preferred?

A surgical procedure is planned for the patient. The following investigation is performed immediately before the operation (Figure 9.2).

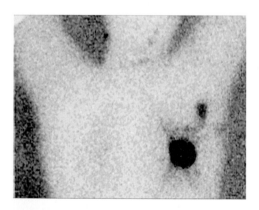

Figure 9.2

Q.7   What is this investigation, how is it performed, and what does it show? What treatment options are available for management of the axilla?

The patient undergoes wide local excision, specimen X-ray and sentinel node biopsy. Histopathology demonstrates a 22 mm grade II ductal carcinoma with focal vascular invasion. Tumour excision is complete with the closest resection margin being 5 mm from the inferior edge. Of the three sentinel lymph glands removed, two demonstrated metastatic tumour deposits. The patient subsequently underwent completion axillary dissection. Histopathology of the axillary fat demonstrated 1/13 further lymph glands with metastatic tumour. The cancer stained strongly for oestrogen receptor and progesterone receptor but was negative for HER-2 (human epidermal growth factor receptor-2).

Q.8 What is the patient's prognosis? What factors determine prognosis and what additional treatments are recommended? How are these recommendations made?

The patient underwent chemotherapy followed by sequential breast radiotherapy and hormone treatment using an aromatase inhibitor. Regular follow-up was arranged to include clinical examination and annual mammography.

Answers

A.1 The two most obvious risk factors are that the patient is female and over the age of 50 years. Breast cancer is a disease almost exclusively affecting women although approximately 1% of all breast cancers affect men.

Family history is an important breast cancer risk factor. The nature of the family history is important whereby closely related relatives, bilaterality, age of onset and the number of affected relatives all play a role in determining breast cancer risk. The presence of other organ-specific cancers (i.e. ovarian, soft tissue malignancies) is also important and may indicate a hereditary form of the disease involving breast cancer-specific genes such as BRCA1 or BRCA2.

Hormonal factors also affect breast cancer risk. Women who start menstruating early in life, have a late menopause or have a late age of first pregnancy are at increased risk of developing breast cancer. Current users of hormone replacement therapy (especially combined preparations using both oestrogen and progesterone) are also at increased risk of breast cancer.

The risk increases with longer duration of hormone replacement therapy use. The risks associated with HRT disappear 5 years after stopping this treatment.

A.2 The following features on the mammogram would suggest malignancy:
• a mass of increased density
• ill-defined margins
• spiculated stellate architecture
• distortion of adjacent breast architecture
• the presence of associated pleomorphic microcalcifications.

The following features are more suggestive of a lesion being benign:
• well-defined lesion
• smooth border.

This woman's mammogram shows:
• Fatty involution of breast, consistent with the patient's age.
• A 2 cm dense, ill-defined solitary mass with spicules extending into the surrounding tissue in the upper outer quadrant.
• No areas of calcification.
• No other abnormal tissue.

Answers *cont.*

These features are suggestive of a malignant lesion and the patient will require further investigtion.

A.3 The woman should be formally assessed by a medical practitioner using the triple test. This includes:
- clinical examination
- further radiological assessment (ultrasound or other imaging)
- pathological assessment.

In this particular clinical scenario, an ultrasound of the area is helpful and will add further information. High frequency (≥7.5 Mhz) ultrasound has a high sensitivity and distinguishes most solid and cystic lesions and can differentiate benign from malignant lesions with a high degree of accuracy. Ultrasound is indicated for focal breast lesions at all ages. For women under the age of 35 years, ultrasound is usually the only imaging technique required. Ultrasound is less sensitive than mammography in the early detection of breast cancer at a population-based screening level and is therefore not recommended for such purposes.

A.4 While cytological examination of a fine needle aspirate has a sensitivity for breast cancer of approximately 90% a negative finding does not exclude breast cancer. In some cases, the cytology may demonstrate atypical cells suspicious of malignancy, without confirming the diagnosis. In other cases, the fine needle aspiration may not be representative of the lesion. Under these circumstances, the fine needle aspiration could be repeated or a core biopsy may be performed.

A.5 The diagnosis needs to be given clearly and sympathetically. As with breaking any bad news, the following principles should be observed:
- Break the news in a place that will be free from interruptions.
- It is helpful to have a close relative or friend present.
- Establish the patient's understanding of her condition and that of any previous experiences with breast cancer.
- Give a gentle indication that the news may be bad.
- Use words the patient understands, and avoid ambiguous terms and euphemisms.
- Explain what further tests will be done: for instance, blood tests, bone scan, CT scans.
- Outline in broad terms the different treatment options available such as surgery, radiotherapy, hormonal therapy and chemotherapy.
- Remember the two issues that the patient will most likely be concerned about are: 1) will she have to have her breast removed, and 2) is she going to die?
- Try and provide a positive tone to the conversation as much as possible. Reassure her that most early breast cancers can be treated with a high chance of cure with current treatment strategies. Many cancers can be treated using breast-conserving surgical techniques. Explain that you will counsel her further once you have the results of the additional studies that will help determine if the cancer has spread. Explain that further recommendations will be made after the pathology report is obtained.
- Allow for silence and give opportunities to ask questions.
- The patient should be given the opportunity to speak with a trained breast nurse. Access to a specialist breast nurse has been shown to improve patient

Answers *cont.*

outcomes by reducing psychological morbidity and providing women with adequate information about breast cancer diagnosis and treatment.

• Make arrangements for a prompt follow-up appointment.

A.6 Current breast cancer treatment may involve a combination of surgery (breast conserving surgery or mastectomy), radiotherapy or systemic treatments including chemotherapy, hormonal therapy or targeted treatments such as Herceptin.

Breast-conserving treatment (involving wide local excision of the tumour with complete resection margins and the subsequent use of breast radiotherapy) is the most common procedure undertaken for breast cancer. This type of treatment is suitable for unifocal cancers (usually less than 3 cm in diameter) where the volume of breast tissue to be resected will still leave a satisfactory cosmetic outcome. Options for patients with tumours considered too large (relative to the size of the breast) for breast-conserving treatment include neoadjuvant systemic therapy (i.e. chemotherapy or hormone therapy) to shrink the tumour, an oncoplastic procedure which involves transfer of tissue into the breast defect from elsewhere (i.e. latissimus dorsi miniflap) or reconstructing the breast using various modifications of breast reduction techniques, to achieve a more satisfactory cosmetic outcome. Contraindications to breast-conserving treatment include large tumours, clinically evident multifocal/multicentric disease, the presence of an extensive duct carcinoma in-situ (DCIS) component or where the patient specifically prefers mastectomy. Patients with a previous history of collagen vascular disorders may not be suitable candidates for breast-conserving therapy

due to the adverse tissue effects following radiotherapy. Under these circumstances, mastectomy is recommended.

For cancers which are not clinically palpable, preoperative localization is undertaken to help the surgeon identify the site of the cancer and facilitate its excision. Various techniques include hookwires or the use of carbon particles which are injected into the breast under ultrasound or mammographic guidance. At the time of surgery, the excised breast specimen is orientated using sutures and metallic marker clips and submitted for intraoperative specimen X-ray using mammography to demonstrate the presence of the lesion within the specimen. If the lesion is located close to a designated resection margin, the surgeon can then immediately re-excise breast tissue from that margin to help obtain tumour clearance. Approximately 1 in 6 women who undergo breast-conserving surgery may require a further operation to obtain tumour clearance due to the presence of tumour at one or more resection margins. In some circumstances, mastectomy may be required.

A.7 This is a lymphoscintigram, demonstrating two sentinel lymph glands in the axilla. The sentinel lymph glands represent the first glands that drain lymph from a tumour-bearing site. After injecting the breast with radioactive colloid (in this case, technetium-99-labelled antimony trisulphide colloid) around the tumour or beneath the areola, a lymphoscintigram is undertaken to identify the location of the sentinel lymph gland(s). These are usually located in the axilla but may be identified in other sites such as the internal mammary region or supraclavicular area. At the time of surgery, a lymphotropic blue dye is also

63

Answers *cont.*

injected into the breast to assist the surgeon in identifying the sentinel lymph gland(s). A handheld gamma probe is used by the surgeon to confirm the presence of radioactivity in the sentinel lymph gland(s) which are also stained blue. The premise of sentinel node biopsy means that in cases where there is no spread of cancer to the sentinel lymph gland(s), the likelihood of cancer in the remaining lymph glands is small (<3%), thus obviating the need for axillary dissection. Randomized controlled studies have demonstrated a significant reduction in arm morbidity and lymphoedema and an improvement in quality-of-life for patients undergoing sentinel node biopsy-based treatment in early breast cancer. It is currently offered as the preferred option in staging the axilla for women with clinically node-negative breast cancer. In women where there is clinical lymph node involvement, axillary dissection is recommended.

A.8 This patient has a relatively poor prognosis. The likelihood of breast cancer recurrence and death from breast cancer in this particular case is approximately 60% and 40% respectively.

The important pathological prognostic factors currently used to determine prognosis are:
- tumour size in millimetres (increasing size associated with a worsening prognosis)
- tumour grade I–III (a measure of differentiation and 'aggressiveness' of cancer biology)
- lymph node status
- lymphovascular invasion
- age at diagnosis (where age<40 is often associated with a poorer outcome).

These factors are often used in various prognostic calculators such as the Nottingham Prognostic Index (which defines

four separate prognostic categories – excellent, good, moderate and poor) or ADJUVANT ONLINE (an online prognostic calculator that provides absolute disease-free survival or breast cancer survival specific for individual cases and the perceived benefit with various adjuvant treatments).

Several molecular predictive factors are important in predicting response to systemic treatments. These include oestrogen receptor and progesterone receptor (predict response to hormonal treatment) and HER-2 (human epidermal growth factor receptor-2, which predicts for a more aggressive tumour phenotype, less responsive to hormone treatment alone).

Hormonal treatments are usually recommended for oestrogen receptor-positive tumours. For postmenopausal women, anti-oestrogens (e.g. tamoxifen) or aromatase inhibitors are now offered. Recommendations about specific hormonal treatments depend on a number of tumour-related factors and co-morbidities of the patient. For example, tamoxifen is associated with certain side-effects including an increased risk of thromboembolic disease and stroke whereas aromatase inhibitors place women at increased risk of osteoporosis and fracture. Recent clinical trials suggest that aromatase inhibitors are associated with a reduction in breast cancer recurrence compared with tamoxifen, particularly for high-risk cancers. Adjuvant chemotherapy is recommended for moderate or high-risk breast cancers that do not express oestrogen receptor. Chemotherapy is sometimes recommended for women with moderate or high-risk oestrogen receptor-positive cancers where the prospects of disease control are improved with the addition of chemotherapy to hormone

Answers *cont.*

therapy. Cancers that over-express HER-2 respond to monoclonal antibody therapy using Herceptin.

Gene expression profiles are currently being assessed in various clinical trials. These techniques use fresh or paraffin-embedded breast cancer tissue using a number of PCR reactions for specific gene sequences to subdivide patients into various prognostic subgroups with the aim of individually tailoring prognosis and treatment. Although gene expression profiles are not routinely used in clinical practice, it is envisaged that in the future,

these will guide decisions on the choice of hormonal or chemotherapy agents for each patient.

Treatment recommendations following breast cancer surgery are preferably undertaken at a multidisciplinary meeting attended by surgeons, medical oncologists, radiation oncologists, breast care nurses and geneticists. Recent studies have demonstrated benefits to both the patient and treating specialists in terms of breast cancer outcomes, entry into clinical trials and an understanding of the various treatments between specialties.

Revision Points

Breast Screening

The sensitivity of mammography for breast cancer is age-dependent (>90% in women aged ≥60 years, <50% in women under the age of 40 years). Breast density tends to be higher in younger women and breast density obscures the early signs of breast cancer. This is the reason why population-based mammographic screening programmes have demonstrated a 20–30% reduction in breast cancer mortality for women aged 50–70 years of age.

Triple Test

The triple test (clinical examination, imaging, pathological assessment) is one of the most accurate tests in current medical practice. Although the individual components of the triple test have variable sensitivity, specificity and predictive values for determining benign from malignant conditions, when used together, the triple test has an accuracy approaching 99.5%. In some circumstances, the lesion may not be palpable such that breast imaging and pathological assessment are required to complete the test. Pathological assessment

by FNA has a 90% sensitivity and if carcinoma is strongly suspected and the FNA is negative, a core or open biopsy is required.

Sentinel Node Biopsy

The role of sentinel node biopsy is established for small breast cancers (≤3 cm) but its role for larger cancers or multicentric cancers is less clear. In cases where the sentinel lymph glands confirms the presence of metastatic tumour deposits, axillary dissection is usually recommended. There are some circumstances where the likelihood of non-sentinel node involvement is minimal when the sentinel node contains metastatic tumour. This principally relates to the size of the metastasis and the extent of lymphatic invasion of the primary breast cancer. Various nomograms have been designed to assist clinical decision-making whether to proceed with axillary dissection or omit this procedure for cases where the sentinel node is positive. Current clinical trials are also assessing this issue.

Issues to Consider

- Does sentinel node biopsy have a role in the management of any other diseases?
- Why does male breast cancer have a worse prognosis than the disease in women?
- Have any other screening programs shown the same positive outcomes as that for breast cancer?

Further Information

www.cancer.gov *An excellent website from the US National Cancer Institute covering many aspects of cancer including consensus statements on the management of breast cancer.*

www.cancerscreening.nhs.uk An interesting website covering various aspects of cancer screening including for breast cancer in the UK.

www.nbocc.com The website of the National Breast and Ovarian Cancer Centre. Australia's most significant breast cancer website providing consumer information, regular breast cancer updates and recommendations to medical practitioners about best clinical practice.

Dixon, J.M. (Ed.), 2006. Breast surgery – a companion to specialist surgical practice, third ed. Elsevier Saunders, London.

A 54-year-old man with a high-voltage electrical conduction injury

John E. Greenwood

A 54-year-old man with a severe burn injury is brought into the emergency department by an emergency response medical retrieval team. The man had been standing on a mobile metal platform when it struck overhead power cables while elevating.

The man was standing on the platform of a rising 'scissor lift'. As the platform struck overhead cables, eye-witnesses reported a loud bang, sparks and arcing of electrical current. The patient was wearing steel toe-capped boots and was trapped for approximately 2 minutes, before co-workers pushed the platform away from the cables with a wooden pole. The incident occurred at 14.00. He was taken to his local hospital by ambulance before transfer to a level 1 trauma hospital by an airborne medical retrieval team. He arrived at the trauma centre at 20.45.

Q.2 Describe the important points of your initial assessment and calculate his initial intravenous fluid requirements.

The patient was intubated and ventilated and a urinary catheter inserted in preparation for transport. His blood pressure was 125/80 mmHg with a pulse rate of 130/min. His clothes were removed to allow an accurate assessment to be made of the extent and severity of his injuries. The photographs show the burned areas of his buttocks, left knee and right foot (Figures 10.1–10.3). There was a 6 cm burn on the scalp with a similar appearance to those on his buttocks. His back had four similar burns. The changes to the left foot resembled those seen on the right foot. Five similar-sized burns were present on the upper limbs. Blood samples were collected for haemoglobin estimation, cross-matching, serum electrolytes and creatinine kinase.

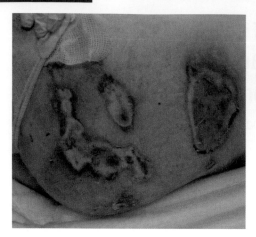

Figure 10.1

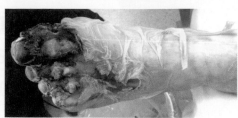

Figure 10.3

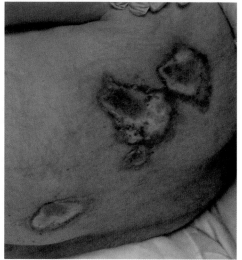

Figure 10.2

Figure 10.4

Q.3 Describe his burns.

The left calf was 'rock hard' on palpation; the left foot was white, cool to touch and displayed a capillary refill time of 5 seconds. His right foot was pink but there were severe burns to the digits with bone and joint exposure. There was a deep defect, an arcing 'blow-out' hole, lateral to the left knee. The compartments of the left forearm were 'tight'. Some surgical interventions are required.

Q.4 What emergency surgical interventions are required here? Describe the difference between escharotomy and fasciotomy.

His urine output was 1 mL/kg/hour (appropriate for an adult); its appearance is shown in Figure 10.5.

Figure 10.5

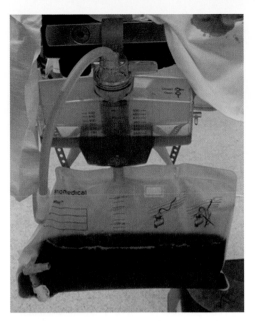

Q.5 Comment on the appearance of the urine, the likely cause, and state what measures need to be taken.

The patient attended the operating theatre as soon as trauma clearance was completed (21.30). A full assessment of his burns was possible after an aggressive scrub debridement of all skin lesions. The surgeon confirmed left lower leg compartment syndrome and that the hole over the anterolateral aspect of the left knee communicated with the knee joint. The left 1st to 4th toes were non-viable, the sole was cold and white. The right calf compartments were soft. There was a full-thickness burn (~1% total body surface area (TBSA)) over the lateral right ankle. The right 1st to 3rd toes were deeply destroyed and 'burst' open to reveal damaged joints and bones. The distal right foot was deeply burned. The left forearm compartments were swollen and tight. Full-thickness burns were noted over the right lateral thigh, lateral to the right knee, left elbow, radial and ulnar left forearm and on the scalp. Fasciotomies were performed medially and laterally to the left lower leg, lateral left thigh and radial and ulnar left forearm. Clearly demarcated non-viable tissue was excised at its visible margins effectively requiring a left forefoot amputation and an equally radical debridement of the right distal foot. Fascial excision of burn over the anterolateral left knee defect was performed and the knee joint was washed out (arthroscopy two days later would show the cartilages to be undamaged). Tangential excision of all deep burns was performed. The scalp burns were debrided down to galea aponeurotica. Superficial burns were recorded at left thigh and right lateral calf. All wounds were dressed.

The terminology for burns has changed and 'first', 'second' and 'third degree' burns are no longer described. The term 'fourth degree burns' persists.

> **Q.6**   What is meant by 'fourth degree' burns?

Two days later there had been a sharp declaration of the left calf and foot necessitating below-knee amputation – if the arthroscopy had shown severe damage to the left knee joint, an above-knee amputation would have been likely, since this joint was open and the defect required complex free flap repair. This surgery would not have been merited if the knee joint was unlikely to be functional later. Necrosis of deep foot muscles was noted on the right and further debridement was performed. All wounds were redressed. A VAC (vacuum assisted dressing) was applied to the right forefoot debridement.

> **Q.7**   What is meant by a 'free flap'?

The patient began to recover physiologically and 4 days after his injury he was extubated. He was transferred to the burns unit 2 days later. He underwent skin grafting to the scalp, left forearm, hip and back wounds which healed well, but the right foot tissues deteriorated and further deep necrosis was evident. He returned to theatre for right below-knee amputation. Prior to amputation, some of the lateral right calf tissue (including the peroneal artery as its blood supply) was used to create a free flap which was used to close the left knee defect (with the flap peroneal artery anastomosed to the artery to the vastus medialis of the left leg).

> **Q.8**   What are the important early complications that must be considered in the management of this patient?

The patient continued to improve, aided by strong support from family and friends. Approximately 6 weeks after his injury, he was transferred to a rehabilitation facility where he remained for a further 6 weeks. The patient today walks on bilateral below-knee prostheses, is independent and happy. No late sequelae had developed at 6 months post-injury.

Answers

A.1   Since the patient arrived intubated and ventilated, no direct history is available. In any trauma case it is important to interview witnesses, ambulance officers, members of the retrieval team, etc. to obtain as much information as possible about the incident leading up to the injury and what has happened in the time between the injury and arrival at the hospital. The following information is important:

- The circumstances of the burn injury and whether the mechanism increases the likelihood of associated injury.
- The time of the incident (thus the time elapsed since injury).
- The nature of the burn (electrical conduction) raises specific questions:
  - What voltage drove the injuring current? Differentiating between high voltage (>1000 V) and low voltage (<1000 V, usually domestic 240 V or small

Answers *cont.*

industrial 415 V) is extremely important in predicting deep tissue damage since high voltage injuries are much more severe.

- The duration of contact (this is the other major parameter in predicting severity).
- Any ignition of clothing?
- Any loss of consciousness at the scene?
- Any violent movement, jactitation or fall associated with the injury?

- What clothing/footwear/personal protective equipment was the patient wearing at the time of the injury?

Some information may have to wait until family arrive, or may necessitate a phone call to the patient's family doctor, such as:

- Does the patient have any pre-existing medical or surgical problems?
- Is the patient taking any medicines?
- Drug or other allergies?
- Tetanus status?

A.2 The initial assessment (primary survey) must assess:

1. **A**irway and cervical spine – since this patient is intubated, laryngoscopy may give some idea of the upper airway (above the vocal cords) which may have been affected if clothing ignition had occurred since the incident was in a closed environment (a factory shed). Per-endotracheal tube bronchoscopy can be performed using a flexible laryngoscope/fine bronchoscope to assess the lower airway. Muscular jactitations, being 'thrown' or falling from a height, are very common as a result of current conduction. In any situation the cervical spine can be disrupted. A hard collar, sandbags and tape or spinal board immobilization must be employed until radiological clearance of the cervical spine. The staff of the intensive care unit

(ICU) were informed before arrival that the patient was intubated and would be housed on ICU post-admission.

2. **B**reathing – there was no immediate evidence of respiratory disease or penetrating chest trauma. Rate and depth of breathing were controlled by ventilator. A chest X-ray is mandatory in trauma patients.

3. **C**irculation

- general issues: the pathophysiological response to major burn injury (25% of the total body surface area or TBSA) involves a whole-body capillary vasodilatation as well as recruitment of closed capillary loops. Major extravasation of plasma occurs into all the interstitial tissues (not just where the burns are) for the first 8–12 hours. This process then ceases in non-burned areas but persists under the burn for a further 12–16 hours. This results in a fall in circulating volume and hypovolaemic shock. Additionally in areas of deep burn, there is loss of whole blood which was circulating in the skin at the time of the burn. Also, conduction of electrical current causes deep tissue death and vascular thrombosis, destroying more blood and causing capillary extravasation into affected muscular compartments. Finally, blood loss may accompany bony fractures sustained during the incident. Major intravascular access (two large-bore cannulae at least) should be obtained (if not already done) and blood samples sent for complete blood count and electrolytes, group and save, etc.

- local issues: muscular death and injury within tight fascial compartments in the limbs. As swelling occurs, the pressure within these compartments

Answers *cont.*

rises – the tissues become tense ('woody') and very painful to passive stretching of the local joints (in the conscious). The capillary pressure supplying the muscles is ~40 mmHg and the muscles will become ischaemic once this pressure is exceeded in the compartment. Muscle death therefore occurs long before the pulses disappear (which happens when the compartment pressure exceeds the systolic pressure). The peak creatinine kinase result in this man was 150 000 indicating *severe* muscle damage. The skin overlying the compartment MAY NOT APPEAR INJURED or may appear stretched/ shiny or reddened and 'angry'. Early fasciotomy (incisions through skin, fat and muscular fascia of ALL compartments in the affected limb) is essential.

4. Disability – conduction of enormous currents though nervous tissues designed to function at microvoltage-driven currents can result in severe and permanent disruption. With this patient unconscious, only a cursory initial assessment could be performed. The presence of arc or contact wounds on the scalp is ominous.

5. Environment – the skin is the major thermoregulatory organ and loss of large amounts of it predispose to rapid cooling with exposure. Additionally first aid manoeuvres such as cooling with water, or the application of burn hydrogels, can lead to profound hypothermia. Such agents should be discontinued, the room temperature raised and active warming devices and techniques employed. Burn patients do not respond well to hypothermia. Exposure is of course necessary to

perform a full primary and secondary survey as well as to assess burn severity and extent. Burn assessment can be done serially.

A secondary survey can now be performed looking for joint disruptions or dislocations, bony fractures and to fully assess the burn size, burn sites and burn depth. The standard techniques for assessing burn size (Wallace rule of nines, Lund and Brouder charts, etc.), while good at assessing cutaneous injuries, tend to underestimate fluid requirements since electrical conduction causes deep tissue injury which cannot be measured with any accuracy. However, skin injury calculation can at least provide a 'starting' volume for fluid resuscitation using an approved formula. The modified Parkland formula suggests that the fluid volume (in Hartmann's solution) needed in the first 24 hours can be calculated by multiplying the patient's weight in kilograms by the percentage of the total body surface area which has been burnt by 3 or 4 mL. In this case it would be prudent to err on the 4 mL factor, to account in part for the underestimation mentioned above. Thus, with the 25% TBSA cutaneous burn in this 80 kg patient, the fluid requirement in the first 24 hours is $4 \times 25 \times 80 = 8000$ mL, half (4000 mL) to be given in the first 8 hours after injury and the second half over the next 16 hours. All formulae are merely guidelines to be increased or decreased according to the patient's physical response picked up by monitoring (particularly urine output).

A.3 The burns occupy around 25% of the patient's total body surface area and are, as usual, heterogenous in depth. The estimation is not easy from the photographs because the burns on the

Answers *cont.*

trunk, head and upper limbs were caused by arcing at multiple sites separated by uninjured skin. The burns to the skin of the toes of both feet are 'fourth degree' (involving non-skin deep tissue such as vessels, tendons, bones, ligaments and joints). The burn over the lateral left knee is similarly fourth degree since deep tissue disruption to the knee joint capsule is evident). These injuries are devastating and are the commonest reason for amputation in burns practice. More proximally on the feet, the burns are white and dry – these are full thickness (although venous thrombosis is visible below the burn). The burns over the shins and anterior ankles are deep dermal. The only superficial/mid-dermal burns (which could be treated conservatively) are over the anterior thighs. The left buttock, hip, flank and scapular burns are deep full thickness (involving subcutaneous fat), as are the scalp burns.

A.4 Escharotomy is division or 'opening' of circumferential full-thickness burns of the limbs or trunk. An escharotomy does not extend through the subcutaneous fat. An escharotomy is performed through incisions running down the midaxial lines but avoiding important superficial structures (ulnar nerve at elbow, common peroneal nerve as it winds around the neck of the fibula, etc.). Fasciotomy is division of the muscular fascia of all affected compartments in a limb injured by severe crush or, in this case, electrical conduction. Skin incisions are designed to afford best exposure of the muscular fascia. The clinical findings mandate fasciotomy release of the left calf muscular compartments and those of the left forearm. Radical debridement of severely disrupted and non-viable tissue of both feet was also performed early (within a few hours). Close

and frequent operative review of tissues obviously having conducted large current is necessary. The electrical injury has damaged the left foot to such an extent that the patient is likely to require a left below-knee amputation.

A.5 The urine has a maroon colour which is almost certainly due to the presence of haemochromogens – most likely to be myoglobin, although haemoglobin usually accompanies it. These large proteins are released by damaged muscle and vessels and can result in sluggish blood flow (especially where hypovolaemia is allowed to co-exist). The main problem is the challenge they pose to the kidneys leading to acute renal failure. Intravenous fluid administration should be increased to raise the urine output up to 2 mL/kg/hour rather than the 1 mL/kg/hour normally optimal in adult burn patients during resuscitation; 25 g of mannitol (an osmotic diuretic) can be administered immediately intravenously followed by the addition of 12.5 g to each litre of administered fluid. Finally, intravenous administration of bicarbonate (2 vials stat) alkalinizes the urine, making the pigments more water-soluble and facilitating their excretion. With these manoeuvres, the urine colour lightens from black/dark purple through purple, plum, maroon, dark red/brown, rose, pink, orange and dark yellow on its way to a normal straw colour.

A.6 'Fourth degree' burns involve tissues deep to the subcutaneous fat such as deep vessels (including large arteries), tendons, bones, ligaments and joints. They are devastating and the commonest cause of amputation in burns practice.

A.7 A 'free flap' is a composite piece of tissue, which can be made up of skin, fat,

Answers *cont.*

fascia, tendon/muscle and bone (in any combination depending on the origin and the defect to be repaired), which is raised with the arterial inflow and venous drainage intact. The vascular pedicle is then divided (usually as far from the flap as possible, giving the greatest pedicle length possible), separating the tissue from its donor site. The artery and vein(s) within the vascular pedicle are then anastomosed to vessels at the recipient site (the defect to be repaired) and the flap inset to fill the defect. The tissue is thus technically a flap because it has an immediate blood supply but a 'free' flap because the blood supply has to be established by surgical anastomosis. In this case a composite piece of tissue was raised from tissue planned to be discarded as part of the right below-knee amputation, its blood supply was the peroneal artery which was anastomosed into the vastus medialis artery so the flap could repair the left knee defect.

A.8 The immediate complications of an electrical injury include cardiac arrhythmias (which can cause instant death), skin burns and compression fractures. Important early complications include hypovolaemia secondary to inaccurate assessment of burn size (failing to account for the hidden internal injury), vascular compromise, nerve destruction (muscular paralysis/loss of sensation), muscle breakdown and myoglobinuria leading to acute renal failure, other injuries (including compression fractures of the vertebrae), compartment syndrome and sepsis secondary to inadequate debridement of necrotic tissue.

Revision Points

Principles of Treatment

- Immediate aid (stop the injurious process, cool the burnt area, minimize systemic cooling).
- Primary survey (**a**irway, **b**reathing, **c**irculation, neurological assessment).
- Secondary survey (history, overall examination and examination of head, neck, chest, abdomen and perineum, limbs).
- Assessment of burns (areas involved, percentage of total body surface area, depth).
- Fluid resuscitation.
- Management of the burn wounds.

Classification of Burns

- Electrical.
- Thermal.
- Chemical.

Complications of Electrical Conduction Injury

Immediate
- Arrhythmias.
- Skin burns.
- Compression fractures.

Early (Days)
- Hypovolaemia.
- Vascular compromise.
- Nerve destruction.
- Muscle breakdown.
- Acute renal failure.
- Sepsis.

Intermediate (Weeks)
- Cataracts.
- Peripheral neuropathy.
- Ischaemic tissue loss.

Revision Points *cont.*

Late
- Psychiatric disturbances.
- Paresis and paralysis.
- Guillain-Barré syndrome.
- Transverse myelitis.
- Amyotrophic lateral sclerosis.

The mechanisms of fluid loss and consequent hypovolaemia are multifactorial and in electrical injury involve:

- Direct destruction and fluid loss at the burn site.
- Capillary extravasation.
- Soft tissue and bony injury.

Issues to Consider

- What is the role of skin substitutes in the management of burn injuries?
- What are the criteria that determine hospital admission for a patient with burns?
- How would the presence of an associated inhalation injury alter the management of this patient?

Further Information

Enoch, S., Roshan, A., Shah, M., 2009. Emergency and early management of burns and scalds. British Medical Journal 338, 937–941. *A review on the current management of burns.*

http://www.burnsurgery.org/ *A detailed website covering many aspects of burns management. Harvard Medical School.*

Reflux in a 35-year-old man

Chris Deans and Andrew C. DeBeaux

A 35-year-old man presents with symptoms of epigastric bloating and heartburn. He also describes a retrosternal burning sensation, particularly at night, which may wake him from sleep. He has experienced 'stomach' symptoms for most of his adult life and has used over-the-counter antacids periodically with some relief. In the past few months his symptoms have become more frequent. His job has become more stressful recently, and he thinks the increased stress is related to his worsening symptoms. His symptoms have now reached a level that has made him report to his general practitioner.

He has no other past medical history and takes no regular medications. He smokes between 5 and 10 cigarettes per day and only drinks alcohol at the weekend, when he often drinks in excess of 10 pints of beer. He is overweight with a body mass index (BMI) of 32. His general examination is otherwise normal.

Q.1 What is the most likely diagnosis and what is your initial management plan?

The patient is given some counselling on lifestyle measures and encouraged to use over-the-counter medications as required. He returns for a follow-up visit 3 months later. He has stopped smoking and has reduced his alcohol intake. He has also managed to lose 5 kg in weight. He feels healthier than ever before but many of his dyspeptic symptoms persist.

Q.2 What is your next management plan? Which investigations might you request?

Q.3 Which pathogen is associated with reflux and dyspepsia symptoms? What investigations are available to test for it?

You adopt a 'test and treat' management strategy. You refer the patient for a breath test which comes back positive. You prescribe a 10 day course of triple therapy (esomeprazole, amoxicillin and metronidazole) and arrange to see him back for review in 6 weeks. At his review you find that after an initial improvement his symptoms have recurred in the preceding week.

Q.4 What is the appropriate management plan for the patient?

A repeat breath test is positive and the patient is given a further course of triple therapy which gives him good symptomatic relief. Two years later the patient returns. His dyspepsia-type symptoms have settled, but his main complaint now is heartburn. Also, when he bends over he can reflux gastric content into his mouth, making him cough. Six months previously he was started on pantoprazole but every time he stops the medication his symptoms worsen. He does not like the idea of taking tablets long term and wishes to discuss other treatment options. He has heard about endoscopic methods for 'fixing the valve'.

Q.5 What treatment options would you discuss with this patient?

The patient has already tried increasing the dosage of his PPI, but to no effect.

Q.6 What investigations might you consider performing before undertaking surgery?

Your patient decides not to opt for surgery and he continues on his PPI therapy. A few years later he returns. Despite deciding to continue on medical therapy his compliance with acid suppression has been poor. For the past few months his reflux symptoms have worsened and he had been feeling increasingly tired. You think he looks pale and you perform some blood tests.

His haemoglobin is 102 g/L, white cell count 6.7×10^9/L, platelet count 275×10^9/L and mean cell volume 72 fL.

Q.7 What do these blood tests reveal and what do they suggest?

You are concerned by his anaemia and arrange for him to undergo an urgent upper GI endoscopy. (Remember, in iron deficient anaemia, if the upper GI endoscopy is normal, a colonoscopy may be indicated.) The view in Figure 11.1 shows the lower oesophagus.

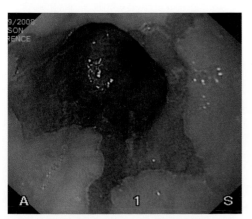

Figure 11.1

What is the pathological condition seen at endoscopy and what should be done?

Biopsies are reported as showing Barrett's metaplasia with features of high-grade dysplasia. There are no features of malignancy on the samples analysed. You commence the patient on high-dose PPI and reinforce the importance of compliance. Another endoscopy is arranged for 6 weeks' time with repeat biopsies.

Despite good compliance with drug therapy, the repeat endoscopy identifies a small area of raised Barrett's mucosa which is biopsied, along with multiple other sites. These repeat biopsies now show low-grade dysplasia, except for the biopsies from the raised area, which identify localized high-grade dysplasia with features of carcinoma in situ.

Q.9 What is your next management strategy?

Endoscopic ultrasound confirms a small nodular area which is staged as T1 disease at most. No other mucosal abnormality is identified and the surrounding lymph nodes are not suspicious of metastatic disease. The staging CT scan is reported as normal.

Q.10 How would you further manage this patient?

Your patient is treated by endoscopic mucosal resection (EMR) and the abnormal area is completely excised. He will need to continue on lifelong PPI therapy and he will need regular endoscopic surveillance to monitor his Barrett's segment.

Answers

A.1 Dyspepsia or reflux disease.

- Dyspepsia is a term often used for many upper gastrointestinal symptoms such as epigastric discomfort and heartburn and is poorly defined. Some pathological conditions may be found as the cause of these symptoms, but in many cases no abnormality is identified and the condition is described as functional dyspepsia.
- Reflux disease, more correctly termed gastro-oesophageal reflux disease (GORD), is the reflux of gastric contents back into the oesophagus.

Patients with alarm symptoms, such as weight loss, recurrent vomiting, anaemia or dysphagia, should be referred for urgent investigation by upper gastrointestinal endoscopy. For most patients with uncomplicated dyspepsia the initial management is aimed at symptomatic treatment. Initially, general lifestyle changes are recommended, including smoking cessation, weight loss, minimizing alcohol and caffeine intake, reducing food intake before going to bed, and sleeping with the head of the bed raised. Over-the-counter antacid preparations and mucosal

Answers *cont.*

protecting agents may also provide some symptomatic relief. These measures alone may be sufficient to provide symptomatic control.

A.2 Patients with persistent symptoms require further evaluation. Patients older than 50 years should be considered for referral for an upper gastrointestinal endoscopy as the risk of an underlying malignancy is higher in this age group. For younger patients without alarm symptoms, an endoscopy is probably not indicated at this stage. A trial of acid suppression therapy may be advised. Proton pump inhibitors (PPIs) and histamine-2 receptor antagonists are widely used worldwide with a good safety profile, although the effects of long-term use are still not fully determined. Prokinetic agents, such as metoclopramide, may be also used to aid gastric emptying particularly when associated with gastro-oesophageal reflux.

A.3 *Helicobacter pylori* (*H. pylori*) is a Gram-negative bacillus that favours the conditions found within the gastric antrum. The organism promotes acid hypersecretion within the stomach and induces gastric inflammation and has been associated with dyspepsia and reflux symptoms.

Several methods have been developed to test for the presence of *H. pylori*.
- Serology is the least useful test as a positive result denotes only previous exposure and does not necessarily indicate a current or active infection.
- Stool antigen test.
- The carbon urea breath test (CUBT) is the non-invasive test of choice. The patient drinks C-13 or C-14-labelled urea which the bacterium metabolizes to produce labelled carbon dioxide. This is absorbed

by the gut, incorporated in the body's metabolism and then exhaled as labelled CO_2. The CUBT should not be performed within 2 weeks of PPI therapy as a false negative result may be obtained.
- Antral biopsy. This invasive test is the most reliable – but not the most convenient. An endoscopic biopsy is taken from the gastric antrum and the sample placed into a culture medium that contains an indicator dye, such as phenol red. *H. pylori* hydrolyses urea to ammonia which raises the pH of the medium and changes the indicator colour. This is called a CLO test Figure 11.2. Direct microscopy may also show the presence of the microbe on histological sections.

A.4 It is essential that all patients are reviewed following eradication therapy to assess their response to treatment. Patients who are asymptomatic following treatment may be discharged and advised to continue with general healthy lifestyle recommendations. Patients with recurrent or persistent symptoms following eradication therapy should be re-tested for *H. pylori* infection. First-line eradication therapy successfully treats *H. pylori* infection in 70–80% of patients. If the repeat test is positive, a further course of second-line antimicrobial therapy would be indicated. If the repeat test was negative several options should be taken into account. Firstly, the diagnosis may be wrong. Consideration should be given to other causes of the symptoms, such a gallstone disease or bowel-related disorders. In older patients, for example 50 years or older, further thought should be given to whether the patient warrants an endoscopy if this has not already been performed. Finally, if all other factors have

79

Answers *cont.*

been considered and in an otherwise healthy young adult, the patient may be managed as functional dyspepsia.

A.5 In the first instance this patient should be encouraged to persist with medical therapy and use a higher dose of PPI. While the vast majority of patients with gastro-oesophageal reflux disease are managed quite satisfactorily with medical treatment a small proportion of patients will opt for surgical management. The usual reasons are a persistence of heartburn despite high dosage PPI therapy and/or volume reflux. A number of non-operative (endoscopic) procedures for the control of reflux have been promoted (e.g. radio-frequency scarification at the lower oesophageal sphincter, stapled fundoplication). Although some short-term success has been reported with these techniques none has yet shown any durability.

The advantages and disadvantages of other options should be discussed. The standard surgical approach currently offered to patients with troublesome GORD is laparoscopic fundoplication. The principles of the procedure include reduction and repair of any hiatal hernia combined with a partial or total fundoplication (a wrap of the fundus of the stomach around the intra-abdominal component of the oesophagus). The majority of patients who undergo fundoplication will have improvement or abolition of their symptoms and a recent randomized trial reported both improved symptom control and general well-being following anti-reflux surgery consistent with that achieved by best medical therapy. The potential side-effects following fundoplication of dysphagia, gas bloat and inability to belch or vomit must be discussed.

A.6 An endoscopy allows identification of any oesophagitis that may be present along with confirmation by histological analysis. The presence of an associated hiatus hernia can also be assessed and any co-existent disease, such as peptic ulceration, may be identified. In selected cases a barium swallow and meal allows assessment of upper gastrointestinal tract function, particularly with respect to the assessment of swallowing propagation and volume reflux. A contrast study is particularly helpful in delineating the anatomy of large paraoesophageal hernias.

Oesophageal manometry and pH studies are commonly performed investigations prior to surgery. Manometry allows analysis of oesophageal contractions, both resting and on swallowing, and measurement of the lower oesophageal sphincter (LOS) pressure. It may be possible to identify abnormal oesophageal contractions which have developed secondary to acid-induced irritability of the oesophagus. Poor oesophageal motility might indicate a partial rather than a total fundoplication would be the preferred option to reduce the risk of postoperative dysphagia. High resting LOS pressures and poor peristalsis may suggest a motility disorder and may influence surgical suitability. Twenty-four-hour ambulatory pH recordings provide information on the amount of acid exposure in the lower oesophagus. In the 24-hour period, those who have an oesophageal pH of less than 4 for more than 5–7% of the time are deemed to have significant reflux. Correlation between symptoms and low pH strengthens the diagnosis.

Answers *cont.*

A typical history of reflux, endoscopic evidence of oesophagitis, and symptomatic response to acid suppression are strong indicators for a good surgical outcome.

A.7 These tests demonstrate anaemia with a low MCV, in keeping with iron deficient anaemia. With his past history of heartburn and dyspepsia he may be bleeding from somewhere in the upper digestive tract.

A.8 The endoscopic photograph demonstrates a tongue of columnar-lined epithelium running up the oesophagus. The patient has Barrett's oesophagus. This is a well-recognized complication of chronic gastro-oesophageal reflux, occurring in around 10% of patients. Other complications of reflux include peptic strictures and iron deficiency anaemia.

The area of Barrett's should be biopsied and carefully examined for evidence of dysplasia. Barrett's oesophagus is considered a pre-malignant disease. Surveillance in such patients is, however, controversial. There is no good evidence to support the concept that the prevention of acid reflux reverses the metaplasia or malignant risk. However, current thinking suggests that if no dysplasia is present then 5-yearly endoscopy is reasonable. If dysplasia is detected, then more frequent endoscopy at 3–6-month intervals is indicated, depending on the degree of dysplasia. PPIs should be prescribed for such patients.

A.9 Treatment with high dose acid suppression therapy may have contributed to the overall improvement from high grade dysplasia to low grade dysplasia (or this might represent sampling error). However,

the nodular area is a worrying feature and histology has identified carcinoma in situ. The patient should be staged to assess the extent of the disease. Initial staging investigations would include endoscopic ultrasound (EUS) and a CT of the chest and abdomen. EUS is the best staging modality for the loco-regional assessment of oesophageal tumours (T and N stage). CT is used to identify distant metastatic disease, especially lung and liver (M stage). Additional staging modalities, such as bone scans and positron emission tomography (PET), may be used in selected cases.

A.10 Without further treatment the nodular lesion will likely progress to invasive carcinoma. Further management is therefore concerned with removing the diseased area. In this scenario, this could involve either a local resection or undertaking an oesophagectomy. Endoscopic mucosal resection (EMR) allows localized removal of the abnormal area (Figure 11.2). Saline or adrenaline is injected into the submucosal layer to elevate the abnormal mucosal segment. A suction cap is then applied and cautery is used to remove the abnormal nodule. The specimen is sent for histological evaluation to ensure complete resection. This option is favourable in terms of morbidity and potential mortality that is associated with oesophagectomy. However, in some patients the option of oesophagectomy may be preferred if there are multiple areas of high-grade dysplasia, there is invasion into the submucosa on the EMR specimen, or the suspicion of invasive carcinoma with nodal involvement is high.

Radiofrequency ablation and photodynamic therapy are treatments under investigation for Barrett's oesophagus.

Answers *cont.*

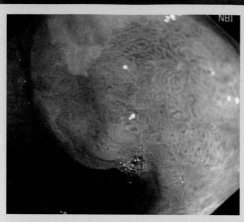

Figure 11.2

Revision Points

Principles of Treatment of Gastro-Oesophageal Reflux

- Lifestyle measures.
- *Helicobacter pylori* eradication.
- Acid suppression.
- Surgery:
  - correction of any hiatal defect
  - increasing lower oesophageal sphincter pressure.

Acid Suppression

- Effective acid suppression in 90% of patients.
- Unknown long-term effects.
- Theoretical increased risk of adenocarcinoma of the oesophagus.

Surgery

The two main mechanisms to minimize reflux are the integrity of the lower oesophageal sphincter and the intra-abdominal oesophagus. As the abdominal pressure rises, as long as there is intra-abdominal oesophagus, there is no pressure gradient across the gastro-oesophageal junction (GOJ).

Once the GOJ enters the chest (e.g. a sliding hiatus hernia) then only the lower oesophageal sphincter can prevent reflux. The principles of surgery are to repair any hiatal defect, reduce the intra-abdominal oesophagus back into the abdominal cavity, and to fashion a fundoplication where the fundus of the stomach is wrapped partially or completely around the intra-abdominal part of the distal oesophagus to hold it within the abdominal cavity.

Complications of Gastro-Oesophageal Reflux Disease

- Iron deficiency anaemia.
- Peptic stricture.
- Barrett's oesophagus.

Barrett's Oesophagus (Columnar-Lined Epithelium)

- Long-term complication of GORD.
- Occurs in 10% of patients with GORD.
- A pre-malignant condition.

Issues to Consider

- Should screening programmes be developed to identify people with Barrett's oesophagus?
- What is the effect of obesity on gastro-oesophageal reflux disease and the risk of adenocarcinoma of the oesophagus?
- What is narrow band imaging and what are its roles in clinical medicine?

Further Information

Grant, A.M., Wileman, S.M., Ramsay, C.R., et al., and the REFLUX Trial Group 2008. Minimal access surgery compared with medical management for chronic gastro-oesophageal reflux disease: UK collaborative randomised trial. British Medical Journal 337, a2664.

www.asge.org *The website of the American Society for Gastrointestinal Endoscopy includes guidelines on Barrett's oesophagus and the management of the patient with dysphagia.*

www.bsg.org.uk *The website of the British Society of Gastroenterology, including guideline for the diagnosis and management of Barrett's columnar-lined oesophagus.*

www.gerd.com *A pharmaceutical company sponsored website covering all aspects of reflux disease.*

www.nice.org.uk *Guideline for the management of dyspepsia, 2004.*

www.sign.ac.uk *Guideline 87 – Management of oesophageal and gastric cancer, 2006.*

Dysphagia and weight loss in a middle-aged man

Sarah K. Thompson

A 55-year-old man presents with a 3-month history of dysphagia and weight loss. He reports that his initial problem was with solid foods only, but he has had to switch to a minced diet for the past month. His wife uses a blender to prepare all of his meals. He has lost almost 15 kg in weight. He has never been diagnosed with gastro-oesophageal reflux disease, and he does not have any medical problems that he is aware of. He used to smoke a pack of cigarettes per day but quit 5 years ago. He drinks between 6 and 12 beers per week and is not on any medication. In the past he has had an appendicectomy and a right inguinal hernia repair with mesh.

On examination he appears to have lost some weight recently but the rest of the physical examination is unremarkable. He does not have any palpable lymphadenopathy.

Q.1 What are the worrying features in the history? What are your differential diagnoses?

You realize that his symptoms warrant investigation, even in the absence of any physical signs, and you go on to arrange some investigations.

Q.2 What investigations would you order?

Blood results are as follows:

Investigation 12.1 Summary of results			
Haemoglobin	106 g/L	White cell count	8.3×10^9/L
MCV	77 fL		
MCH	29.5 pg		
MCHC	230 g/L		
Platelets	180×10^9/L		
Sodium	141 mmol/L	Calcium	2.16 mmol/L
Potassium	3.7 mmol/L	Phosphate	1.15 mmol/L
Chloride	104 mmol/L	Total protein	69 g/L

Investigation 12.1 Summary of results—cont'd			
Bicarbonate	29 mmol/L	Albumin	33 g/L
Urea	7.1 mmol/L	Globulins	36 g/L
Creatinine	0.08 mmol/L	Bilirubin	7 µmol/L
Uric acid	0.24 mmol/L	ALT	26 U/L
Glucose	4.4 mmol/L	AST	50 U/L
Cholesterol	3.5 mmol/L	GGT	17 U/L
LDH	127 U/L	ALP	65 U/L

Q.3 What do the blood tests show?

A further investigation is performed and a representative film is shown (Figure 12.1).

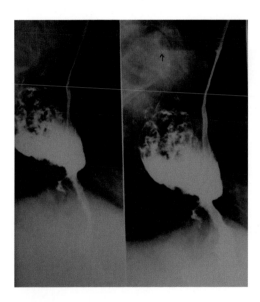

Figure 12.1

Q.4 What is this investigation? What does it show?

Based on the radiological findings, the patient is referred for another investigation (Figure 12.2).

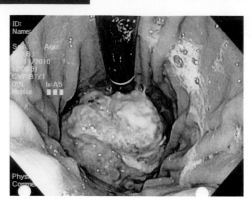

Figure 12.2

Q.5 What is this investigation and what does it show?

The lesion is biopsied and confirmed to be a moderately differentiated adenocarcinoma. The patient is referred for further staging investigations (Figure 12.3 and Figure 12.4.).

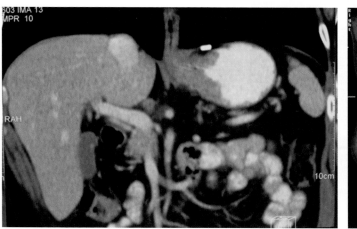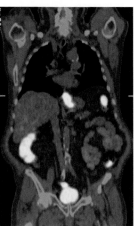

Figure 12.3

Figure 12.4

Q.6 What are these two investigations? What do they show?

Q.7 What further investigations (if any) are required?

Various imaging investigations are performed and do not show any evidence of tumour dissemination. The tumour appears to be confined to the stomach wall, although there may be some thickening in the immediately adjacent tissues.

Q.8 Describe the treatment options available to patients with gastric cancer.

The patient and his diagnostic tests are discussed at a multidisciplinary meeting. The treatment recommendation is for neoadjuvant chemotherapy before and after surgical resection.

Q.9 While treatment is ongoing, how can one prevent further weight loss and malnutrition?

Following three cycles of chemotherapy (over 3 months) and 4 weeks of stabilization, the patient underwent surgery. Figure 12.5 shows the operative view of the upper abdomen.

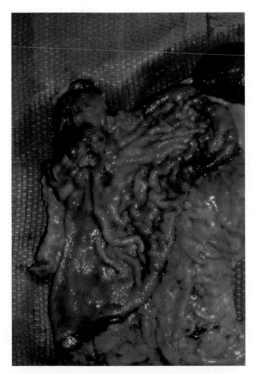

Figure 12.5 Operative specimen.

Q.10 Describe this operative specimen. What is the prognosis for this malignancy?

The tumour showed extensive transmural infiltration by a moderately differentiated adenocarcinoma with involvement of the lymph nodes along the left gastric artery. The patient underwent three more cycles of chemotherapy 2 months following his gastrectomy. He initially did very well but died of disseminated disease 18 months later.

Answers

A.1 From the history there are several features which point to a diagnosis of a gastrointestinal malignancy. Dysphagia and weight loss appearing for the first time in someone over 50 should cause concern and prompt investigation. This patient also has risk factors (alcohol and smoking) for both oesophageal and gastric cancer.

Other diagnoses to consider include:
- achalasia
- peptic stricture or ulceration
- oesophageal dysmotility (e.g. diffuse oesophageal spasm)
- benign oesophageal lesion (e.g. oesophageal leiomyoma)
- extrinsic compression from mediastinal lymphadenopathy/lung lesion.

A.2 Investigations should include:
- complete blood picture (anaemia)
- serum biochemistry (disturbance of liver function with metastatic disease)
- imaging of the upper digestive tract.

A.3 The blood results show a mild microcytic anaemia with a low MCV and MCHC. This is typical of iron deficiency anaemia and consistent with bleeding from occult gastrointestinal pathology. The other blood tests are normal.

A.4 The contrast study is a barium meal and this shows narrowing at the junction of the oesophagus and stomach. There is hold-up of contrast in the distal oesophagus, and the oesophagus appears dilated above the gastro-oesophageal junction. These appearances are typical of either achalasia or pseudoachalasia (i.e. a distal oesophageal cancer, or a lesion in the proximal stomach).

This man needs an endoscopic examination of his upper gastrointestinal tract. In most circumstances the imaging investigation of choice for a patient with these symptoms would be an endoscopy. However, barium meal examinations are still frequently performed by general practitioners as the initial investigation of upper digestive tract symptoms.

A.5 The patient has undergone an endoscopic examination of the upper digestive tract. This image shows a polypoid tumour extending from the squamo-columnar junction into the proximal stomach (the endoscope has been retroflexed to obtain this view). These tumours are classified according to their location in relation to the squamo-columnar junction:

Answers *cont.*

- Type I: adenocarcinoma of the distal oesophagus which may infiltrate the junction from above.
- Type II: true carcinoma of the cardia arising from cardiac epithelium or short segments with intestinal metaplasia at the junction.
- Type III: subcardial gastric carcinoma infiltrating the gastro-oesophageal junction from below.

The patient therefore has a Type III tumour.

A.6 The first image shows a CT scan of the abdomen (with intravenous and oral contrast). There is thickening of the wall of the proximal stomach and no evidence of metastatic deposits. CT scans of the chest, abdomen and pelvis (particularly spiral scans) are capable of providing highly accurate information on:

- the primary tumour (size, position and spread into adjacent tissues)
- presence of metastatic disease in lymph nodes, liver or lungs
- presence of ascites.

The CT is less helpful in the detection of peritoneal deposits. If there is evidence of metastatic disease then no further investigations are required. CT has limitations in detecting nodal disease (N stage) and is not very accurate at assessing the depth of penetration of tumours through the stomach wall (T stage). CT will generally under-stage both the T and N stage in gastric cancer.

The second image is a positron emission tomography (PET) scan which demonstrates a hot spot in the proximal stomach, corresponding to the proximal gastric cancer.

Positron emission tomography (PET) scans have become increasingly useful in gastric cancers. They are more sensitive than CT scans and EUS in detecting distant metastases, such as bony metastases. This nuclear medicine imaging technique detects uptake from a positron-emitting radionuclide tracer (commonly fluorine-18) that is introduced into the body on fluorodeoxyglucose (FDG) molecules prior to the scan. Fluorine-18 is a glucose analogue that is preferentially taken up by rapidly growing malignant tumours. PET scans will not detect primary gastric cancers in up to 30% of cases (usually those with signet ring cell features), and in these select cases may not be useful in detecting the presence of any metastatic disease.

A.7 Further investigations are needed to accurately stage the disease and then determine the best treatment options. These include: Staging laparoscopy to rule out the presence of small peritoneal deposits. These are common in gastric cancer and cannot be easily detected by CT or EUS. Endoscopic ultrasound scanning (EUS) can give accurate information about depth of penetration of the tumour through the stomach wall and also on the extent of any lymph node involvement. Where available, EUS is a useful adjunct to CT in preoperative staging of gastric cancer.

A transthoracic echocardiogram and pulmonary function tests (arterial blood gas and spirometry) will help determine the patient's general state of health.

A.8 The treatment of gastric cancer depends on:

- histopathology on biopsy
- stage of the disease after investigations
- general state of health of the patient
- need to palliate symptoms related to the primary tumour (such as anaemia, obstruction).

Answers *cont.*

Curative treatment may be considered for:
- early gastric cancers
- gastric lymphomas
- some advanced gastric adenocarcinomas which have no evidence of local or distant spread.

Treatment options include:
- endoscopic resection of early gastric cancers
- chemotherapy for lymphomas
- surgical intervention (with or without neoadjuvant chemotherapy) for more advanced adenocarcinomas:
  - radical resection for 'cure'
  - resection or bypass for palliation
- palliative care measures.

Very early and localized cancers that have not invaded the gastric submucosa (early gastric cancer) can be removed endoscopically. These sorts of tumours are rare outside of Japan.

In most parts of the world the majority of patients with gastric cancer have incurable disease at the time of presentation. In contrast, gastric cancer is relatively common in Japan where screening programmes are used to detect the disease at a much earlier stage and a high percentage of patients are cured by surgery.

While some individuals can be cured of more advanced cancers, the role of surgery is usually to relieve symptoms and palliate obstruction or bleeding. Improved methods of palliation have decreased the need for surgical intervention. These procedures include endoscopic ablation of the tumour by laser or argon beam coagulation, palliative chemotherapy and palliative radiotherapy. Self-expanding metal stents can be used to relieve obstruction.

A.9 The location of cancers of the oesophagus and stomach may directly interfere with the patient's nutritional status. While treatment is ongoing, it is important to ensure the patient is capable of meeting his/her nutritional requirements. The advice of a dietician should be sought prior to the commencement of treatment. In many cases, supplementation with high energy and protein drinks will be sufficient (e.g. Sustagen). If the tumour has partially occluded the lumen of the oesophagus or stomach, placement of a naso-gastric feeding tube (or naso-enteric feeding tube for a distal gastric tumour) will prevent further weight loss and malnutrition while the patient is undergoing treatment. For more advanced tumours (i.e. those with complete occlusion of the lumen), a surgically placed feeding tube into the proximal jejunum may be necessary.

A.10 This is a total gastrectomy specimen in which all of the stomach has been removed along with the omentum and spleen. There is thickening of cardia and fundus from tumour infiltration. The mucosa in the body/distal stomach looks relatively normal while in the proximal stomach, ulceration is evident (in the centre of the tumour) and this probably represents transmural infiltration (T3).

The prognosis for gastric cancer remains poor with overall 5-year survival of 10–15% in most Western countries. This reflects the advanced stage of the disease at presentation and the increasing age of the population; many patients with gastric cancer are elderly and frail and not suitable for curative surgical treatment. In Japan the overall 5-year survival is 50% or above. This reflects diagnosis at an earlier stage and more effective surgical treatment.

The incidence of gastric cancer is decreasing dramatically in the West. In

Answers *cont.*

developing countries the incidence remains high and is particularly so in Japan, China, East Asia and Latin America. The reason for the fall in incidence in the West is related to environmental factors. *Helicobacter pylori* is associated with gastric cancer. The prevalence of *Helicobacter* in Western communities has steadily declined as public health and hygiene have improved. This has coincided with the reduction in gastric cancer. Dietary changes with an increase in protein relative to carbohydrate, increasing food hygiene and refrigeration and increasing consumption of fresh fruit and vegetables have probably also decreased the incidence of gastric cancer.

The distribution of gastric cancer in the West is changing. Cancers used to be prevalent in the distal stomach. It is these cancers that are becoming less common whereas, for reasons unknown, the incidence of cancers of the cardia (together with adenocarcinoma of the distal oesophagus) has increased dramatically over the last two decades.

In surgical series in the West survival for potentially curative surgery is around 50%. Early gastric cancer (confined to the mucosal layer of the stomach) can be cured by surgery but as the tumour spreads through the gastric wall and involves lymph nodes the likelihood of a cure lessens.

Revision Points

Gastric Cancer

Incidence
- 15–17 : 100 000 in the Western world.

Risk Factors
- Male sex.
- *Helicobacter pylori* infection.
- Dietary factors (smoked foods, etc.).
- Pernicious anaemia.
- Previous partial gastrectomy.
- Cigarette smoking and alcohol intake.

Histology
- Adenocarcinoma (90%).
- Lymphomas (6%).
- Gastrointestinal stromal tumours (GIST) (4%).

Presentation
Depends on the location of the tumour. If in the proximal stomach, patients often present with dysphagia and weight loss. Tumours in the mid to distal stomach present with symptoms of epigastric pain, indigestion, early satiety, weight loss, vomiting, anaemia and abdominal mass. Patients over 50 with new-onset symptoms should be investigated immediately.

Clinical Features
Patients with early disease have no obvious signs but patients with advanced disease are often thin (or even cachetic) and pale. Supraclavicular lymph node enlargement, an epigastric mass or ascites are signs of advanced disease.

Revision Points *cont.*

Prognosis

The overall prognosis for adenocarcinoma is poor with only 10–15% surviving 5 years. Five-year survival rates for those who undergo surgical resection range from 0 to 50%, depending on the extent of disease.

Investigation

• Endoscopy and biopsy for diagnosis.
• Imaging for staging.

Treatment

• Resection for cure (gastrectomy) with or without neoadjuvant chemotherapy.
• Surgery, endoscopic intervention or radio/chemotherapy for palliation.

Issues to Consider

• What are the complications associated with gastric resection?
• Why is gastric cancer more common in Japan? Are there any screening tests or preventative strategies which could be useful?
• How may the changing incidence of *Helicobacter pylori* infection be affecting the changing incidence of proximal and gastric cancers?

Further Information

www.cancer.gov/cancertopics/wyntk/stomach *A web page from the National Cancer Institute with links providing current information on many different aspects of gastric cancer (in the form of a web-based information booklet).*

www.surgical-tutor.org.uk *A surgical resource with extensive up-to-date information on gastric cancer.*

www.helico.com *The website of the Helicobacter Foundation, founded by Dr Barry Marshall.*

PROBLEM
13

Abdominal pain in a young woman

Peter Devitt

A 28-year-old woman presents to the emergency department with upper abdominal pain. The pain starts in the epigastrium and radiates to the right and left upper quadrants. She rates the pain as 7 out of 10. She has had several similar episodes over the last 6 weeks. During each episode, the pain was of rapid onset and resolved spontaneously after several hours. On each occasion she was nauseated but did not vomit. She is significantly overweight with a body mass index of 36.

Q.1 What further information would you like from the patient? What are the possible diagnoses?

The patient is otherwise in good health with an unremarkable medical history. She is considerably distressed by the pain, but the physical examination is normal apart from some tenderness in the right upper quadrant. She is overweight with a BMI of 34. Arrangements are made for her admission.

Q.2 What investigations does this patient require?

An ultrasound examination of the upper abdomen is performed (Figures 13.1 and 13.2).
There is bilirubin + on urinalysis. Her serum biochemistry is shown below.

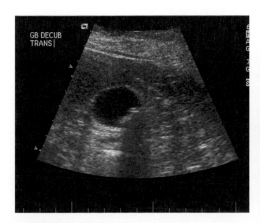

Figure 13.1

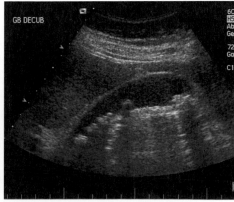

Figure 13.2

Investigation 13.1 Summary of results			
Haemoglobin	145 g/L	White cell count	14.9×10^9/L
Platelets	354×10^9/L		
Sodium	148 mmol/L	Calcium	2.16 mmol/L
Potassium	4.3 mmol/L	Phosphate	1.15 mmol/L
Chloride	106 mmol/L	Total protein	58 g/L
Bicarbonate	27 mmol/L	Albumin	38 g/L
Urea	15.2 mmol/L	Globulins	20 g/L
Creatinine	0.13 mmol/L	Bilirubin	45 µmoL/L
Uric acid	0.24 mmol/L	ALT	118 U/L
Glucose	4.6 mmol/L	AST	123 U/L
CholesteroL	3.5 mmol/L	GGT	297 U/L
LDH	212 U/L	ALP	254 U/L

Q.3 What do the investigations show?

The day after admission the patient is feeling much better and is pain-free.

Q.4 What is the appropriate advice to give the patient?

Her liver function tests are improving. She listens to your advice and agrees to a plan of ERCP followed by elective cholecystectomy. Her weight has not previously been mentioned as a problem. Should it be added to the introduction if it is used her? She is discharged home with arrangments for an ERCP the following week.

Five days later you are asked to see the patient in the emergency department. She has had further bouts of pain on and off for 2 days and has vomited a number of times. She also reports that her urine has darkened and that her stools are pale. She has not slept well the past 2 nights because of drenching sweats and she reports two violent shivering attacks this morning. She is uncertain of the date or day.

On examination she looks ill, distracted and has a temperature of 39.5°C. She is flushed and has yellow sclera. Her pulse is 110 bpm and her blood pressure is 90/50 mmHg. She has dry mucous membranes. Examination of her cardiorespiratory system is unremarkable. Her abdomen is soft and there is no localized area of tenderness.

Q.5 State the diagnosis and describe an appropriate plan of management.

With prompt resuscitation the patient improves and an ERCP is performed once she is stable. In preparation for this procedure, informed consent must be obtained.

Q.6 What risks would you inform the patient of when seeking consent?

The ERCP is performed and the image shown in Figure 13.3 is obtained.

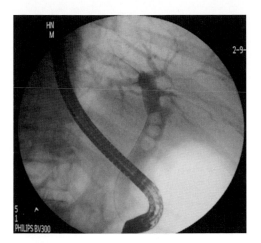

Figure 13.3

Q.7 What does the image show?

The patient makes a rapid recovery from her illness and her liver function tests return to normal. She is discharged home, manages to lose 20 kg and subsequently undergoes an elective laparoscopic cholecystectomy.

Answers

A.1 Further information must be sought on:
- The pain:
  - its nature (constant or colic)
  - radiation (round or through to the back, retrosternal, shoulder, down into abdomen)
  - its severity, did it disturb her normal activities, her sleep or stop her going to work
  - any relieving or exacerbating features.
- Any associated urinary or gastrointestinal symptoms.

- Any evidence of biliary obstruction during these episodes such as overt jaundice (friends and family may notice), pale stools and dark urine.
- Any past history of gastrointestinal or renal tract problems.

These severe episodes of right upper quadrant pain requiring opiate analgesia are characteristic of biliary colic (stones in the gallbladder or bile duct). The pain will often radiate around the costal margin to the back. Biliary colic may result from obstruction of the cystic duct, which typically occurs when a gallstone becomes impacted in Hartmann's pouch. The pain – which is typically unremitting and constant – lasts until the gallstone falls back into the gallbladder and the obstruction is relieved.

Other diagnoses to consider include:

- Renal stones or ureteric colic. Stones in the renal tract can produce severe upper abdominal and back pain.
- Peptic ulcer disease. The pain is not usually so rapid in onset and is not usually of such severity.
- Oesophageal spasm. Oesophageal pain is usually retrosternal, but this source should always be considered in cases of upper abdominal pain.
- In an older patient myocardial ischaemia or infarction must be considered in those who present with acute epigastric pain.

A.2 The following investigations are required:

- An ultrasound examination of the upper abdomen. The prime objective is to look for gallstones. The examination is performed following a fast, otherwise the gallbladder will be contracted and any stones difficult to see. The thickness of the wall of the gallbladder will also be assessed (thickening may suggest inflammation). The liver parenchyma can be studied and any dilatation of the biliary tree visualized. Stones may occasionally be seen in the biliary tree (the sensitivity of ultrasonography for this is less than 50%). Renal stones may also be detected, together with any ureteric obstruction.
- Liver function tests looking for evidence of recent or ongoing biliary obstruction.
- Urinalysis to check for haematuria and bilirubinuria.

A.3 This is an image from an ultrasound of the gallbladder showing a thin-walled gallbladder with several small echogenic foci which cast acoustic shadows beyond. These are gallstones. The biliary system does not appear to be dilated and no stones can be seen outside the gallbladder. The serum biochemistry results show deranged liver function with moderate elevation of the transaminases, alkaline phosphatase and bilirubin. All these would be in keeping with the patient's current problem being related to duct stones.

A.4 This patient needs to be advised that her current episode of pain is almost certainly biliary in origin, as were the previous ones. Left untreated she will most likely have further problems.

She needs a cholecystectomy. The frequency and severity of her symptoms suggests that this should be done relatively soon. The standard of care would be to offer her a laparoscopic cholecystectomy during the current admission. Two things mitigate against this: her obesity and the high likelihood of duct stones. These two factors would increase the risk of conversion from a laparoscopic to an open operation. Opinion is divided on optimum treatment. Some surgeons might elect to proceed to laparoscopic cholecystectomy, cholangiography and intraoperative duct clearance – knowing that this might involve conversion to open surgery. An alternative approach would be endoscopic retrograde cholangiopancreatography (ERCP), duct clearance and weight reduction prior to planned laparoscopic cholecystectomy.

A.5 She has the classical triad that describes cholangitis: fever, right upper quadrant pain and jaundice. Of greater concern, she is hypotensive and is

Answers *cont.*

becoming confused. In this life-threatening situation of biliary sepsis the patient requires rapid resuscitation. She must be given intravenous fluids, supplemental oxygen and broad-spectrum antibiotics. Once intravenous access has been established blood samples must be sent for laboratory investigations, including blood cultures and coagulation studies. One litre of isotonic saline can be run in rapidly and further infusion judged on the response. Suitable antibiotic regimens would include gentamicin/amoxicillin/metronidazole or a second-generation cephalosporin such as cefoxitin. Initial management should be in a high-dependency unit with pulse oximetry, blood pressure and cardiac monitoring.

The ultrasound should be repeated, looking for biliary obstruction. She will likely need an urgent ERCP to relieve the obstruction and achieve biliary drainage so you should contact the gastroenterologists or biliary surgeons.

A.6 In obtaining informed consent for ERCP, you need to explain the rationale for the procedure and its potential risks and benefits. The aim of the procedure is to decompress the common bile duct and get sepsis under control. The endoscopist may place a stent into the common bile duct and/or may be able to retrieve the stone. The benefit of the ERCP in the present circumstances is that, if successful, the patient may be able to avoid major and hazardous open surgery to her common bile duct. The main risks of ERCP are pancreatitis (1–5%) and haemorrhage (1–2%). Both of these complications can be life-threatening and are more common when there is prolonged instrumentation of the biliary tree as in complex cases like these. There is a also a small risk of a retroperitoneal perforation following sphincterotomy and the patient must be informed of these risks in addition to the risks of sedation or anaesthesia needed to carry out the ERCP. In the present circumstances, the potential benefits of ERCP far outweigh the risks.

A.7 The image shows opacification of the biliary tree with contrast in the common bile duct and the intrahepatic system. There are three filling defects in the common bile duct. These are gallstones. A guidewire has been passed up the duct above the stones. This will allow a catheter with a balloon tip to be introduced in order that the stones may be extracted. In preparation to removing the calculi, the endoscopist will have made a cut through the sphincter of Oddi using diathermy. This procedure is known as a sphincterotomy. A stent will be placed after the stones have been removed to facilitate drainage.

Revision Points

Gallstones

Incidence
- Common worldwide (except Africa). Rates vary from 5 to 36%.
- Increasing in the Western world possibly due to diet, obesity and an ageing population.

Risk Factors
- Female sex (3×).
- Obesity.
- Hyperlipidaemia.
- Diabetes mellitus.
- Ileal disease.
- Haemolysis.

Revision Points cont.

Intraductal parasites are an important cause in some parts of the developing world.

Types

- Most stones are a mixture of cholesterol and bile pigment. Pure cholesterol or pure bile pigment stones are uncommon but do occur.
- Most stones in developed countries are predominantly cholesterol.
- The exact mechanism of cholesterol stone formation is unknown but may involve mucous proteins from the gallbladder wall promoting crystal formation.
- Predominant bile pigment stones are found in patients with haemolysis and parasitic infection.

Clinical Presentation

Problems may relate to:

- Stones in the gallbladder:
  - biliary colic
  - acute cholecystitis
  - carcinoma (rare).
- Stones in the ductal system:
  - jaundice
  - cholangitis
  - acute pancreatitis.
- Stones in the small intestine:
  - gallstone ileus (rare).

The vast majority of gallstones are asymptomatic. Fifteen per cent of patients with gallstones will also have duct stones. Stones in the common bile duct tend to produce symptoms. What is sometimes labelled 'chronic cholecystitis' is more likely to represent something within the spectrum of functional gut disorders and the gallstones found on investigation of these patients are merely coincidental.

Imaging Studies

- Gallstones:
  - abdominal ultrasonography (90% sensitivity)

- Duct stones:
  - abdominal ultrasonography (50% sensitivity)
  - ERCP
  - magnetic resonance cholangiopancreatography (MRCP).

Cholangitis and Management of Duct Stones

- Prompt resuscitation with intravenous fluids and antibiotics.
- If mild and improving – elective ERCP.
- If severe or not responding to resuscitation – urgent duct decompression. If this cannot be done by ERCP, percutaneous drainage may be required.

Treatment of Gallstones

- Laparoscopic cholecystectomy.

A balance must be reached between the risk of surgery and the potential benefit to the patient. The patient must be fully involved in the decision-making process. Treatment should be recommended for patients who have developed symptomatic gallstones.

In acute cholecystitis, initial treatment should be conservative with pain relief, intravenous rehydration and, if not settling, antibiotics. Cholecystectomy should then be performed at the earliest opportunity.

- If identified preoperatively bile duct calculi can be managed with ERCP and subsequent laparoscopic cholecystectomy.
- If identified at the time of surgery, duct stones can be removed by choledochtomy or transcystically – or left for ERCP at a later date.

Issues to Consider

- What other conditions apart from gallstone disease should be treated by cholecystectomy?
- In what circumstances might ERCP not be a feasible procedure for duct stone retrieval?
- Are there any circumstances where patients with asymptomatic gallstones should be advised to have a cholecystectomy?
- Are there any other feasible alternatives to cholecystectomy to get rid of gallstones?

Further Information

http://www.quackwatch.com/ *One practitioner's efforts to expose many of the fraudulent claims made by the proponents of alternative medicine. Search for 'gallstones'.*

http://www.gastro.org/patient-center/ digestive-conditions/gallstones *Up-to-date information on gallstones with a patient slant, from the American Gastroenterological Society.*

A woman with acute upper abdominal pain

Duncan J. Stewart and Roger Ackroyd

A 57-year-old woman is admitted with a 2-day history of increasingly severe upper abdominal pain, radiating through to the back. Although initially colicky in nature, the pain is now constant. She has lost her appetite and has vomited on several occasions. Over the preceding months she has suffered with intermittent bouts of colicky upper abdominal pain that have lasted a few hours at a time. She has no allergies and is a non-smoker. She has no other significant past medical history, including no previous abdominal surgery. On examination she is overweight and looks unwell and dehydrated, although she is apyrexial. Her heart rate is 115 bpm and regular and her blood pressure is 130/90 mmHg. Respiratory examination reveals decreased air entry and dullness to percussion at the left base. Her abdomen is mildly distended and tender in the epigastrium and peri-umbilically. There are no palpable masses and although present, bowel sounds are infrequent.

Q.1 Based on the history and examination, briefly discuss the differential diagnoses.

To refine your list of differential diagnoses you order some investigations.

Q.2 Which initial investigations would you order and why?

The patient's ECG reveals a sinus tachycardia and no other changes. Her chest X-ray is shown in Figure 14.1 and her blood test results are shown in Investigation 14.1. Her BMI is calculated to be 34 kg/m².

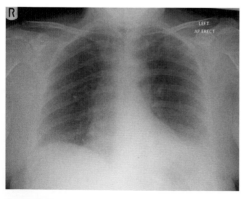

Figure 14.1

Investigation 14.1 Summary of results

Hb	151 g/L	Sodium	142 mmol/L		T Prot	62 g/L
WCC	17.2 × 10⁹/L	Potassium	3.7 mmol/L		Alb	35 g/L
Plts	350 × 10⁹/L	Urea	6.8 mmol/L		Glob	27 g/L
Creatinine	110 μmol/L	Bilirubin	27 μmol/L			
Gluc	11 mmol/L	Chloride	101 mmol/l		ALT	29 U/L
Chol	3.7 mmol/L	Bicarb	20 mmol/L		AST	44 U/L
Amy	2105 U/L	Calcium	2.1 mmol/L		GGT	115 U/L
Lac	2.8 mmol/L	Lipase	4200 U/L		ALP	185 U/L
					LDH	550 U/L

Q.3 What do the investigations show, what is the likely diagnosis and what other investigations would you like at this point?

The results of the arterial blood gas analysis on inspired room air and the C-reactive protein (CRP) are shown in Investigation 14.2.

Investigation 14.2 Summary of results

pH	7.36	CRP	139 mg/L
pCO_2	34 mmHg		
pO_2	70 mmHg		
Bicarb	20 mmol/L		
Base deficit	3		
Saturations	95%		

Q.4 How would you initially manage this patient? How would you assess potential disease severity?

Overnight, she remains stable and begins to feel better.

Q.5 What is the likely underlying cause of the pancreatitis and what investigation should be performed to investigate this?

An ultrasound scan shows gallstones in a distended gallbladder, with dilatation of the intrahepatic bile ducts. The extrahepatic biliary tree and the pancreas are obscured by bowel gas.

Over the next 24 hours the patient deteriorates. She develops a pyrexia of 38.8°C and becomes jaundiced. She is transferred to the high dependency unit and her repeat blood results are shown in Investigation 14.3.

Investigation 14.3 Summary of results					
Hb	139 g/L	T Prot	47 g/L	CRP	376 mg/L
WCC	22.7 × 10⁹/L	Alb	25 g/L		
Plts	498 × 10⁹/L	Glob	20 g/L		
		Bilirubin	97 µmol/L		
Sodium	136 mmol/L	ALT	72 U/L		
Potassium	3.5 mmol/L	AST	63 U/L		
Urea	10.7 mmol/L	GGT	210 U/L		
Creatinine	168 mmol/L	ALP	460 U/L		
Calcium	1.97 mmol/L	LDH	610 U/L		

Q.6 What radiological investigation(s) would now be appropriate?

The magnetic resonance cholangiopancreatogram is shown in Figure 14.2. The MRCP shows dilated intra- and extrahepatic ducts and a solitary stone (*arrow*) impacted at the bottom of the common bile duct. The pancreatic duct is also visible passing to the right of the picture.

Figure 14.2

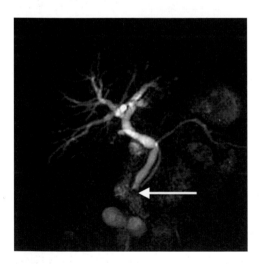

Q.7 Given the clinical deterioration and the radiological findings, what is the next management step?

She has a successful sphincterotomy, duct clearance and stent insertion at ERCP and makes a prolonged, but otherwise uneventful recovery over the next 10 days.

Q.8 What are the remaining steps in the management of this patient?

Answers

A.1 The diagnoses to consider include acute pancreatitis, perforated peptic ulcer and acute cholecystitis. It is possible that she has been suffering with attacks of biliary colic for some time and, given the progressive nature of her pain and its radiation through to the back, acute pancreatitis would be the most likely clinical diagnosis. Although not always the case, you may expect the patient to have a rigid abdomen if the cause were a perforated peptic ulcer. It is important to consider the possibility of a myocardial infarction or a lower lobe pneumonia giving rise to similar symptoms, especially considering the findings on respiratory examination.

Other diagnoses to consider are ischaemic gut and intestinal obstruction. Ischaemic gut is a difficult diagnosis to make but may be more likely in those with pre-existing vascular disease or cardiac dysrythmias, particularly atrial fibrillation. There are few, if any, features to suggest the possibility of intestinal obstruction.

A.2

- Full blood count – an elevated white cell count would support the hypothesis of an inflammatory or infective process.
- Serum biochemistry – to gauge the degree of electrolyte disturbance from vomiting and also assess renal function and degree of dehydration. With upper abdominal pain and the possibility of biliary disease or obstruction, liver function tests are also important.
- Chest X-ray – to evaluate the findings on respiratory examination and to look for free sub-diaphragmatic gas.
- 12-lead electrocardiogram – the patient has what clinically appears to be a sinus tachycardia – and further evaluate the possibility of a cardiac cause for the pain.

- Serum amylase and lipase – grossly elevated levels would confirm acute pancreatitis.

A.3 The chest X-ray shows a small left-sided pleural effusion. The white cell count is elevated, as are the serum lipase and amylase estimations. Given the degree of hyperamylasaemia and hyperlipasaemia this patient almost certainly has acute pancreatitis. The clinical picture and the raised white cell count and blood glucose are certainly in keeping with this. A rise in the serum amylase to at least three times the upper limit of normal would be expected. Hyperamylasaemia to a lesser degree can, however, be associated with alternative intra-abdominal conditions such as acute cholecystitis and intestinal ischaemia. In situations of diagnostic difficulty, measurement of the serum lipase has a higher sensitivity and specificity than serum amylase.

She has deranged liver function tests, with an elevated alkaline phosphatase and a slightly raised bilirubin, although this is unlikely to be detectable clinically. It would be prudent to check the clotting profile in this circumstance.

She needs arterial blood gas analysis and a C-reactive protein measurement.

A.4 This patient needs careful management. Initially, she should be fluid resuscitated with intravenous crystalloids. She may require a considerable volume of fluid over the next few days because of the acute inflammatory response leading to fluid sequestration around the inflamed pancreas, within bowel loops and in the interstitial fluid compartment. She needs close monitoring of fluid input and output and will need a urinary catheter connected to an hourly drainage bag.

Answers *cont.*

If vomiting is a problem, she may benefit from a nasogastric tube, although patients with acute pancreatitis may, if tolerated, benefit from oral intake and nasogastric feeding in an attempt to reduce the incidence of septic complications.

She will require opiate analgesia.

Given the presence of a small pleural effusion at presentation and oxygen saturations of 95% on air, she should have supplemental oxygen, although at this stage nasal cannulae with 2–4 L/minute will probably suffice. She will require regular measurement of oxygen saturations by pulse oximetry.

She will need regular monitoring of serum electrolytes, calcium and blood sugar. She may require supplemental calcium and intravenous sliding scale insulin therapy.

The Atlanta classification (1992) is the most widely used clinically based scoring system that stratifies patients as having either mild or severe disease depending largely on the severity of associated organ dysfunction, combined with the presence or absence of local and systemic complications. However, numerous attempts have been made to develop scoring systems with the aim of predicting which patients will go on to develop severe pancreatitis to allow early intensive monitoring and therapy. On admission, a BMI of >30 and the presence of a pleural effusion are predictive of severe disease. The acute physiology and chronic health evaluation (APACHE) II scoring system has been used in pancreatitis and can be applied to patients with acute pancreatitis from the time of admission. A score of >8 predicts severe disease. The modified Glasgow score consists of eight variables applied after 48 hours of admission. Each positive variable scores 1, with a total of ≥3 predicting severe pancreatitis (see revision

points). A CRP of >150 IU after the first 24 hours is indicative of severe disease. However, much still depends on clinical impression of severity, especially if there is persistent or deteriorating organ failure extending beyond 48 hours after admission.

A.5 The most common cause of acute pancreatitis in Western medicine is gallstones. Every patient diagnosed with acute pancreatitis should have an abdominal ultrasound scan within 24 hours.

A.6 Given the presence of gallstones and dilated intrahepatic bile ducts on ultrasound, in conjunction with a rising serum bilirubin, a rising WCC and pyrexia, the most useful investigation is magnetic resonance cholangiopancreatography (MRCP) to confirm the presence of a stone within the bile duct.

Your patient is at risk of developing severe pancreatitis. With a BMI >30, she had a left pleural effusion at presentation, her CRP has risen to >150 mg/L and her modified Glasgow score is 5 (age > 55, WCC >15 × 10⁹/L, calcium <2 mmol/L, LDH >600 U/L and albumin <32 g/L).

A.7 She needs urgent endoscopic retrograde cholangiopancreatography (ERCP), with sphincterotomy and stone extraction +/− removable stent insertion to ensure relief of biliary obstruction, ideally with 72 hours.

A.8 This patient needs a cholecystectomy. This should ideally be arranged within the same hospital admission and as a laparoscopic procedure. The biliary stent should be removed endoscopically once her gallbladder has been removed.

Revision Points

Causes

The more common causes are listed below, with gallstones being responsible for approximately 50% of cases.

- Gallstones.
- Alcohol.
- Iatrogenic (ERCP/surgery).
- Drugs.
- Trauma.
- Hypercalcaemia.
- Hyperlipidaemia.
- Viral illness (e.g. mumps).
- Idiopathic.

Presentation

Upper abdominal pain, nausea, vomiting and anorexia. Jaundice occurs less frequently.

Diagnosis and Investigations

- Serum amylase to confirm diagnosis.
- Chest X-ray to exclude visceral perforation.
- ECG to exclude cardiac causes of pain.
- Abdominal ultrasound scan within 24 hours to look for gallstones as a cause.
- Consider CT to assess for pancreatic perfusion, necrosis and peripancreatic fluid collections. This may be of limited management value within the first 4 days of the illness.

Prediction of Disease Severity

- Obesity (BMI > 30 kg/m^2).
- Presence of pleural effusion on admission.
- CRP > 150 mg/L.
- APACHE score > 8.
- Modified Glasgow score (assessed at 48 hours after admission):
  - Age >55 years.
  - WCC >15×10^9/L.
  - pO$_2$ <60 mmHg on air.
  - Albumin <32 g/L.
  - Unadjusted calcium <2 mmol/L.
  - LDH >600 U/L.
  - Glucose >10 mmol/L (in absence of diabetes).
  - Urea >16 mmol/L.

Management

- Usually supportive only. Fluid resuscitation, monitoring electrolytes, analgesia, ensuring adequate nutrition and determining cause. May need ERCP in the acute phase if gallstones the cause, especially with jaundice or cholangitis, to ensure adequate biliary drainage.
- Surgical necrosectomy occasionally required if necrotic, non-perfusing areas of pancreas and clinically deteriorating patient. If gallstones are the underlying cause, the patient will need a cholecystectomy.

Complications

Up to 85% of cases are mild and self-limiting with few complications. However, multi-organ failure can occur, with upper gastrointestinal haemorrhage, pancreatic abscess/necrosis and formation of pseudocyst.

Prognosis

Overall mortality 5–10%, although in severe haemorrhagic pancreatitis mortality may approach 90%.

Issues to Consider

- How would the management of this patient differ if the cause of the pancreatitis was alcohol related?
- What are the symptoms and signs associated with pseudocyst formation and how is this complication treated?

Further Information

Ayub, K., Slavin, J., Imada, R., 2004. Endoscopic retrograde cholangiopancreatography in gallstone-associated acute pancreatitis. Cochrane Database of Systematic Reviews 2004, Issue 3. Art. No.: CD003630. DOI:10.1002/14651858.CD003630.pub2. *Provides the evidence base for endoscopic intervention in patients with severe acute pancreatitis due to gallstones.*

Banks, P.A., Freeman, M.L., 2006. Practice guidelines in acute pancreatitis. American Journal of Gastroenterology 101, 2379–2400. DOI: 10.1111/j.1572-0241.2006.00856.x *The most recent American guidelines published.*

Advocate abandonment of the Ranson scoring system due to unacceptably poor predictive power.

Bollen, T.L., van Santvoort, H.C., Besselink, M.G., et al., 2008. The Atlanta classification of acute pancreatitis revisited. British Journal of Surgery 95, 6–21.

Mofidi, R., Patil, P.V., Suttie, S.A., et al., 2009. Risk assessment in acute pancreatitis. British Journal of Surgery 96, 137–150. *Two very informative reviews of the various scoring systems available for use in the management of acute pancreatitis.*

UK Working Party on Acute Pancreatitis, 2005. UK guidelines for the management of acute pancreatitis. Gut 54, 1–9. DOI:10.1136/gut.2004.057026 *Provide a comprehensive management strategy for patients with acute pancreatitis. Represent the most recent European guidelines published. Updates available at* http://gut.bmjjournals.com/cgi/content/full/54/suppl_3/iii1.

Flank pain in a 60-year-old man

Darren Foreman

A 60-year-old man presents with an 8-hour history of left flank pain. This had a sudden onset and the pain 'comes in waves'. Over the last couple of hours, the pain has worsened, and in the last hour he feels nauseated and describes uncontrollable shivers and shakes.

Q.1 What further history would be appropriate?

The patient has never had pain like this before and is usually in good health apart from type II diabetes for which he takes metformin. His past history is unremarkable. On examination, he looks ill, is pale and diaphoretic, and the pain makes him appear uncomfortable. His temperature is 38.7°C, and he has a heart rate of 95/min, blood pressure of 90/60 mmHg, respiratory rate 23/min and an SaO_2 91% breathing room air. His BMI is 30. His abdomen is soft to palpation, with no localizing signs.

His white cell count is 21 (91% neutrophils), creatinine 380 mmol/L, potassium 4.5 mmol/L and blood glucose 12 mmol/L. Urinalysis shows large amounts of red and white blood cells, and nitrites. An ECG is performed and confirms sinus tachycardia with no acute ST changes.

Q.2 What is your diagnosis and immediate management?

Two large-bore intravenous cannulae are inserted and a broad-spectrum antibiotic (ceftriaxone) is administered after blood and urine cultures have been obtained. Opiate analgesia and an antiemetic are given. A fluid balance chart and insulin sliding scale is commenced. After an hour and 2 litres of isotonic saline the patient is comfortable and his vital signs have stabilized. You can now turn your thoughts to looking for the cause of the sepsis.

Q.3 In general, what are the risk factors for sepsis?

Q.4 What are the possible underlying causes for sepsis in this man?

Now that the patient's condition has stabilized some further investigations can be considered.

Q.5 What imaging would be appropriate at this stage?

A non-contrast CT scan is performed and two representative slices are shown in Figure 15.1A, B.

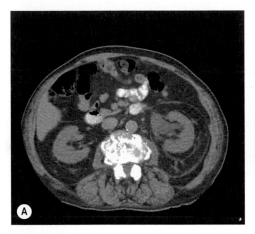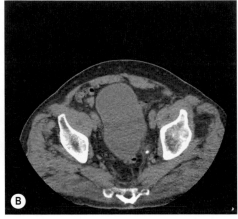

Figure 15.1A   **Figure 15.1B**

Q.6 What do these CT images show?

The CT scan findings confirm the clinical impression of urosepsis with a stone obstructing the left renal tract.

Q.7 How does a ureteric stone cause renal colic, and what other urinary symptoms may be present?

Q.8 How do you manage his pain?

Q.9 What factors are important in determining whether a stone will pass spontaneously?

Q.10 What are the indications for urgent procedural intervention?

Once the patient is stabilized, a ureteric stent is inserted under general anaesthetic via cystoscopy and frank pus drains from the left kidney. A specimen is sent for microscopy and culture and grows *Escherichia*.

The pain resolves rapidly and within 24 hours the patient's temperature, creatinine and potassium are all within normal limits. Antibiotics are continued intravenously for 5 days total, and the patient is discharged with 10 days of oral antibiotics.

He is readmitted 2 weeks later for a ureteroscopy after his urine is confirmed to be sterile.

Q.11 What is being performed in the following photographs (Figure 15.2A, B)?

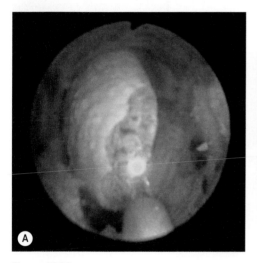

Figure 15.2A

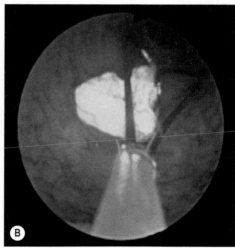

Figure 15.2B

The stone fragments are sent to the laboratory for analysis, and are confirmed to be of calcium oxalate composition. The patient is encouraged to maintain a high oral fluid intake to increase his urine volume and reduce the urinary concentration of calcium oxalate. He is given dietetic advice to avoid foods with high oxalate concentrations. The patient was discharged the day following ureteroscopic stone extraction and remained stone-free when reviewed 12 months later.

Answers

A.1

- Further details about the pain are required. What is the location, is it colicky in nature, what is the severity, does it radiate anywhere and are there any aggravating or relieving factors?

- Are there any other associated symptoms, in particular symptoms of the gastrointestinal (vomiting, diarrhoea) and urinary tracts (dysuria and haematuria)?
- It is important to ascertain relevant medical history, including diabetes, gout,

Answers *cont.*

previous surgery and any history of renal stones or gastrointestinal disease. Current medications and allergies should be noted.

A.2   This man is about to go into septic shock and requires urgent resuscitation with intravenous fluids and supplemental oxygen in a close observation area, such as a high dependency unit. In the absence of any abdominal tenderness or evidence of peritonitis and the finding of microscopic haematuria, the patient is likely to have urosepsis.

A.3   The most common risk factors for sepsis are immunosuppression, malignancy, multiple trauma, diabetes mellitus, malnutrition, elderly age, renal or liver failure.

A.4   The patient almost certainly has an obstructed and infected renal system. A ureteric stone is the likely underlying cause, but the problem could be the result of a sloughed renal papillae, blood clot or acute retroperitoneal pathology. Other non-obstructive urinary tract conditions to consider include pyelonephritis and renal abscess.

Other problems to be considered should include biliary tract sepsis, perforated peptic ulcer disease, pancreatitis and diverticulitis, but these are less likely in the absence of abdominal signs. Aneurysmal disease must always be considered in these circumstances but a leaking or ruptured abdominal aortic aneurysm is not usually accompanied by a fever.

A.5   A non-contrast CT urogram is the investigation of choice for renal colic. This can be performed rapidly and all the required information obtained within a single breath hold. Oral and intravenous contrast materials are not required as virtually all renal tract stones appear densely opaque. In this case two other (and critical) reasons for not using contrast include the renal impairment and the patient's use of metformin. The use of contrast in such circumstance would risk worsening the renal function. A CT scan will give clear definition of the renal tract and show stones within the system and/or any obstruction. The investigation will also provide information on structures and pathological processes outside the renal tract, such as non-urological causes of flank pain including appendicitis, diverticulitis and dissection of an abdominal aortic aneurysm.

A.6   These are axial views of a non-contrast CT demonstrating (1) a grossly dilated left renal pelvis with surrounding perinephric stranding, and no renal stones are seen; (2) a 6 mm distal left ureteric stone with periureteric oedema and stranding, approximately 1 cm from the vesicoureteric junction.

A.7   Complete ureteric obstruction causes a sudden increase in pressure within the collecting system (ureter, renal pelvis, calyces), which stretches nerve endings resulting in severe, sharp flank pain. Hyperperistalsis of the ureter is responsible for intermittent changes in the intraluminal pressure and subsequent waxing and waning of pain severity. Stones located in the upper ureter tend to radiate pain to the flank and costovertebral angle, and more distal stones radiate pain to the distribution of the ilioinguinal nerve (groin) and genital branch of genitofemoral nerve (inner thigh, scrotum, labia). Stones adjacent to the bladder, such as in this patient, may cause

Answers *cont.*

local irritation, which is experienced as urinary frequency and urgency. Haematuria may be present.

A.8 A combination of anti-inflammatories and opioids is effective for renal colic.

NSAIDs are readily administered intramuscularly, intravenously or as a suppository, and are less likely to cause nausea and vomiting than opioids. Recurrent stone forming patients can easily self-administer an indomethacin suppository prior to presenting to an emergency department. Subcutaneous or intravenous morphine is commonly used in conjunction with an antiemetic. Regular assessment of the patient's pain score is required to ensure adequate analgesia.

A.9

- Size – smaller stones are more likely to pass. Approximately 75% of stones with diameter < 4 mm pass spontaneously, and only 35% with diameter > 7 mm.
- Location – there are three anatomical locations where the ureter tends to narrow: at the pelviureteric junction (PUJ), where the ureter crosses the iliac artery, and at the vesicoureteric junction (VUJ).

A more distal location of the stone predicts a higher rate of spontaneous passage.

- Duration and grade of obstruction – prolonged symptoms and signs of high-grade obstruction (hydronephrosis, perinephric stranding, extravasation of urine) make spontaneous passage very unlikely.

A.10

- Fever, urinary infection, deteriorating renal function and pain that is difficult to control are indications to intervene early to relieve the obstruction. This can be performed by a ureteric stent or percutaneous nephrostomy tube.
- All these indications relate to the medical condition of the patient, and are not related to stone size or position.

A.11 These are ureteroscopic photographs demonstrating Figure 15.1A after (1) the ureteric stone during LASER lithotripsy, and Figure 15.1B basket extraction of stone fragments.

Revision Points

Sepsis

- Risk factors include immunosuppression, malignancy, multiple trauma, diabetes mellitus, malnutrition, elderly age, renal or liver failure.

Ureteric Stones

Presentation

- Detailed history may reveal stone location, depending on the nature and site of the pain.

Risk Factors

- Dehydration, dietary excess, gout, hypercalcaemia, family history, hormonal imbalances and causes of infection and urinary stasis.

Investigations

- Urine culture, complete blood picture, renal function, CT urogram (non-contrast).

Revision Points *cont.*

Treatment
- Supportive care with fluid resuscitation, correction of electrolyte abnormalities, antibiotics, blood sugar control, analgesia and antiemetics.
- Early relief of obstruction by insertion of ureteric stent or percutaneous nephrostomy.

Stone Composition
- Calcium-containing stones (calcium oxalate and calcium phosphate) 75%.
- Infected stones (struvite or magnesium ammonium phosphate) 15%.
- Uric acid stones 10%.
- Cystine stones 1%.

Factors Predisposing to Stone Formation
- Environmental – dehydration, dietary excess.
- Metabolic – gout, hypercalcaemia, family history, hormonal imbalances, drug-induced.
- Anatomic – any abnormality leading to urinary stasis or infection, e.g. bladder outflow obstruction, ureteric stricture, PUJ obstruction, calyceal diverticulum.

Prevention of Calcium Oxalate Stones
- Maintain a high oral fluid intake to increase urine volume and decrease the urinary concentration of calcium oxalate.
- Avoid foods rich in oxalate – chocolate, tea, rhubarb, strawberries.
- No restriction in calcium intake is required, but maintain moderation.
- Low salt and fat diet with increased fibre may be beneficial.

Issues to Consider
- What is a PUJ obstruction and what are the causes?
- Are there any instances of presumed ureteric colic where an intravenous pyelogram might be used in preference to a CT urogram?

Further Information

http://en.wikipedia.org/wiki/Kidney_stone

http://emedicine.medscape.com/article/437096-overview

http://kidney.niddk.nih.gov/Kudiseases/pubs/stonesadults/

Lower abdominal pain in a 77-year-old woman

Naseem Mirbagheri and Stewart Skinner

A 77-year-old woman presents to the emergency department with acute abdominal pain. She had been feeling unwell over the previous 2 days with left iliac fossa discomfort and constipation. This morning she woke from sleep with worsening acute lower abdominal pain, mainly on the left lower side of her abdomen, constant in nature and aggravated by movement. The pain was associated with some nausea and vomiting. There had been no bowel action for 3 days. There was no rectal bleeding.

Q.1 What is the most likely diagnosis and what other conditions must be considered?

There is nothing else from the history that helps towards a diagnosis. Her past history is unremarkable apart from hypertension for which she takes perindopril. The patient is unwell and dehydrated. Her heart rate is 120 bpm and regular, blood pressure 90/70 mmHg and temperature 38°C. Her abdomen is soft apart from an area of localized tenderness in the left iliac fossa. Rectal examination is normal with some soft faeces present.

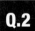

Q.2 What is the clinical problem, what should your initial management plan be and what investigations should be arranged?

You decide to perform arterial blood gases to determine the pH and lactate levels as you are worried about the possibility the patient may have ischaemic bowel. The results are shown below (the normal range is in parentheses).

Investigation 16.1 Summary of results	
pH	7.2 (7.38–7.43)
pCO_2	36 mmHg (35–45)
HCO_3	16 (20–24)
Lactate	1.42 (0.50–2.00)
Base excess	−9.3 (−3.3–1.2)
K	3.5 (3.8–5.0)

Q.3 Based on the above findings, do you think ischaemic bowel is likely and how would this change your management plan?

The patient's condition responds rapidly with the intravenous fluid replacement and after 2 litres of intravenous fluid her blood pressure is 120/85 mmHg. The chest and abdominal X-rays do not show any abnormalities.

Q.4 What further investigation should now be undertaken?

A CT scan of the abdomen is performed. Two representative films are shown in Figures 16.1 and 16.2.

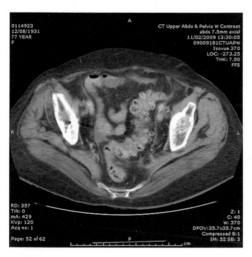

Figure 16.1

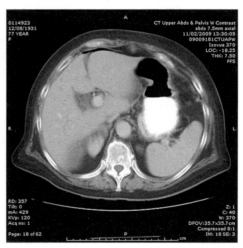

Figure 16.2

Q.5 What do the above CT images show and what management is most appropriate?

Q.6 What are the most common infective organisms involved in this disease process and what antibiotics would you use to treat such infection?

The patient continues to improve and it is decided to pursue a course of conservative management. After 4 days of intravenous fluids and antibiotics her condition is judged satisfactory for her to be discharged home.

Q.7 How would you manage this patient after discharge and what advice would you give with respect to long-term management?

Q.8 What is likely to happen to a patient in the long term after presenting with an attack of acute diverticulitis. What complications may occur in the future?

Answers

A.1 The story fits well for acute diverticulitis. Other gastrointestinal problems to consider include intestinal obstruction and appendicitis. Pancreatitis may sometimes present with a similar clinical picture. Urinary infection, vascular and gynaecological problems must also be considered although with the nausea, vomiting and constipation, they are less likely. The sudden worsening of her pain raises the possibility of perforation – a well-recognized complication of diverticulitis.

A.2 The patient is hypotensive, probably due to dehydration and sepsis. She has a localized peritonitis and this suggests an inflammatory process, perhaps with abscess formation or free perforation. This would all fit for acute diverticulitis with a possible related complication. The initial management plan and investigations should be as follows:

* Resuscitation: insert an intravenous cannula and rehydrate with colloid solution or isotonic saline (e.g. 250–500 mL of a colloidal solution immediately, then 1 litre of isotonic saline over 1–2 hours). Fluids are essential to support the circulatory system prior to addressing the source of her problem. An indwelling urinary catheter should be inserted to measure urine output and adjust fluids accordingly. An arterial line and a central venous line maybe necessary if patient

fails to respond or there is evidence of associated cardiac failure. A nasogastric tube may ease the nausea and vomiting.
* Antibiotics: those with broad-spectrum activity should be started.
* Investigations: bloods should be collected for full blood count, urea and electrolytes, liver function test and lipase. Arterial blood gas analysis should be performed to assess the pH and lactate level.
* Plain chest and abdominal radiographs: to look for evidence of pneumoperitoneum or intestinal obstruction. (Note: free air under a diaphragm is a very specific but not a sensitive finding. In other words, not all patients with a perforated viscus will have free air under a diaphragm and a CT scan of the abdomen is a more sensitive investigation.)

A.3 The blood gas results indicate a metabolic acidosis, but the normal lactate level makes ischaemic bowel less likely. Metabolic acidosis in this case is probably due to poor tissue perfusion from dehydration and sepsis. Management still lies in urgent resuscitation and rehydration.

A.4 With diverticulitis as the most likely diagnosis a CT scan of the abdomen will be helpful looking for localized thickening of the colonic wall (over 4 mm) in association with any diverticuli and inflammation ('stranding') of adjacent pericolic fat and

Answers *cont.*

mesentery. Evidence of abscess or fistula formation or the presence of free perforation would also be sought. Intraluminal contrast enemas are now outdated in light of the increased sensitivity and specificity of the CT scan in the detection of a disease process which focuses more on the outside rather than the inside of the bowel lumen. Barium enemas are contraindicated in the acute setting because of the risk of spillage of irritant barium into the peritoneal cavity in cases of perforation.

A.5 The CT images show signs of complicated diverticultis with perforation. In Figure 16.1 multiple diverticuli in the sigmoid colon are present, and free air is visible between the liver and diaphragm in Figure 16.2. Other views show inflammation of the pericolic fat and mesentery of the sigmoid colon with locules of free air in the paracolic gutter.

The CT confirms the suspected diagnosis of diverticulitis with perforation.

In some cases where the perforation is contained and the patient is stable, conservative management with intravenous antibiotics and bowel rest may be undertaken. However, most cases of perforated diverticular disease require surgical intervention as a life-saving measure and the safest procedure would be a Hartmann operation where the sigmoid colon containing the perforation is resected, the rectum is oversewn and an end colostomy formed. Formal resection, bowel washout and primary anastomosis with a covering stoma is an acceptable alternative in those patients without gross peritoneal contamination. When consenting a patient for operation, the need for a creation of a stoma should be emphasized. At some later stage the stoma may be

reversed but in reality less than half of these patients are suitable for any further surgical intervention because of their poor general state of health.

A.6 Enteric organisms including enterococcus, Gram-negative bacilli (e.g. *Escherichia coli*) and anaerobes (such as *Bacteroides fragilis*) are common. Amoxicillin should be used for enterococcus, gentamicin or a third-generation cephalosporin for Gram-negative bacilli and metronidazole for anaerobic organisms.

A.7 The patient will require colonoscopy to confirm the diagnosis and to exclude any colonic malignancy. Normally this is done 4–6 weeks after the acute episode to allow the inflammation to settle and reduce the risk of bowel perforation during colonoscopy.

A.8 The majority of patients will have no further problems and will not need any further treatment. Colonic resection has been advocated for those patients who have had two or more episodes of uncomplicated diverticulitis, but there is little firm evidence to support this approach. Patients are often advised to adhere to high fibre diet and avoid nuts and seeds but there is no evidence to suggest that this strategy will reduce the complications associated with established colonic diverticulae.

Elective resection for diverticular disease is rarely indicated. Patients will uncommonly have recurrent attacks and require elective or emergency surgery. Indications for elective surgery are stricture formation, colovesical fistula or recurrent attacks of diverticulitis. Indications for emergency surgery are perforated diverticular abscess or perforation causing purulent or faecal peritonitis.

Revision Points

- In Western countries, about 60% of people over the age of 60 will develop colonic diverticular disease. Low fibre diet is identified as a risk factor for such an incidence.
- Colonic diverticula are the result of raised intraluminal pressure and segmentation of the colon from abnormal motility. As a consequence, colonic mucosa herniates at the point of colonic wall weakness where nutrient blood vessels penetrate through to the mucosa. These diverticula are pseudodiverticula as they are lined by mucosa only and do not contain a muscle layer.
- The sigmoid colon is the most common site for diverticular disease in Western communities while right-sided colonic diverticula are more common in Asian people. Diverticular disease may be present throughout the entire colon.
- The term diverticular disease refers to the presence of diverticula in the colon and has largely replaced the older term diverticulosis. In diverticulitis (i.e. inflammation of the diverticuli), an obstructing faecolith results in microperforation of the diverticulum and a secondary, mainly extraluminal, infection of the colon. The extent of perforation and contamination will determine the severity of presentation. The severity of an episode of acute diverticulitis is graded according to the Hinchey classification:
  - Stage I: diverticulitis with pericolic abscess
  - Stage II: distant abscess (retroperitoneal or pelvic)
  - Stage III: purulent peritonitis secondary to rupture of a pericolic or pelvic abscess
  - Stage IV: faecal peritonitis secondary to gross perforation of the colon.

The CT scan can rapidly assess the severity of complicated diverticulitis.
- Acute diverticulitis most commonly affects the sigmoid colon and presents with lower abdominal pain localizing to the left side, usually associated with anorexia, nausea, fever and altered bowel habit (diarrhoea or constipation). If the inflamed segment of the affected colon has a long mesentery and lies on the right side then it can mimic appendicitis or urinary tract infection if it is adjacent to the bladder.
- Men and women are affected equally with colonic diverticula. Only 10–20% of those affected will have symptoms of diverticular disease. Complications are relatively uncommon and the majority of patients will have no symptoms at all.
- Diverticular complications include: abscess formation, fistula formation (colovesical/colovaginal/enterocolic or colocutaneous), colonic stricture, bleeding and perforation which may lead to a generalized purulent or faecal peritonitis. Colovesical fistulae are the most common fistulae associated with diverticular disease and are more common in men since in women the uterus acts as a barrier organ between the sigmoid and bladder.
- The management of acute sigmoid diverticulitis has evolved over the past 25 years in favour of non-operative management. Antibiotics are the mainstay of conservative management. CT-guided drainage of an abscess may be necessary especially if the abscess is larger than 5 cm.
- The majority of patients with diverticulitis will respond to conservative management such as bowel rest and antibiotics. Indications for surgery in diverticulitis include: failure to respond to conservative management, complicated diverticulitis

Revision Points *cont.*

with gross peritoneal sepsis (Hinchey stages III and IV), fistula formation, severe obstructing stricture, severe bleeding or inability to exclude carcinoma. Many patients presenting with complicated diverticulitis have no history of diverticular disease.

- Hartmann's procedure is the most common operation for perforated diverticulitis as it has been shown to be safe and to have a better outcome than other procedures such as defunctioning colostomy or three-stage procedure. The aim of surgery is to remove the diseased bowel segment, control sepsis and restore bowel continuity when possible. Hartmann's procedure involves resection of the diseased segment, leaving a health rectal stump and fashioning an end colostomy. Many of these patients will never have bowel continuity restored – mainly because of the risks associated with another major abdominal procedure and attendant co-morbidities.

- Laparoscopic lavage of peritoneal cavity alone with no resection for generalized peritonitis secondary to perforated diverticulitis has recently been shown to be feasible with a low recurrence in the short term and is likely to become popular in the near future.

- Elective surgery is now uncommon as recent evidence suggests that subsequent attacks of uncomplicated diverticulitis do still respond equally well to conservative management. Also the probability of readmission with each subsequent attack diminishes. Thus elective surgery is now based on individual circumstances: disease factors such as the severity and frequency of the disease and patient factors such as psychosocial impact of the disease, ability to cope and willingness to accept the risk of anastomotic leak with associated morbidity and mortality.

Issues to Consider

- What is the place of laparoscopy and lavage in the management of perforated diverticular disease?
- Why do Europeans develop left-sided colonic diverticula and Asians right-sided diverticula?

Further Information

Myers, E., Hurley, M., O'Sullivan, G.C., et al., 2008. Laparoscopic peritoneal lavage for generalized peritonitis due to perforated diverticulitis. British Journal of Surgery 95, 97–101.

Ooi, K., Wong, S.W., 2009. Management of symptomatic colonic diverticular disease. Medical Journal of Australia 190, 37–40.

Shaikh, S., Krukowski, Z.H., 2007. Outcome of a conservative policy for managing acute sigmoid diverticulitis. British Journal of Surgery 94, 876–879.

Nausea and constipation in an older woman

Robert Ludemann

A 68-year-old woman presents with a 2-day history of nausea and constipation. She has not been able to eat or drink anything in the last 2 days because of the nausea. Her co-morbidities include obesity (BMI=41), type II diabetes, hypertension, sleep apnoea and carcinoma of the rectum treated 2 years previously by abdoperineal excision and end colostomy. Her medications include simvastatin, perindopril and gliclazide. The patient has now developed colicky and generalized abdominal pain and has vomited once.

On examination the patient appears uncomfortable and in pain. Her pulse is 90 bpm and blood pressure 148/88 mmHg. The cardiopulmonary examination is unremarkable. Her abdomen is obese and appears distended with mild tenderness to palpation. She has a lower midline scar from umbilicus to pubis and a left iliac fossa colostomy. There is no palpable mass in the abdomen or either groin. The stoma appears healthy.

Q.1 What is your preliminary diagnosis for this patient and what are the most common causes?

Q.2 What investigations would be appropriate at this stage?

The results of the investigations are shown below and in Figures 17.1 and 17.2.

Investigation 17.1 Summary of results			
Haemoglobin	160 g/L	White cell count	8.6×10^9/L
PCV	0.53		
Platelets	379×10^9/L		
Sodium	145 mmol/L	Calcium	2.16 mmol/L
Potassium	4.6 mmol/L	Phosphate	1.15 mmol/L
Chloride	105 mmol/L	Total protein	62 g/L
Bicarbonate	27 mmol/L	Albumin	35 g/L
Urea	9.1 mmol/L	Globulins	27 g/L
Creatinine	0.12 mmol/L	Bilirubin	16 µmol/L
Uric acid	0.24 mmol/L	ALT	28 U/L
Glucose	9.5 mmol/L	AST	24 U/L
Cholesterol	4.5 mmol/L	GGT	17 U/L
LDH	212 U/L	ALP	51 U/L

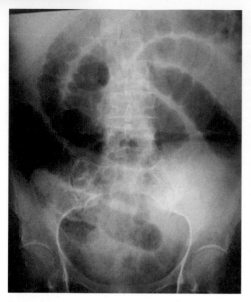

Figure 17.1

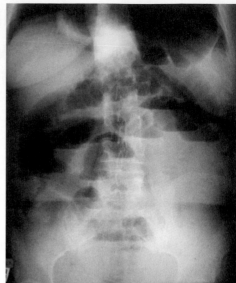

Figure 17.2

Q.3 What is your interpretation of the investigations?

Q.4 What is your initial management plan for this patient?

Over the next 2 days there is no apparent improvement in the patient's condition. The nasogastric losses exceed 2 L of brown turbid material each day.

Q.5 What should the next steps in the patient's management be?

A CT scan of the abdomen is performed. Two representative images are shown in Figures 17.3 and 17.4.

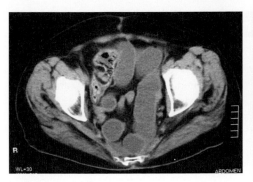

Figure 17.3

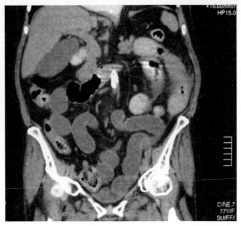

Figure 17.4

Q.6 What is your interpretation of the CT scan?

Q.7 What are the surgical options and how should the patient be managed in the immediate postoperative period?

At operation a knuckle of small bowel is found prolapsed and obstructed through a defect in the pelvic floor. The segment of obstructed bowel is reduced into the abdominal cavity and shown to be viable. The defect is closed. After surgery the patient recovers well with return of gastrointestinal function. Her wound is closed in a delayed fashion on postoperative day 5. With the resumption of her diet post surgery, the patient is transitioned to a subcutaneous insulin regimen and is ready for discharge on postoperative day 6.

Q.8 This patient is classified as morbidly obese with the complications of diabetes, hypertension and sleep apnoea commonly seen with morbid obesity. Describe the surgical therapies that have been shown to be of benefit for morbidly obese patients.

Answers

A.1 The patient's presentation is consistent with small bowel obstruction. Since there is little vomiting with this patient, her obstruction is likely to be in the distal small bowel. The most common cause of small bowel obstruction in the developed world is surgical adhesions. The next most common cause is an abdominal wall hernia. Rarer causes include neoplasms and intussusception. Large bowel obstruction may be the result of volvulus, neoplasia or diverticular disease.

Answers *cont.*

The patient's prior bowel surgery suggests adhesive obstruction or possible cancer recurrence.

A.2 A complete blood count and basic chemistry panel will help assess the patient's degree of dehydration. Abdominal films will confirm your diagnosis of a bowel obstruction.

A.3 An elevated haematocrit and blood urea confirm the patient's dehydration. Elevated blood glucose suggests need for improved diabetes management. The upright and supine abdominal films show dilated loops of small bowel and air–fluid levels. No gas is seen in the colon or stoma confirming the diagnosis of a small bowel obstruction. It is also noted there are no gas shadows overlying the hernial orifices, nor is there gas in the biliary tree which would suggest a rare cause of small bowel obstruction, gallstone ileus.

A.4 Intravenous rehydration with an isotonic solution supplemented with potassium and – if vomiting – intestinal decompression with a nasogastric tube are the mainstays of initial therapy (see Problem 1). Intravenous fluid replacement must take into consideration that lost through nasogastric decompression. Analgesia is prescribed for any discomfort. Because of her elevated blood glucose and a history of poor diabetes control, the patient is started on an insulin infusion. The patient will require close and regular assessment to alert the managing physician to any changes that would alter the conservative plan. These changes include a change in the nature of the pain (colicky to constant), localized tenderness and tachycardia. In addition the patient's need for analgesia might increase.

A.5 The patient has now been obstructed for at least 3 days and there are no apparent signs of resolution with this plan of conservative management. A CT scan of the abdomen might help define the site and nature of the obstruction. With her past history of bowel cancer she could have recurrence of the disease. It is likely the patient is now going to require surgical intervention.

A.6 There are numerous dilated and fluid-filled loops of small bowel. These loops descend into the pelvis and there appears to be a transition point in the right iliac fossa. No mass lesions are seen.

A.7 The midline wound should be reopened and a careful laparotomy undertaken looking for the site and nature of the obstruction. Any evidence of recurrence of the malignancy should be sought. The viability of the bowel must be carefully assessed. Patients with adhesion-obstruction frequently have areas of ischaemia, either at the site of obstruction or in a closed loop. Since the woman is obese and is diabetic, consideration must be given to delayed primary closure of the superficial layers of the wound to reduce the chance of wound infection.

For determination of wound management in general surgery a simple scoring system can be used that includes the type and complexity of operation, whether the surgery is considered contaminated, the clinical history of the patient including factors of age, smoking and alcohol abuse, steroid use and preoperative albumin level. The greater the score, the more delayed primary wound closure can be considered. Stringent blood glucose in the postoperative patient has been shown to reduce wound infection rates and the best

Answers *cont.*

way to achieve this tight blood glucose control is by the use of an insulin infusion with a change to long-acting insulin when appropriate. It should be noted that prior undiagnosed diabetes mellitus is a common problem in patients hospitalized for other reasons.

A.8 Bariatric surgery has seen a dramatic increase over the last decade as obesity-related problems have reached epidemic proportions in a number of Western countries. The surgery has been shown to be effective in producing weight loss in this patient group and also in correcting the complications of diabetes, hypertension and sleep apnoea associated with morbid obesity. There are several different types of operations that are currently employed and these are either restrictive (e.g. gastric band) or malabsorptive (e.g. gastric bypass). Patients with BMIs in excess of 45 are probably best treated with a malabsorptive procedure where success is less dependent on dietary compliance. For those with lesser degrees of obesity and better motivation to modify their dietary habits the reversible laparoscopic band procedure may be a better option.

Revision Points

The important causes of small bowel obstruction include:
- Adhesions.
- Abdominal wall hernia.
  All other causes are uncommon:
- Tumours (primary, secondary, polyps).
- Internal hernias.
- Crohn's disease.

Most cases of adhesion-obstruction develop secondary to previous abdominal surgery. There is no temporal relationship between the date of the original operation and onset of obstruction and 80% of cases will resolve spontaneously. While a plain abdominal film will confirm the presence of dilated loops of obstructed small bowel, the CT scan is used with increasing frequency in the management of these patients to define the nature and site of the obstruction.

Conservative management consists of gut rest, intravenous fluid replacement and close observation looking for evidence of bowel ischaemia:

- Change in the nature of the pain (from colicky to constant).
- Localization of the pain and development of spot tenderness.
- Fever and tachycardia.
- Leucocytosis.

After an episode of adhesion-obstruction about 30% of patients will have recurrent episodes. Small bowel obstruction secondary to a hernia requires prompt surgical correction. Likewise, most cases of obstruction due a cause other than adhesion will also require surgical intervention.

Emergency surgery always carries increased risks and these risks are magnified in the presence of other co-existing problems which include:
- Cardio-respiratory disease.
- Immunosuppression (e.g. diabetes).
- Renal disease.
- Obesity.

Abdominal wall hernias are the common cause of obstruction in developing

Revision Points *cont.*

countries. Hernias should be treated by prompt surgical correction.

It is estimated that in the USA about 25% of the population is obese and the prevalence of morbid obesity is increasing at twice the rate of the prevalence of obesity. Other countries, including Australia, have figures approaching these levels. The impact of obesity on health is considerable and overweight patients are more likely to have problems related to:

- Diabetes.
- Hypertension.
- Arthritis.

Obesity also appears to be a risk factor in a number of malignancies such as carcinoma of the pancreas and oesophagus.

At present surgery offers the only effective medical therapy to control weight and to bring about sustained weight reduction. Evidence is emerging that gastric bypass may prolong the lives of the morbidly obese.

Bariatric Surgery

Bariatric surgery can be a safe and effective tool for weight loss in the morbidly obese and can help in the control of the co-morbidities of morbid obesity. Weight loss from bariatric surgery can be a result of both induced calorie restriction and calorie malabsorption developing from the surgical procedure. Most bariatric surgery is offered as a laparoscopic procedure with a mortality of less than 1%. Long-term effective weight loss with bariatric surgery still requires acceptance of a sensible diet and a dedicated exercise programme.

Issues to Consider

- What other investigation(s) might be considered to assess the likelihood of complete or incomplete obstruction in the early management of a patient with intestinal obstruction?
- What are the potential perioperative problems faced by this patient that might be a direct consequence of her obesity?

Further Information

Dronge, A.S., Perkal, M.F., Kancir, S., et al., 2006. Long-term glycemic control and postoperative infectious complications. Archives of Surgery 141 (4), 375–380; discussion 380.

Maglinte, D.D.T., Howard, T.J., Lillemoe, K.D., et al., 2008. Small-bowel obstruction: state of the art imaging and its role in clinical

management. Clinical Gastroentology and Hepatology 6 (2), 130–139.

Mallo, R.D., Salem, L., Lalani, T., et al., 2005. Computed tomography diagnosis of ischemia and complete obstruction in small bowel obstruction: a systematic review. Journal of Gastrointestinal Surgery 9 (5), 375–380.

Needleman, B.J., Happel, L.C., 2008. Bariatric surgery: choosing the optimal procedure. Surgical Clinics of North America 88 (5), 991–1007.

Neumayer, L., Hosokawa, P., Itani, K., et al., 2007. Multivariate predictors of postoperative surgical site infection after general and vascular surgery: results from the patient safety in surgery study. Journal of the American College of Surgeons 204 (4), 1178–1187.

A lady with diarrhoea and abdominal pain

Jonathan Mitchell and Philip Clelland

A 23-year-old lady attends your surgery. She gives a 2-month history of worsening diarrhoea. She is opening her bowels eight times a day and twice at night. The stools are loose with mucus but no blood. She has lost 4 kg in weight and has not eaten properly for 2 weeks. The diarrhoea is associated with cramping abdominal pains and malaise. She has spent 6 months in India working for a charity and returned 2 months ago. She had several short spells of diarrhoea while there.

She has previously been diagnosed with irritable bowel syndrome by her GP. She takes the oral contraceptive pill only but was prescribed antibiotics 10 weeks ago for a chest infection. She smokes four cigarettes per day and drinks 10 units of alcohol each week. She is currently working in a care home but has had to take time off due to her current symptoms. She is not in contact with her family.

Q.1 What are the differential diagnoses for her current symptoms?

Q.2 What other questions would you ask?

Observations are within normal limits. Examination reveals mild right-sided abdominal tenderness only. Rigid sigmoidoscopy is unsuccessful due to patient discomfort.

Q.3 What initial tests would you perform as her GP?

You prescribe loperamide. Blood tests are shown below. An abdominal X-ray is shown in Figure 18.1. Stool microscopy and culture are negative.

A lady with diarrhoea and abdominal pain

Investigation 18.1 Summary of results

Haemoglobin	115 g/L	White cell count	15.6×10⁹/L
MCV	80 fL	Neutrophils 70%	10.9×10⁹/L
Platelets	395×10⁹/L		
Sodium	134 mmol/L	Calcium	2.40 mmol/L
Potassium	2.7 mmol/L	Phosphate	0.90 mmol/L
Chloride	99 mmol/L	Total protein	62 g/L
Bicarbonate	20 mmol/L	Albumin	35 g/L
Urea	16.8 mmol/L	Globulins	27 g/L
Creatinine	0.14 mmol/L	Bilirubin	16 µmol/L
Uric acid	0.24 mmol/L	ALT	44 U/L
Glucose	4.4 mmol/L	AST	32 U/L
Cholesterol	3.5 mmol/L	GGT	45 U/L
LDH	212 U/L	ALP	54 U/L

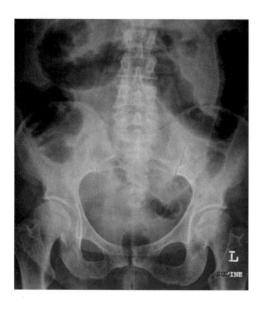

Figure 18.1

Q.4 What is your interpretation of the blood tests? What does the X-ray show?

Three days later her symptoms are worse. She is now pyrexial and although her abdomen is soft she is much more tender in the lower abdomen. She also has a tender rash on her lower legs.

Q.5 What is the likely unifying diagnosis?

You discuss her case with the on-call gastroenterologist who advises urgent admission to hospital. On arrival she has acute abdominal pain, is pyrexial and tachycardic.

Q.6 As the admitting doctor, what treatment would you initiate?

She is transferred to the gastroenterology ward later that day. A flexible sigmoidoscopy without bowel preparation is performed and biopsies taken. This shows severe colitis with mucosal granularity and loss of vascular pattern, contact bleeding and aphthous ulceration.
  She is reviewed by the gastroenterologist and started on steroids.

Q.7 What dose, type and route of steroid would you give? What else should be measured while taking high-dose steroids?

She is monitored closely with daily blood tests and a scan is performed of her abdomen. She is also reviewed by the on-call surgical team.
  She is reviewed by a dietician who starts a feeding programme.

Q.8 What routes of feeding do you know? Which would be the best option for this patient?

She improves and after 5 days is discharged home on oral prednisolone. This is to be tapered by 5 mg each week. She is followed up 2 weeks after discharge in the outpatient clinic. Biopsies taken at the time of the sigmoidoscopy show transmural inflammation and non-caseating granulomata. The features are consistent with Crohn's disease.
  When she is reviewed in clinic her stool frequency has increased to five times and her cramping abdominal pain has returned on reducing her prednisolone dose.

Q.9 What treatments may be discussed with her?

She is commenced on azathioprine and an appointment made for 2 months' time. She is told to have her blood tests monitored closely.

Q.10 What blood tests should she have and why?

She is followed up for several years and her symptoms remain controlled. At a clinic appointment 3 years later she has developed abdominal pain and bloating after eating. This is sometimes accompanied by vomiting. The gastroenterologist sends her for a scan (shown in Figure 18.2).

Figure 18.2

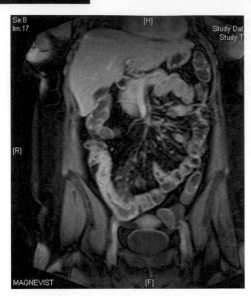

Se:8
Im:17
[H]
Study Dat
Study T
[R]
[F]
MAGNEVIST

Q.11 What type of scan is this? What complication has developed? How can this be managed?

Answers

A.1 Diarrhoea means different things to different people. A working definition is >3 loose stools in a 24-hour period.

Diarrhoea can be divided into acute or chronic. Acute is classified as lasting less than 14 days. It is usually secondary to infection which can be further subdivided by the presence of blood as shown in Table 18.1 below.

Infections are often self-limiting and rarely require antibiotics.

Chronic diarrhoea can be classified by its pathophysiology. There is overlap between aetiologies (Table 18.2):
- Osmotic: poorly absorbed osmotically active solute in faecal matter.
- Secretory: abnormal intestinal epithelial cell ion transport.
- Inflammatory: inflammation and ulceration of mucosa impairing absorption and causing loss of proteins and solutes.

- Altered motility: theoretically, enhanced intestinal motility is implicated in diarrhoea but there is a limited evidence base.

A.2 Key questions when assessing patients with diarrhoea are:
- Patient age.
- Duration*.
- Frequency.
- Type of motion: steatorrhoea (pale and fatty stools seen in malabsorption), volume.
- Presence of blood in stool.
- Incontinence.
- Nocturnal symptoms*.
- Systemic symptoms*.
- Vomiting.
- Loss of weight*.

*<3 months and presence of these features suggest organic cause more likely.

Answers *cont.*

Table 18.1 Infectious causes of diarrhoea

Acute Diarrhoea With Blood	Acute Diarrhoea Without Blood
Shigellosis	Viruses
Escherichia coli 0157	*Escherichia coli*
Campylobacter	Cholera
Salmonella	Protozoa
Amoebic dysentery	*Strongyloides*
Antibiotic associated diarrhoea	Food toxins
Schistosoma (rarely)	Malaria
	Milder infection with *Shigella/Salmonella/Campylobacter*

Table 18.2 Types and causes of diarrhoea

Osmotic	Secretory	Inflammatory	Altered Motility
Congenital carbohydrate malabsorption: e.g. pancreatic insufficiency secondary to cystic fibrosis	Congenital defect in ion absorption	Infection: *Giardia* and *Yersinia*	Irritable bowel syndrome
Acquired carbohydrate malabsorption: coeliac disease, post enteritis, post bowel resection	Bacterial enterotoxins	Inflammatory bowel disease	Diabetes
	Laxatives	Radiotherapy	Post surgery
	Drugs	Hypersensitivity	Bile salts
	Toxins	Autoimmune	Hyperthyroidism
		Diverticular disease	Prokinetic drugs
		Ischaemia	
		Neoplasia	

- Presence and location of abdominal pain.
- Contact with potentially infected food/water.
- Systemic disease, e.g. diabetes mellitus, hyperthroidism.
- Immune deficiency, e.g. HIV/AIDS.
- Previous GI surgery.
- Travel history.
- Unwell contacts.
- Medications, e.g. recent antibiotics raise the possibility of *Clostridium difficile* infection.
- Food sensitivity.
- Family history.
- Sexual history.

A.3 After a full examination, three stool samples for culture, microscopy and *Clostridium difficile* toxin should be sent. The stool can also be tested for faecal elastase (low in pancreatic insufficiency), calprotectin (a marker of intestinal inflammation and raised in inflammatory bowel disease) or fat quantification (high in malabsorption).

Blood should be sent for full blood count, C-reactive protein, urea and electrolytes, liver function tests, coeliac serology, thyroid function tests, glucose, magnesium, calcium, folate and vitamin B_{12}.

Answers *cont.*

Table 18.3 Differentiating ulcerative colitis and Crohn's disease

Feature	Crohn's Disease	Ulcerative Colitis
Symptoms	Diarrhoea, abdominal pain, weight loss	Bloody diarrhoea with mucus, urgency, tenesmus
Signs	Fever, fistulae, perianal disease,abdominal masses	Fever, abdominal tenderness
Extra-intestinal	Oral ulceration, erythema nodosum, pyoderma gangrenosum, scleritis, episcleritis, uveitis, gallstones, pauciarticular arthropathy, DVT	Oral ulceration, erythema nodosum, episcleritis, uveitis, gallstones, pauciarticular arthropathy, DVT, primary sclerosing cholangitis

A plain abdominal X-ray can reveal constipation (unreliable), dilated bowel, pancreatic calcification and colonic wall oedema in the context of diarrhoea.

A.4 She is anaemic with a high white cell count. Anaemia is a common finding and should be classified according to the mean cell volume into microcytic (generally iron deficiency), normocytic (often chronic disease) and macrocytic (most commonly deficiency of vitamin B_{12} or folate). The electrolytes show a low potassium and raised urea. Hypokalaemia is common in prolonged diarrhoea. The elevated urea indicates dehydration.

This is an abdominal X-ray. It shows dilated large bowel and mucosal oedema in keeping with colitis. Mucosal oedema is identified by thickening of the bowel wall and loss of the haustral pattern. The haustra are seen as intermittent ridges arising from the bowel wall and are due to the arrangement of the circular muscle fibres.

A.5 She is most likely to have inflammatory bowel disease. The chronicity of her symptoms make infection less likely. Pain, weight loss and diarrhoea are classical features of Crohn's disease. Her rash is a typical presentation of erythema nodosum. She is a smoker which is linked to Crohn's disease.

It is often difficult to distinguish between ulcerative colitis and Crohn's disease clinically. Clues in the clinical presentation are given in Table 18.3.

A.6 The immediate issues are her dehydration and pain. She should be given intravenous normal (0.9%) saline with supplemental potassium and probably magnesium. The rate of fluid administration is dependent on the degree of dehydration and any co-existing conditions, e.g. heart failure. She should also be given analgesia. She may require morphine which should be given with an antiemetic but cautiously. Dehydration in addition to Crohn's disease increases thrombotic tendency. She should receive prophylactic subcutaneous anticoagulation (e.g. enoxaparin) to avoid thrombotic complications. Her loperamide should be stopped as it will make it difficult to monitor stool frequency. A stool chart should be commenced to assess response to treatment.

A.7 The options are:
- Prednisolone 40 mg od orally.
- Hydrocortisone 100 mg qid intravenously.

Intravenous therapy is given to patients with severe symptoms (bowels open >6 times/24 hours, fever, weight loss, abdominal pain and tenderness, intermittent nausea or vomiting, or anaemia) or who are

Answers *cont.*

systemically unwell. Oral treatment is reserved for patients with milder symptoms. If patients respond to IV steroids (falling bowel frequency and CRP), they are converted to oral steroids after 5 days and the dose is tapered by reducing by 5 mg weekly.

It is important to measure the blood glucose regularly while patients are taking high-dose steroids to monitor for steroid-induced diabetes mellitus. Patients should also be given a calcium supplement to protect against osteopenia. If steroids are to be used in the longer term then consideration should be given to starting a bisphosphonate to prevent osteoporosis.

A.8 Artificial feeding should be given if inadequate oral nutritional intake has persisted for more than 7–14 days.

Artificial feeding can be given directly into the bowel (enterally) or into a vein (parenterally). Enteral feeding is generally preferred as feeding into the bowel helps to maintain intestinal structure and function. It is also associated with fewer complications than parenteral routes.

The enteral route is contraindicated in ileus, bowel obstruction and persistent vomiting. Enteral feeds are delivered via a nasogastric (NG) tube. Parenteral feeds should be administered via a central line. Complications of parenteral feeding include infection of the central line and refeeding syndrome.

A.9 Medical treatments for Crohn's disease include:
- Aminosalicylates, e.g. mesalazine.
- Azathioprine/6-mercaptopurine (6-MP).
- Metronidazole.
- Corticosteroids.
- Methotrexate.
- Anti-TNF therapies/biologicals.

She has been treated with steroids but on tapering the dose her symptoms have flared. This is not uncommon. Alternative treatments should therefore be discussed. The usual approach is to increase the steroid dose again and initiate azathioprine or 6-MP treatment. Steroids, though effective, should not be used long term due to their side-effects and so another immunomodulator is introduced. Azathioprine/6-MP has a 60–70% response rate within 3–6 months. An alternative approach would be induction of remission with infliximab.

Slow-release oral aminosalicylates are better than placebo in treating colonic Crohn's disease although their efficacy is less impressive than other treatments. Their main side-effects are gastrointestinal (heartburn, diarrhoea, abdominal pain) which can limit their utility in this group of patients.

Metronidazole is thought to be of modest benefit in colonic Crohn's but its long-term use is limited by the risk of peripheral neuropathy. It is most effective in healing perianal complications.

Corticosteroids are mainly used as the initial treatment in Crohn's disease. This is because 60–80% of patients respond within 10–14 days. An alternative for patients with ileitis and right-sided colonic disease is controlled ileal release budesonide which has high hepatic metabolism and therefore fewer systemic side-effects.

Methotrexate can be used as an alternative to azathioprine/6-MP. It may be most beneficial in patients with associated arthritis. Folic acid should be given daily to limit bone marrow suppression. Other potential side-effects include liver and pulmonary toxicity.

Answers *cont.*

Anti-TNF therapies are established for the treatment of Crohn's disease. Infliximab is the preparation most commonly used for inflammatory bowel disease. It is a monoclonal antibody against TNF-alpha which is human and mouse in origin. Levels of TNF-alpha correlate with the disease activity of Crohn's disease.

Infliximab is used to induce and maintain remission in patients with severe active Crohn's disease and also to treat fistulating Crohn's disease when treatment with immunomodulating drugs and corticosteroids has failed or is not tolerated and when surgery is inappropriate. It is usually given in a dose of 5 mg/kg at 0, 2, and 6 weeks, followed by 5 mg/kg every 8 weeks. Some patients will develop antibodies to infliximab and this can reduce their clinical response to treatment. Recommended approaches to this are:

* reduce the 8 week reinfusion interval OR
* double the dose to 10 mg/kg.

If the above fail, use both approaches.

Adalimumab is an alternative anti-TNF treatment which is fully human and is given subcutaneously. It is therefore easier to give on an outpatient basis.

If a patient is taking another treatment agent for Crohn's disease, e.g. 6-MP/ azathioprine/methotrexate, when commenced upon anti-TNF therapy this is generally continued for up to 6 months. This is thought to help reduce the chance of developing antibodies. Dual therapy should not be continued long term due to the potential risks of malignancy such as lymphoma or serious atypical infections.

Adverse effects of these agents include:

* Infusion reactions.
* Infections – reactivation of latent TB is a particular concern and so a chest X-ray should be performed prior to commencing treatment.
* Demyelinating disease.
* Skin reactions.
* Heart failure.
* Liver toxicity.
* Malignancy.

A.10 Patients treated with azathioprine are at risk from dose-related bone marrow suppression and hepatotoxicity. They should have a thiopurine methyl transferase (TPMT) level taken prior to initiation of treatment. This enzyme metabolizes azathioprine and low levels help predict patients at risk of developing bone marrow toxicity. A full blood count should be performed weekly for the first 4 weeks and following this period at least every 3 months. Liver function tests should also be performed at these times.

A.11 An MRI small bowel study or enteroclysis. MRI can detect small bowel disease in areas of the small intestine that are inaccessible to endoscopy. In studies of children with suspected Crohn's disease, MRI detected ileitis with high sensitivity and specificity. It is being used with increasing frequency to diagnose small bowel Crohn's disease. It is particularly of use in younger patients as it does not expose them to large doses of radiation. An alternative is a small bowel barium follow through. The patient drinks contrast containing barium and X-rays are taken periodically, highlighting the outline of the small bowel. Typical radiological findings in Crohn's disease include mucosal irregularity, cobblestoning, stricturing or the presence of fistulae.

This scan shows extensive Crohn's disease in the terminal ileum, with luminal narrowing.

Answers *cont.*

There are multiple complications that can develop in a patient with Crohn's disease. These can be separated into problems affecting the bowel secondary to chronic inflammation, extraintestinal conditions, malabsorption and malignancy. Problems affecting the bowel include obstruction secondary to strictures, haemorrhage, fistulae, abscesses, perforation and toxic megacolon.

Malabsorption can result in deficiency of the following:

- Bile salts – resulting in fat malabsorption. This can cause impaired absorption of the fat-soluble vitamins and malnutrition.
- Vitamin B_{12} – causing pernicious anaemia.
- Vitamin D and calcium – causing bone loss. This, associated with steroid use, puts these patients at risk of osteoporosis.

There is also an increased risk of colon cancer in patients with longstanding Crohn's colitis.

Revision Points

Crohn's Disease

Incidence
- 3–14 : 100 000 in the Western world.

Risk Factors
- Higher rates in Caucasians.
- Lower rates in Asia, Africa and South America.
- Increased risk if first-degree relative has Crohn's.
- Positive association between smoking and Crohn's.

Histology
- Inflammatory changes involving the full thickness of the bowel wall.
- Focal ulceration.
- Non-caseating granulomas, lymphoid hyperplasia.
- Acute and chronic inflammatory cell infiltration.
- Any part of GI tract from mouth to anus may be involved.

Clinical Features
- Onset 15–40 years with a smaller second peak 50–80 years.
- Colicky abdominal pain/subacute obstruction.
- Sequelae of malabsorption and chronic diarrhoea (e.g. weight loss, low vitamin B_{12}, hypocalcaemia, anaemia, hypomagnasaemia).
- Fistulae.
- Perianal disease.
- Extraintestinal features include arthritis, episcleritis, erythema nodosum and gallstones.

Diagnosis
- Histological diagnosis is the gold standard.
- Small and large bowel imaging helps identify extent of disease and complications.

Treatment
- Goal is to induce remission.
- Corticosteroids/5-aminosalicylic acid derivatives/azathioprine/methotrexate/anti-TNF-alpha antibodies (infliximab).
- Surgical resection.
- Omeprazole for gastric and duodenal Crohn's.

Issues to Consider

- How is giardiasis diagnosed and what are its clinical features?
- What are the possible implications of this diagnosis in a 23-year-old woman?
- What steps can be taken in hospitals to minimize the incidence of *Clostridium difficile* infection?

Further Information

www.nacc.org.uk

www.bsg.org.uk

www.gastro.org

Rectal bleeding in a 45-year-old woman

James Sweeney

A 45-year-old woman is referred with a 3-week history of rectal bleeding. She has noticed bright red blood on the toilet paper. The bleeding is associated with defaecation and is not mixed with the stool. Over the last 4 months she has suffered increasing constipation and tiredness. She has a good appetite, her diet has not altered recently, and her weight is stable. Her general health is good and she has had no major illnesses in the past. She describes troubles with 'haemorrhoids' since the birth of her chldren, and had some injection treatment for them. She smokes 10 cigarettes a day (and is trying to quit) and is not taking any medications.

On examination she looks well and there is no obvious evidence of recent weight loss. Her cardiorespiratory system is normal. On abdominal examination there are no abnormal findings. A rectal examination is performed which shows she has two anal skin tags and some prolapsed internal haemorrhoids.

Q.1 What should be done next?

A sigmoidoscopic examination to 20 cm is normal. Proctoscopy confirms the presence of large internal haemorrhoids, which bleed easily on contact.

Q.2 What is the likely explanation for the bleeding? What is the next step?

You explain to the patient that while the bleeding is most likely to be due to her haemorrhoids, a complete investigation of the large bowel is indicated. You arrange a colonoscopy. A lesion is found (Figure 19.1).

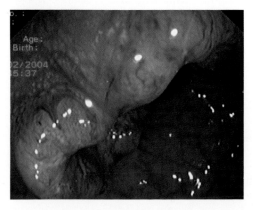

Figure 19.1

Q.3 What does Figure 19.1 show?

The tumour is indentified in the ascending colon. The colonoscopy was otherwise normal. The biopsy shows moderately differentiated adenocarcinoma.

Q.4 What should you do after the colonoscopy and why?

Her haemoglobin is 100 g/L, her liver function tests and biochemistry are normal. A CT abdomen and chest is normal.

Q.5 How would you counsel this patient?

At operation a carcinoma of the ascending colon is found and a right hemicolectomy is performed. There is no evidence of adjacent or distant spread of the tumour. Apart from the tumour, there was nothing else abnormal in the resected specimen of bowel. There was no indication to perform a defunctioning ileostomy and she makes a good recovery. The histology is confirmed and the carcinoma involves the muscularis propria and extends into the pericolic fat. There is no perineural, vascular or lymph node involvement.

Q.6 What further advice is the patient going to require?

The patient understands that you will keep her under surveillance. She would like to know what this will involve.

Q.7 What is the aim of the follow-up programme? What kind of surveillance will you employ?

Q.8 What is your counsel?

The patient wants to know if any of her children are at risk for developing this cancer.

You explain to the patient that the risk to her children is slightly greater than it would be for the general population. Table 19.1 shows the risks.

The patient's son is with her. He understands that he is at slightly increased risk and would like to know what screening you would recommend for him. He is aged 23.

Table 19.1 Risk factors in colorectal cancer	
Family History	**Risk**
Category 1	Up to 2 fold
One first-degree or second-degree relative with colorectal cancer diagnosed at 55 or over	
Category 2	3 to 6 fold
One first-degree relative with colorectal cancer diagnosed under 55	
Two first-degree or second-degree relatives on the same side of the family with colorectal cancer diagnosed at any age	
Category 3	1 in 2 lifetime
Proven or suspected HNPCC (hereditary non-polyposis colorectal cancer)	
Suspected or proven FAP (familial adenomatous polyposis)	
Somebody in family in whom the presence of a high-risk mutation in the APC (adenomatous polyposis coli) or one of the mismatch repair (MMR) genes has been identified	

Q.9 What is your advice to the son?

You advise him that if he is symptom free, he does not need any surveillance at this stage. If he does have symptoms, they should be investigated as appropriate. In any patient who has a positive occult blood test, it is recommended they have a colonoscopy. Similarly, you explain to him that any patient who presents with new rectal bleeding needs investigation. As a guiding rule, any patient who presents with an iron deficiency anaemia needs a full colonic investigation unless there are clear alternative causes such as menorrhagia.

The son has heard that 'polyps in the bowel usually turn to cancer'.

Q.10 What kinds of polyps occur in the large bowel and what is their malignant potential?

The patient remains in good health and is kept under regular surveillance.

Answers

A.1 The patient has three symptoms that cause concern: increasing constipation, rectal blood loss and tiredness. You should ask further questions that may indicate why she is constipated. There are many possibilities in addition to colonic pathology, such as dietary changes, use of narcotic analgesia (codeine) or development of hypothyroidism. You should enquire about a personal history of polyps and family history of colon cancer. In the absence of an obvious cause for her constipation (confirmed by impacted faeces in the rectum), such as recent use of a codeine-containing compound, this patient will require examination of all of her large bowel. A sigmoidoscopy may be performed as part of the general physical examination

Answers *cont.*

and might clarify matters and identify a source for the bleeding in the anal canal or lower rectum. Even if the patient does have internal haemorrhoids, which may be the cause of the bleeding, she must be investigated further. Haemorrhoids are extremely common, but it is important to inspect the rest of the large intestine and so not overlook a tumour.

A.2 The most likely cause of bleeding in this type of patient is internal haemorrhoids, but it is essential to exclude a more sinister cause for the blood loss, especially as she has recently become constipated and tired for no obvious reason. Cancer of the colon, although more common in older patients, occurs in this age group and often presents with these symptoms. Despite the haemorrhoids, she must have a colonoscopy. In the absence of other symptoms and the visualization of a bleeding haemorrhoid it would be reasonable to treat the haemorrhoids and only investigate further if the symptoms persist. If a colonoscopy was not available (uncommon) then a barium enema would be an alternative but does not allow any diagnostic or therapeutic manoeuvres such as biopsy and snaring of polyps to be undertaken and if abnormal would require a colonoscopy for assesment and treatment.

A.3 This lesion has the typical appearance of an adenocarcinoma with raised, rolled edges and a central crater. The centre of the ulcer is likely to be ulcerated. The tumour occupies half the circumference of the bowel and is about 3 cm in length.

A.4 As part of the work-up, the following investigations are required:

- Complete blood picture, serum biochemistry, liver function tests and serum CEA (carcinoembryonic antigen).
- CT abdomen and chest.

Iron deficiency anaemia is common in cases of colorectal cancer and must be excluded. The patient may have secondary spread of her disease. Colorectal cancers tend to spread to the liver, but metastatic deposits can also be found in lung and bone. A CT abdomen/chest and liver enzymes may not affect the decision-making of how to manage the primary tumour, but will give an indication of possible spread of the disease. This is often useful knowledge to have before surgery. Staging of the disease will influence adjuvant chemotherapy.

In cases such as this the entire large bowel must be examined. This patient had a negative colonoscopy other than the lesion visualized. However, co-existent disease is often present and patients may have polyps or other primary tumours. Synchronous tumours occur in 5% of patients and polyps may be found in up to 20% of cases. The discovery of polyps or another tumour may influence the extent of surgical resection required.

A.5 You should explain the diagnosis and management to the patient, who needs to understand that she has a cancer of the colon, although at this stage there is no evidence that the disease has spread outside the bowel. Explain that she requires surgery to prevent total obstruction of the colon and attempt to cure her of the disease.

You must explain to the patient in simple language (and be prepared to repeat things several times) what the operation will involve and the risks and benefits of the proposed treatment. You must explain that:

Answers *cont.*

- The surgery will be done under general anaesthetic.
- She is likely to be in hospital for several days.
- Bowel preparation is usually not used for the type of operation she is to undergo.
- Antibiotics will be administered perioperatively to reduce the risk of infection.
- The surgeon will look to see if there is evidence of tumour spread outside the bowel.
- The surgeon will cut out the affected part of the colon including the blood vessels and lymph nodes supplying it and then join the two ends back together.
- If this were not possible she would require an ileostomy. This is when a piece of the bowel is brought out through the abdominal wall to drain into a bag.
- Given the site of her tumour and that the operation is not an emergency, she is unlikely to require an ileostomy.

Risks including infection, anastomotic leakage, thromboembolic risks and operative mortality must be discussed. You can emphasize that these should be kept in perspective, as the patient has little alternative as, untreated, she will develop complete intestinal obstruction.

While not applying to this patient, remember that fears of being left with a 'bag' (colostomy) are common and these concerns must be fully addressed. However, with modern stapling techniques and the realization that the incidence of local recurrence is no greater with a 2 cm margin of clearance than a 5 cm margin, fewer patients now undergo total excision of the rectum with the formation of a permanent colostomy. Most patients with carcinoma of the rectum do not need complete excision of the rectum and anus.

Fifty years ago, only 15% of all rectal cancers were treated with a restorative procedure, whereas that figure currently exceeds 65%. Temporary or defunctioning colostomies are still fashioned, but it is unlikely that the case discussed in this problem would require one. Colostomies (or defunctioning ileostomies) may be required after a difficult dissection deep in the pelvis or after emergency surgery for perforated or obstructed colon. The aim of a colostomy or ileostomy in such circumstances is to reduce the risk of anastomotic leakage, or in the event of established peritoneal contamination, to prevent further soiling.

Surgery remains important in incurable metastatic disease when the primary tumour is producing troublesome symptoms such as bleeding, obstruction or tenesmus. In some circumstances colonic stents can be used to relieve obstruction and avoid surgery in patients with very advanced disease.

A.6 This patient must be given a prognosis. Her tumour has been staged as a Stage ACPS B or $pT_3N_0M_0$ and she will have an approximate 85–90% 5-year survival rate. Expressed simply to the patient, she could be told that all the known cancer has been removed, she has a good chance of cure, but will be monitored to look for recurrence of her disease or development of polyps which might develop into a new cancer. The surveillance will require repeated colonoscopy.

Although chemotherapy has no role in the initial treatment of colorectal cancer, it is well accepted that adjuvant chemotherapy will improve survival for patients with more advanced stages.

Answers *cont.*

A.7 The aim of any cancer follow-up programme is threefold and is to detect:

- Local recurrence.
- Metastatic disease.
- New primary tumours.

Surveillance Strategies

- Estimation of carcinoembryonic antigen (CEA) is of most value if the levels were elevated prior to surgery and then returned to normal following resection of the tumour. Of more value is detection of blood in the stool.
- An immunological faecal occult blood test (FOBT) detects bleeding distal to the terminal ileum. Non-immunological tests (e.g. haematest) are less specific and may detect blood in the stool that could have originated anywhere in the gastrointestinal tract or chemicals related to diet. FOBTs are simple to perform and cause minimum inconvenience to the patient. They are highly sensitive, although not specific. In other words, most cases of occult bleeding will be detected, although the bleeding may be from a benign cause. In patients such as the one described in this case, faecal occult blood testing should be performed every 12 months with colonoscopy if positive.
- Colonoscopic follow-up would be recommended every 3 years if there were no other polyps at initial colonoscopy.

A.8 The cause of colorectal cancer is unknown, but diet is likely to play an important role. In certain instances there may be a genetic predisposition to cancer (e.g. familial adenomatous polyposis (FAP), hereditary non-polyposis colorectal cancer (HNPCC)), or the patient may have a condition such as ulcerative colitis that places them at high risk. It is also apparent that first-degree relatives have a two- to

threefold increase in risk of developing colorectal cancer. A past history of colorectal cancer increases the risk of developing a further carcinoma. However, in most cases no obvious risk factor exists and the cancer is thought to arise from a pre-existing adenoma. Not all adenomas turn malignant but almost all cancers develop in an adenoma. This has led to screening strategies which are based around identification and removal of polyps.

In this instance no particular risk factors can be identified but the young age and right-sided tumour raise the issue of HNPCC. MSI (microsatellite instability) and immunohistochemistry testing and if positive subsequent assessment of the tumour for germline mutations in the DNA mismatch repair (MMR) genes may reveal a strong possibility of HNPCC. These assessments are generally only done when patients meet one of the Amsterdam criteria/Bethesda guidelines. Approximately 10–15% of sporadic colorectal cancers will be MSI positive. The patient should be counselled that her children would be at increased risk over the general population. Use of the chart indicated in the text (Table 19.1) can be helpful.

A.9 On the assumption that the son has no digestive tract symptoms (particularly rectal bleeding), then nothing needs to be done until he is 35 (i.e. 10 years earlier than his mother's diagnosis). The following guidelines should be applied. These recommendations for screening of first-degree relatives of patients with colorectal cancer follow the NH and MRC guidelines (Table 19.2).

A.10 An adenoma is one of four types of polyps that can be found in the colon and rectum. Apart from neoplastic lesions, there

Answers cont.

Table 19.2 Screening guidelines for colorectal cancer

Screening Guidelines	Recommendation
Category 1	Faecal occult blood testing (FOBT) annually from age 50
	Sigmoidoscopy (preferably flexible) every 5 years from age 50
	(Many would argue that if colonic examination is to be undertaken then it should be complete colonoscopy)
Category 2	Colonoscopy every 5 years starting age 50 or 10 years younger than the index case
	FOBT annually
Category 3	Careful surveillance which needs to be tailored to the subgroup
	Consideration for genetic testing

are three benign groups which include hyperplastic and inflammatory polyps and hamartomas. Serrated adenomas are a variant of hyperplastic polyps and may have a faster progression from benign to malignant. All adenomas have malignant potential. Adenomas may be tubular (often pedunculated), villous (usually sessile) or tubulovillous and can be found in any part of the bowel. As with cancers, the most common site for adenomas is the distal colon and rectum. The larger the polyp, the greater the chance of it being malignant. Fifty per cent of all polyps greater than 2 cm contain a focus of malignancy.

Revision Points

Colorectal Cancer

Epidemiology
- One of the most common cancers in developed countries.
- Increasing in incidence (probably a reflection of increasing proportion of older people in the population).

Risk Factors
- Diet.
- Genetic predisposition (e.g. familial adenomatous polyposis).
- Ulcerative colitis.
- Family history (see below).
- A past history of colorectal cancer.
- Pre-existing adenoma.

Symptoms
Will vary with site of tumour.
- Rectum/sigmoid colon (60% of colorectal cancers):
  - change in bowel habit
  - rectal bleeding
  - tenesmus
  - mucorrhoea.
- Right-sided neoplasms:
  - tiredness and lethargy (secondary to an anaemia).

Surveillance
- Screening can reduce the incidence of colorectal cancer.
- Mass screening (FOBT) is not justified.
- 'Average risk' individuals: immunological FOBT for those aged over 50.
- Individuals with a family history of colorectal cancer: see Answer 9.
- Screening of 'at-risk' groups:
  - inflammatory bowel disease
  - familial adenomatous polyps

– adenomatous polyps

– previous colorectal cancer.

  Regular colonoscopy is recommended for the above groups.

Rectal Bleeding

• Will usually be from a benign lesion (e.g. haemorrhoids).

• If bleeding cannot be seen coming from this source, the rest of the bowel must be examined to exclude malignancy.

Change in Bowel Habit

Important causes of constipation include:

• Change in diet.

• Irritable bowel syndrome.

• Diverticular disease.

• Medications.

• Malignancy.

Issues to Consider

• Colorectal cancer is virtually unknown among the indigenous population of southern Africa. Why might this be so?

• If you found a 30-year-old patient with multiple colonic polyps, how would you set about devising a plan of management?

Further Information

National Health and Medical Research Council, Canberra (2005) Guidelines for the prevention, early detection and management of colorectal cancer (CRC).

www.cancer.gov/cancertopics/types/colon-and-rectal *Information about colon and rectal cancer treatment, prevention, genetics, causes, screening, statistics.*

www.gastrolab.net *Endoscopic images presented in an MCQ fashion.*

www.nlm.nih.gov/medlineplus/colorectalcancer.html *Patient-oriented tutorial available via interactive link.*

Haematuria in a 60-year-old man

Darren Foreman

A 60-year-old man presents with a 3-day history of passing blood in his urine. It is painless and he has no other symptoms. His past medical history includes hypertension, and he is on indapamide and perindopril.

Q.1 What are the common causes of gross haematuria to be considered in this case?

Q.2 What further history may help determine the cause?

The patient is obese, with a pulse of 65/min and a blood pressure 130/80 mmHg. There is a large mass palpable in his left abdomen below his costal margin.

Q.3 What investigations should be ordered – and why?

His urine microscopy shows >1000 red blood cells, and culture had no growth. Haemoglobin is 132 g/L, creatinine 128, and liver function tests are normal. A representative slice from the contrast-enhanced CT scan is shown in Figure 20.1.

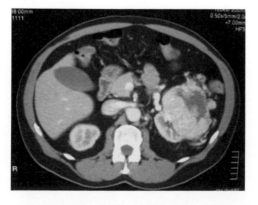

Figure 20.1

Q.4   What does the CT image show?

For tumour staging the CT also assesses for invasion of adjacent structures (renal vein, perinephric fat, adrenal gland, pancreas) and metastases (lungs, bone, liver, adrenal). None of these is identified.

Tumour stage is the most important prognostic factor (Table 20.1).

Table 20.1 Prognosis according to tumour stage	
Renal Tumour	**5-Year Survival**
Confined to kidney	75–90%
Invades perinephric fat, adrenal, renal vein, IVC	50–70%
Lymph node involvement	30%
Distant metastases	5%

Q.5   What management should be recommended?

The histopathology confirms a clear cell RCC which is invading perinephric fat and into the collecting system. There is no local lymph node involvement and the surgical margins are free of tumour. The patient makes an uneventful recovery.

Six months later the patient is reviewed. He has no urinary symptoms, has a good appetite, stable weight and enjoys being back at work. His creatinine is 108, and a CT chest, abdomen and pelvis is performed. This shows enlarged subcarinal nodes. The solitary right kidney appears normal and there are no pulmonary lesions (Figure 20.2).

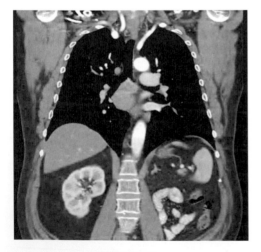

Figure 20.2

Q.6 What is the most likely diagnosis and what should be done?

This location is very difficult to sample due to its deep, central location, and a percutaneous biopsy is not possible. A transtracheal needle aspirate via a bronchoscopy is performed and only yields inflammatory material. A PET/CT scan is arranged and shows the following (Figure 20.3).

Figure 20.3

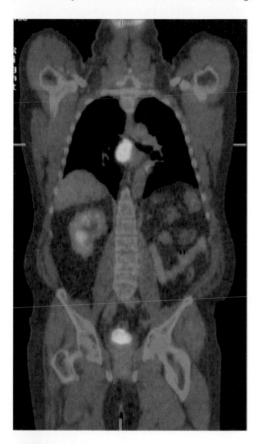

Q.7 What does the PET/CT show and what is the likely diagnosis?

A further attempt at biopsy of this enlarged lymph node is made by transoesophageal aspirate via endoscopy with ultrasound guidance. Cytology confirms malignant clear cells consistent with metastatic RCC.

Q.8 What treatment options are available?

The patient proceeds with treatment using a tyrosine kinase inhibitor and his lymphadenopathy halves in size over 4 months. One year later he continues with the tyrosine kinase inhibitor, and the lymphadenopathy is still present. He remains active and is asymptomatic.

Answers

A.1 Haematuria can arise from upper or lower urinary tract causes.

Upper Tract

- Kidney cancer – renal cell cancer (RCC), transitional cell cancer (TCC).
- Kidney stones.
- Primary renal disorder.

Lower Tract

- Bladder cancer – transitional cell cancer.
- Prostatic hypertrophy.
- Acute bacterial cystitis.
- Radiation cystitis.
- Haemorrhagic cystitis.

Trauma and coagulation disorders must also be excluded.

A.2 Details of the haematuria may help to identify the site of bleeding. Renal bleeding may have associated flank pain if clots are being passed (clot colic). These clots can be elongated due to passage down the ureters. Prostatic bleeding usually occurs at initiation or termination of the urinary stream, and may occur independent to voiding. This often has associated bothersome lower urinary tract symptoms, such as hesitancy, frequency, nocturia and terminal dribbling.

A history of smoking (TCC of kidney or bladder), radiation therapy (radiation cystitis), chemotherapy (haemorrhagic cystitis), occupational exposure to chemicals (TCC bladder), kidney stones, bleeding disorder and anticoagulant use should be elucidated.

The classical triad presentation of RCC with gross haematuria, flank pain and abdominal mass is now rarely seen and is usually indicative of advanced disease. The most common presentation occurs incidentally in asymptomatic patients undergoing radiological imaging for an unrelated condition. Occasionally patients present with systemic symptoms including fever, nausea, loss of appetite and loss of weight. Less commonly patients present with a paraneoplastic syndrome due to cytokine release by the tumour, such as hypercalcaemia, polycythaemia, anaemia, hypertension (HT), Stauffer's syndrome (hepatic dysfunction), neuropathy.

A.3

- Urine microscopy and culture – red blood cells, white blood cells, red cell morphology, casts, bacteria.
- Complete blood picture – anaemia.
- Biochemistry – renal and liver failure, abnormalities may suggest metastatic disease.
- Coagulation studies.

CT urogram is performed before and after intravenous contrast. Contrast should not be given if significant renal impairment is present. This CT carefully assesses the urinary tract and identifies any renal stones, tumours and filling defects of the collecting system (often transitional cell cancers). If no cause is identified, then a cystoscopy is needed to further evaluate the lower urinary tract.

A.4 This is a CT scan of the abdomen after administration of intravenous contrast. There is an 8 cm diameter solid tumour of the left kidney and a normal right kidney. No lymphadenopathy is seen.

A.5 An urgent specialist opinion is required – with a view to left radical nephrectomy.

Radical nephrectomy remains the gold standard for treatment of RCC. This involves excision of the kidney within its enveloping perinephric fat and fascia, and any regional lymph nodes. It can be performed via an open incision or

Answers *cont.*

laparoscopic approach. Nephron-sparing surgery with partial nephrectomy is considered in patients with smaller exophytic tumours, or in patients with renal impairment, a solitary kidney, renal stones or von Hippel–Lindau syndrome. This involves excising the tumour along with overlying fat and leaving the remaining kidney in situ.

A.6 The patient almost certainly has metastatic disease. Clear cell RCCs usually metastasize via haematogenous spread to the lung and lymph nodes. The metastatic behaviour is often unpredictable and may occur early or very late, with deposits often being found in unusual sites. PET scanning may have a role. If the tumour proves to be FDG-avid, this imaging tool may be helpful in subsequent management.

A tissue biopsy will differentiate metastatic RCC from an unrelated malignancy or benign lymphadenopathy. This information is important in deciding on further management.

A.7 This image confirms that the enlarged subcarinal lymph node is metabolically active and the most likely cause is metastatic disease. The radioactive tracer is also taken up by the solitary right kidney and is present within the bladder.

A.8 Metastatic RCC is considered incurable. It is insensitive to chemotherapy and radiotherapy has limited use. Treatment with immune modulators (interferon alpha, interleukin-2) is only available to patients with good performance status, and has a partial response rate of 10–20%. The newest agents available are tyrosine kinase inhibitors (TKIs) such as sunitinib. These block multiple receptor tyrosine kinases which are implicated in tumour growth and angiogenesis. TKIs show an improved partial response rate (20–40%) and longer period of disease stabilization. Referral to a palliative care team may be required in the near future if his disease progresses.

Revision Points

Gross Haematuria

Causes
- Upper tract – kidney cancer (RCC, TCC), stones, primary renal disease, trauma.
- Lower tract – bladder cancer (TCC), acute bacterial cystitis, radiation cystitis, haemorrhagic cystitis, trauma.

Investigation
- Urine microscopy and culture.
- Complete blood picture, biochemistry, coagulation studies.
- CT urogram with contrast.
- Cystoscopy to evaluate lower urinary tract.

Renal Cell Carcinoma (RCC)

Epidemiology
- Accounts for 2% of all malignancies.
- Occurs twice as often in men.
- Usually diagnosed at age 50–70 years.
- Risk factors include cigarette smoking and obesity.

Pathology
- Histological types of include clear cell (80% of all RCC), papillary, chromophobe and collecting duct.
- Prognosis mainly depends on tumour stage.

Revision Points *cont.*

- Multiple or bilateral RCCs occur less than 5% of the time, and may be due to a hereditary cancer syndrome, such as von Hippel–Lindau syndrome, especially with early age of onset.

Presentation
- Can vary and include asymptomatic incidental finding, haematuria, flank pain, abdominal mass, weight loss, fever, nausea and paraneoplastic syndromes.

Treatment
- Treated by surgical excision if the disease is not metastatic.
- Incurable when metastatic, and tyrosine kinase inhibitors are used to slow disease progression.

Issues to Consider

- Under what circumstances would there be a role for nephrectomy in a patient with metastatic RCC?
- What is the genetic basis of von Hippel–Lindau syndrome and what are the syndromal features?

Further Information

http://en.wikipedia.org/wiki/Renal_cell_cancer

http://www.emedicinehealth.com/renal_cell_cancer/article_em.htm

http://www.kidneycancer.org/

http://my.clevelandclinic.org/disorders/kidney_cancer/urology_overview.aspx

The routine check-up

Jimmy Lam

A 65-old-man presents for a routine prostate check. He is otherwise healthy and takes no regular medication. There is no family history of prostate cancer. He has mild lower urinary tract symptoms (LUTS) with slightly reduced flow and mild hesitancy. He looks fit and abdominal examination is unremarkable. On digital rectal examination (DRE) the prostate gland feels enlarged with areas of induration on the right side. Perineal sensation and gross lower limb motor function are intact.

Q.1 What is the significance of his symptoms and physical findings?

It is explained to the patient that while he almost certainly has benign prostate hyperplasia some investigations should be considered. The pros and cons of screening are explained to the patient.

Q.2 What investigations would be appropriate and why?

His PSA is 8.1 ng/mL (normal <4.5 ng/mL) and the serum haematological and biochemical estimations within normal limits. His renal tract ultrasound showed a moderately enlarged prostate and trabeculations within the bladder consistent with chronic outflow obstruction.

Q.3 What is the significance of the results and examination findings and what should be done next?

The patient is advised to undergo a transrectal ultrasound guided (TRUS) biopsy of the prostate. This confirms the presence of a small focus of Gleason 3+3=6 prostate cancer in the right apex, one of the eight areas biopsied.

Q.4 What are the management options and issues?

Q.5 What is the rational for active surveillance?

The patient is reviewed at 3-monthly intervals with repeat PSA and DRE. After 12 months of active surveillance a further TRUS biopsy is performed and shows Gleason 3+3=6 prostate cancer. This time four of the eight areas biopsied show involvement with prostate cancer.

Q.6 What staging tests should be arranged?

A whole body bone scan is performed and is negative.

Q.7 What are treatment options and their side-effects?

Following consultations with the urologist, radiation oncologist and a prostate cancer support nurse, the patient decides to proceed with radical prostatectomy via the robotic approach. Twelve months post surgery, he remains well and his PSA remains undetectable. He is continent and able to achieve erection with the use of phosphodiesterase inhibitors.

Answers

A.1 Benign prostate hyperplasia is a common process in ageing males and accounts for most of the lower urinary tract symptoms in these patients. Incidence of prostate cancer also increases with age but it is unlikely the cause of this patient's lower urinary tract symptoms. Early-stage prostate cancer rarely causes any symptoms and is usually picked up via screening.

Risk factors for prostate cancer include increasing age, family history, long-term exposure to high levels of testosterone as well as a diet high in saturated fat and animal protein. Having one first-degree relative with prostate cancer doubles the risk of developing prostate cancer; having two or more first-degree relatives increases the risk of prostate cancer by as much as fivefold.

A.2 Investigations should include:
- Serum prostate specific antigen (PSA).
- Midstream urine (MSU) – exclude any urinary tract infection.
- Serum biochemistry – to assess baseline renal function given his mild lower urinary tract symptoms (LUTS).
- Renal tract ultrasound – to assess for signs of urinary outflow obstruction.

A.3 About 50% of patients with an abnormal digital examination are subsequently found to have prostate cancer on biopsy and those with an abnormal PSA have about 30% chance of having prostate cancer detected. Because digital rectal examination and PSA testing are complementary, they should be used in combination as a tool for assessing prostate cancer risk.

Answers *cont.*

A.4 His staging investigations have confirmed clinically localized prostate cancer and his options for treatment include radical prostatectomy (via open or laparoscopic/robotic approach), radical radiotherapy (external beam or brachytherapy) or active surveillance. The patient is concerned about the possible side-effects of treatment and elects to defer treatment, opting for regular monitoring with active surveillance.

A.5 The lifetime risk of developing prostate cancer is 1 in 3, the lifetime risk of prostate cancer causing problems is 1 in 10 and the lifetime risk of dying from prostate cancer is 2–3 in 100. Therefore clearly not everyone who develops prostate cancer will die from it. The rationale behind active surveillance is that some patients with low-risk and low-volume cancer may have clinically insignificant or indolent cancer that may not necessarily cause them problems in their lifetime. Provided these patients are appropriately monitored for disease progression and then offered more active treatment, the risk of over-treatment can be reduced and the risks of side-effects of active treatment can be deferred in order to maximize quality of life.

A.6 Staging investigations for prostate cancer generally involve the use of whole body bone scan to detect evidence of bony metastatic disease. In the absence of bone pain and with a PSA <10, the yield of the bone scan is low (<1%). In patients with intermediate and high-risk disease staging with CT/MRI of the abdomen and pelvis may also be appropriate.

A.7 There are no randomized studies comparing radical prostatectomy with either external beam radiotherapy or

brachytherapy for localized prostate cancer. The long-term survival results are similar with either treatment. Hormonal therapy for prostate cancer provides some control but does not cure the patient of the cancer.

Surgical removal of the prostate for cancer can be done via open retropubic, laparoscopic or robotic-assisted laparoscopic approach. The laparoscopic and robotic approaches offers some short-term benefits including reduced blood loss, less postoperative pain, quicker recovery and short hospital stay. Other treatment outcomes such as cancer control, continence and potency are similar to the traditional open approach. Side-effects of surgery include: urinary incontinence (5–15%), erectile dysfunction (30–100%), bladder neck obstruction (<10%) and death (<1%).

Radiotherapy can be given either as external beam radiotherapy (EBRT), low-dose seed brachytherapy or high-dose brachytherapy. EBRT is an outpatient treatment over 6–8 weeks. Side-effects include urinary incontinence (5%), erectile dysfunction (40–80%), long-term bowel and bladder problems (5–10%). Low-dose seed brachytherapy involves the placement of permanent radioactive seeds into the prostate gland. The aim is to deliver a higher dose of radiation more directly to the prostate and reduce radiation damage to the normal surrounding structures. For low-risk cancer it offers similar outcomes to the other treatment but has reduced risks of erectile dysfunction (40%) as well as reduced rectal and bladder morbidity. High-dose seed brachytherapy is usually used in combination with EBRT for higher-risk cancer patients in whom cancer may have spread beyond the prostate.

Hormonal therapy or androgen deprivation is used to slow the growth of prostate cancer. This form of treatment does not cure the cancer but rather suppresses its growth. This can be achieved by surgical castration (bilateral orchidectomy) or chemical castration (anti-androgens or luteinizing hormone-releasing hormone agonists – LHRH agonist). This form of treatment is usually offered to patients who already have cancer spread beyond the prostate or older patients who are not candidates for radical surgery or radiotherapy treatments.

Revision Points

Prostate Cancer

In men, and after skin cancers, carcinoma of the prostate is the most common malignancy in Western communities and the second commonest cause of cancer-related death.

Risk Factors

- Increasing age.
- Family history.
- Diet high in saturated fat and red meats.
- Weak association to cadmium exposure.

Pathology

Most are adenocarcinoma of acinar cell origin. The tumours usually arise from the peripheral zone of the prostate, and 20% are in the transitional zone of the prostate. Eighty-five per cent of cases are multifocal.

Prostatic adenocarcinoma is most commonly graded based on the Gleason grading system which assesses glandular pattern of the tumour at low magnifications. The Gleason pattern ranges from 1 to 5. The Gleason score is the sum of the two most prevalent patterns identified, giving a score between 2 and 10, 10 being the most aggressive.

Natural History

Pattern of spread via direct extension into surrounding tissues, lymphatic spread to region lymph nodes are not uncommon.

Most of the distant metastases are to the bones and visceral metastases are less common.

Staging

Staging is based on the American Joint Committee on Cancer (AJCC) modified TNM system.

Signs and Symptoms

Most patients have few signs in the early stages, but may present with urinary obstructive symptoms or haematuria. Advanced disease may present with signs of metastases such as bone pain. Clinical findings of a palpable prostate nodule or induration may be the only sign.

Diagnosis

Confirmation is usually on transrectal ultrasound-guided prostate biopsy following investigation with PSA and DRE but is sometimes detected incidentally from transurethral prostate resected specimens. Further staging with bone scan, CT and MRI may sometimes be useful.

Treatment

- Watchful waiting – expectant management for those not likely to be affected by the diagnosis of prostate cancer.
- Active surveillance – deferral of active treatment for patients who may have clinically insignificant or indolent disease.

Revision Points *cont.*

These patients are followed up regularly for signs of progression.

- Radical prostatectomy (open, laparoscopic or robotic assisted), radiotherapy (EBRT, brachytherapy) for those with localized prostate cancer.
- Androgen deprivation therapy.

Role of Screening

The Urological Society of Australia and New Zealand (USANZ) currently does not recommend the use of mass population-based PSA screening as public health policy. However, based on recent data from one of two large randomised screening studies, there was a reduced risk of prostate cancer death with PSA testing and treatment in selected patient groups (Aged 55–69 years). Therefore PSA based testing, together with digital rectal examination should be offered to men in his age group, after appropriate counselling about the risks and benefits of such testing. Men over the age of 40 who are concern about their prostate health could have a single PSA test and DRE performed to provide an estimate of their prostate cancer risk over the next 10–20 years based on age-specific median PSA values, with subsequent individualised monitoring according to their risks.

Issues to Consider

- Should an upper age limit be imposed for screening for prostate cancer?
- Why is prostate cancer commoner in developed communities?

Further Information

www.andrologyaustralia.org – Andrology Australia.

www.auanet.org – American Urological Association.

www.cancer.org.au – Cancer Council Australia.

www.prostatehealth.org.au – Australian Prostate Cancer Collaboration.

www.usanz.org.au – Urological Society of Australia and New Zealand.

www.uroweb.org – European Association of Urology.

Acute back pain in a 75-year-old man

Robert Fitridge

You are asked to see a 75-year-old retired electrician who has been brought into the emergency department with an 18-hour history of increasing back pain. He tells you that the pain came on gradually and now goes down into his left groin and thigh. The pain is constant, getting worse. He has never had this pain before. He does not think the pain was precipitated by anything and nothing seems to ease it. In particular, there is no history of trauma, and walking or exertion do not affect it. There are no other associated symptoms.

Eight months ago he suffered a myocardial infarction and since that time has suffered with moderate angina on effort. He takes isosorbide dinitrate 10 mg three times a day for the angina and uses nitrate skin patches at night. He used to smoke 20 cigarettes a day, but ceased after his heart attack. He drinks 20 g of alcohol per day at the weekends. He suffers occasional episodes of indigestion for which he takes an over-the-counter antacid preparation.

The review of systems is otherwise unremarkable apart from symptoms of increasing bladder neck outflow obstruction, which have been worse over the last 2 years. He gets up twice every night to void and says he feels that he can never empty his bladder properly. He has not passed urine since the pain started.

Q.1 What diagnoses go through your mind?

On examination he is thin and in pain. His blood pressure is 140/90 mmHg and he has a regular pulse rate of 100 bpm. His jugular venous pressure is not elevated and his apex beat is displaced 2 cm lateral to the mid-clavicular line and is felt in the fifth interspace. Both heart sounds are normal with no added sounds. His chest is resonant and breath sounds are vesicular. He has a tender, pulsatile mass in the abdomen which feels about 6–7 cm in diameter and is situated at the level of the umbilicus. There is dullness to percussion in the suprapubic region extending four finger-breadths above the pubis. Both femoral pulses are of good volume and pedal pulses are palpable. His legs are neurologically normal and the straight leg raise and sciatic stretch tests are negative. The patient's previous X-rays are available.

The patient recently had an abdominal ultrasound for his urinary frequency (Figures 22.1 and 22.2).

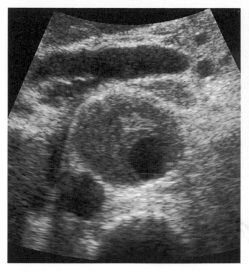

Figure 22.1

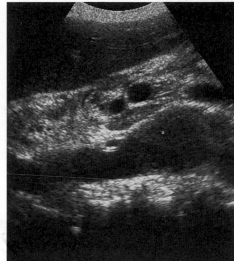

Figure 22.2

Q.2 What does the investigation show?

The ultrasound findings confirm your clinical suspicions.

Q.3 What is your next action?

Q.4 What further investigations may be indicated?

As this patient is haemodynamically stable, a further investigation is performed expeditiously. Two of the images are shown (Figures 22.3 and 22.4).

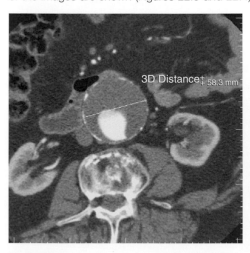

Figure 22.3

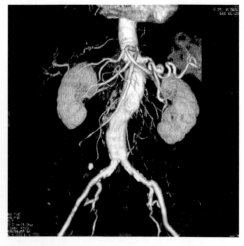

Figure 22.4

Q.5 What type of images are these and what do they show? How do these findings affect your management?

The patient and his family are informed of the diagnosis and the likely outcome if surgery is not undertaken promptly. The aneurysm is in imminent danger of rupture, with a subsequent high mortality. Surgery also has its risks, particularly in this patient with known cardiac disease.

The cardiologists and anaesthesiologists are asked to review the patient, and prepare him for emergency surgery. At surgery, the aneurysm is repaired using a dacron tube graft. Following the procedure he is transferred to the intensive care unit.

Q.6 What complications may follow an aortic aneurysm repair?

The patient makes an uneventful recovery and is home 10 days after the procedure.

Answers

A.1 Acute pain in the back, radiating to the groin, in an elderly male with known atheromatous disease must make you consider a leaking or stretching abdominal aortic aneurysm. This is the diagnosis that needs to be excluded. Other conditions include:
- Aortic dissection.
- Acute pancreatitis.
- Ureteric colic.
- Urinary retention.

This is unlikely to be a musculoskeletal problem (e.g. herniated disc), as the pain is not aggravated by movement.

A.2 The ultrasound shows a large fusiform abdominal aortic aneurysm. The image in Figure 22.1 shows the aneurysm in transverse section and in Figure 22.2 the aorta in longitudinal view. Some thrombus is shown in the posterior wall. The measurement of aneurysm size is taken on the transverse image and is the maximum anteroposterior or transverse diameter. The length of the aneurysm is not important from a management point of view.

A.3 This man has an abdominal aortic aneurysm, which is symptomatic and may now be leaking or about to leak. This is a vascular emergency. Your priority is to insert a wide-bore intravenous catheter, collect blood for electrolytes, full blood count, basic coagulation studies (APTT and INR) and group and match blood. You must alert the vascular surgeons immediately. You must also attach a cardiac monitor and insert a urinary catheter to monitor urine output, and notify the patient's relatives.

A.4 The need for further investigations will hinge on whether the patient is haemodynamically stable. If not stable, further investigations will only delay definitive management. In that case, the patient should go directly to the operating theatre.

As the patient is haemodynamically stable, the surgeons may request a CT scan of the aorta to assess the size of the aneurysm, its relationship to the renal arteries, whether it has leaked and to

Answers *cont.*

exclude any other cause of intra-abdominal pain.

A.5 Figure 22.3 shows a standard transverse cut through the aneurysm sac. Contrast has been administered and the non-enhancing contents of the aneurysm sac represent laminated thrombus. It is these images which provide the surgeon with vital information regarding the presence or absence of a leak. This shows a 5.8 cm abdominal aortic aneurysm which had not leaked. The pain is presumably due to expansion and stretching of the aneurysm.

Figure 22.4 is a spiral CT angiogram reconstruction. The reconstruction gives the surgeon useful information regarding patency/stenoses of renal and iliac arteries, vessel tortuosity and relationship of the aneurysm to the renal arteries. The renal arteries are patent and the iliac vessels are not aneurysmal.

The transverse cuts give the essential diagnostic information regarding size of the aneurysm sac and the presence or absence of leaking blood. The laminated thrombus in the sac does not show up on CTA reconstructions. The spiral CT reconstruction is essential in either the elective situation or in urgent repair when the patient is haemodynamically stable.

A.6 The majority of the mortality (2–10%) and morbidity associated with elective abdominal aortic aneurysm repair is due to pre-existing cardiac disease. The risk of a peri- or early postoperative myocardial infarction in this man will be high.

Other possible complications include:
- Cerebrovascular event.
- Acute thrombotic/embolic events leading to:
  - renal failure
  - bowel infarction
  - acute lower limb ischaemia.
- Sepsis – chest or wound.
- Graft infection.

Revision Points

Abdominal Aortic Aneurysms (AAA)

Incidence
- 5% of males over 65 years of age.
- Less common in women.
- Occur in 10–15% of claudicants.

Risk Factors
- Smoking.
- Hypertension.
- Hyperlipidaemia.
- Genetic predisposition.
  Note: diabetes is not a risk factor.

Pathology
- Degenerative process involving all layers of aortic wall.
- Appears to be caused by increased activity of matrix metalloproteinases (extracellular matrix-degrading enzymes which break down collagen and elastin in the aortic wall). These enzymes seem to be activated by aortic endothelial injury caused by smoking, hypertension or hyperlipidaemia: i.e. aneurysms are not

Revision Points *cont.*

caused by atherosclerosis, although atherosclerosis frequently co-exists.

Clinical Features

- Most frequently asymptomatic.
- May present with abdominal, back or loin to groin pain (if stretching, leaking or ruptured).
- Collapse or cardiac arrest may occur in acute rupture.

Natural History

- Aneurysms less than 5–5.5 cm in diameter rarely rupture (1–2% per year).
- Rupture rate increases exponentially with increasing size over 5.5 cm.

Management

- AAA less than 5 cm in diameter should be treated with aggressive control of risk factors and 6-monthly ultrasound surveillance, unless there is rapid increase in size or development of symptoms, e.g. abdominal or back pain.
- AAA over 5 cm can be considered for repair if risks of surgery (mainly cardiorespiratory) are less than risk of rupture.
- Open surgical repair is most durable technique for fixing AAA.
- Endoluminal stent graft repair is frequently used in anatomically suitable cases. This procedure is associated with lower morbidity and mortality but requires lifelong surveillance with re-intervention rates of 5–10% per year to maintain exclusion of the aneurysm sac.

Issues to Consider

- How might a thoracic aortic aneurysm present?
- How would you diagnose and manage aortic dissection?
- Why do symptomatic patients develop groin and testicular pain?

Further Information

Symons, N.R, Gibbs, R.G., 2009. The management of abdominal aortic aneurysms. British Journal of Hospital Medicine 70, 566–571. *A review of current management.*

United Kingdom Small Aneurysm Trial Participants. 2002. Long-term outcomes of immediate repair compared with surveillance of small abdominal aortic aneurysms. New England Journal of Medicine 346, 1445–1452. www.NEJM.com

www.scvir.org/patient/aaa/ *A website from the Society for Cardiovascular and Interventional Radiology. Patient directed but with good information about endoluminal treatments.*

A 59-year-old man with calf pain

Robert Fitridge

A 59-year-old man presents with a 4-month history of pain in the right calf. The pain occurs only on walking and presents as a cramp-like discomfort, which comes on after he walks about 100 metres. The pain eases off when he stops walking, and he is still able to make his way to the local shops, although he is now reluctant to do so.

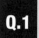

Q.1 What is the likely cause of his symptoms and what other information would you like from the history?

Three years previously he suffered a myocardial infarction and since then has been on enteric-coated aspirin. He takes no other medications apart from a salbutamol inhaler which was prescribed by his general practitioner for 'when he gets a bit tight'. In the past he has had an appendectomy and a prostatectomy. He smokes 20 cigarettes a day and drinks 20 g of alcohol a day. He is 170 cm tall and weighs 85 kg.

Q.2 What will be the important findings to look for on examination and what investigations will you perform?

His blood pressure is 150/85 mmHg and his heart rate is 84 and regular. Examination of his heart is unremarkable. He has a bruit over his right carotid artery. His chest is resonant with decreased breath sounds and a prolonged expiration, but no added sounds. Abdominal examination is normal. His femoral pulses are palpable, as are the more distal pulses in his left leg. His right popliteal pulse is not palpable and neither are the right pedal pulses. Both legs are of similar temperature and there are no other signs of limb ischaemia.

Q.3 What is an ankle–brachial index measurement and what is its significance?

His ankle–brachial index is 0.5 on the right and 0.8 on the left. His lipid profile is reported as being marginally raised and a random blood sugar is within normal limits. His serum biochemistry is unremarkable.

Q.4 How would you explain his condition to him, and what is your advice at this point?

Twelve months later he comes back to see you. He had managed to continue his daily walks down to the local shops until 2 months ago, but despite your advice he has continued to smoke. His pain has worsened recently and now comes on at about 20 metres. He now finds these symptoms interfere with his lifestyle. Most recently he has been woken at night by pain in his leg, which he relieves by dangling the leg over the edge of the bed.

Q.5 What has happened and what do you do now?

Your examination of his cardiorespiratory system does not reveal any new findings. His abdomen is soft, there are no pulsatile masses and both femoral pulses are palpable. His legs and feet are cool to the touch, and the right foot is colder than the left. The toes on his right foot are dusky and there is sluggish capillary return to his big toe. When the leg is lowered over the side of the examination couch it assumes a reddish-purple colour, and when the leg is elevated the foot becomes pale. His popliteal and pedal pulses cannot be palpated on either leg. His Doppler pressures are measured and he has an ankle–brachial index of 0.3 on the right and 0.7 on the left.

On your advice he agrees to see a vascular surgeon, who recommends that an arterial duplex scan is performed. This is shown in Figures 23.1, 23.2 and 23.3. Figure 23.2 demonstrates an occluded segment of superficial femoral artery (SFA). The waveforms above this lesion (23.1) are normal but the waveforms distally (23.3) are damped consistent with the occlusion just proximal to this segment. Subsequently he recommends a CT angiogram (shown in Figure 23.4). These are AP views with the patient's right leg on the left side of Figure 23.1.

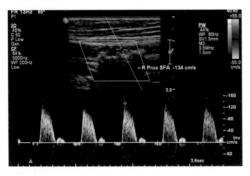

Figure 23.1

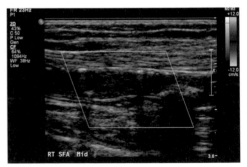

Figure 23.2

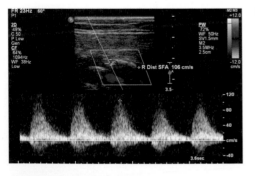

Figure 23.3

Figure 23.4

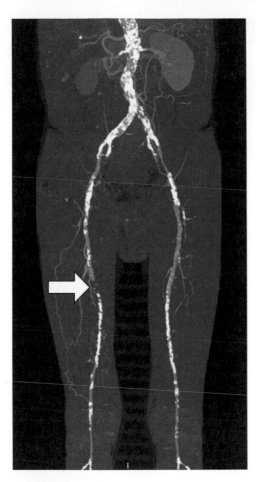

Q.6 What does the angiogram show?

There is diffuse calcification of all vessels. There is an occlusion of the right distal superficial femoral and proximal popliteal artery confirmed with good below-knee vessels.

Q.7 How are you going to manage this problem?

An attempted angiography was unsuccessful and a reverse vein femoropopliteal bypass was performed. This is successful in improving his lower limb circulation but is complicated by a cerebrovascular event involving his non-dominant hemisphere for which he requires 3 months of intensive rehabilitation.

Answers

A.1 His history of calf pain on exercise relieved by rest is typical of intermittent claudication. You may also consider spinal canal stenosis in your differential diagnosis, but relief of the pain by rest points to peripheral vascular disease as the cause of the problem. As such, you would like to know if he has risk factors for cardiovascular disease and any history of other previous or current problems related to his cardiovascular system.

Major risk factors which you must ask about are:
- Hypertension (duration and adequacy of control).
- Diabetes mellitus (duration, Hb A1C).
- Smoking (pack years).
- Hyperlipidaemia.
  Typical cardiovascular co-morbidities are:
- Ischaemic heart disease (especially current but also past symptoms).
- Cerebrovascular accidents or transient ischaemic attacks (TIAs).
- Abdominal aortic aneurysm.

A.2
- The cardiovascular system should be examined for hypertension and evidence of cardiac dysfunction. The carotid arteries should be examined for bruits.
- The respiratory system should be examined for evidence of smoking-related chronic airways obstruction.
- His abdomen should be examined carefully for evidence of aortic aneurysm (present in 10–15% of claudicants).
- His peripheral pulses, including the femoral, popliteal, dorsalis pedis and posterior tibial pulses, should be examined. Provided a pulse can be felt, the quality of the femoral pulse will be assessed (for strength and dilatation) and bruits listened for.

- The legs should be assessed for evidence of ischaemia. This includes the colour and temperature of the limbs. If ischaemia is advanced, the foot will become pale when the leg is elevated and deeply red when it is then lowered to a dependent position. Reduced blood flow through the capillary bed will result in increased uptake of oxygen from the blood by the tissues and this may cause the limb to take on a cyanotic hue. An ischaemic foot tends to be relatively cool.
- The limb should also be examined for areas of ulceration and necrosis – so-called 'dry gangrene' or mummification. There may also be evidence of muscle atrophy. As the ischaemia worsens, atrophy of the skin progresses and it appears shiny and scaly. Loss of hair and thickening of the nails are unreliable signs of ischaemia because they are widely present in the normal population.
- Objective measurement of foot perfusion with Doppler ultrasound is essential – clinical judgement, including palpation of pedal pulse, is fairly inaccurate.
- You should measure the ankle–brachial index (ABI).
  At this stage the patient does not warrant extensive investigation, but the following should be performed:
- Blood sugar.
- Lipid profile.
- Serum biochemistry (looking for any renal impairment).

A.3 By comparing the blood pressures in the brachial (which is assumed to be normal) and the vessels at the ankle (dorsalis pedis and posterior tibial), an estimation can be made of the adequacy of arterial blood flow in the leg. In an individual with normal arteries the ankle–brachial

Answers *cont.*

index is expected to be 0.9–1.2, Most claudicants often have an ABI of 0.5–0.9. A value below 0.5 is often associated with rest pain and when the ratio gets to less than 0.3, viability of the limb may be in jeopardy.

A.4 You should advise him in simple language that:
• The pain in his legs is due to arterial occlusive disease, resulting in insufficient blood getting to the muscles, which is most noticeable during exercise.
• He should continue to walk within his levels of comfort. There is no advantage in walking 'through' the pain. He should stop when pain comes on, wait a minute or two for the discomfort to settle then go on.
• It is absolutely vital that he stops smoking because if he does not the disease will progress and he could develop gangrene or another complication such as a heart attack or stroke.
• He needs to take low-dose aspirin.
• There is evidence that there is some benefit to commencing a statin, even if his lipid profile is normal.
• Apart from Doppler studies, he does not need any other investigations.
• In addition to the Doppler studies previously described, however, it may be worth considering a carotid duplex scan to clarify whether a stenosis is present (bruit heard on initial physical examination).
• He needs to take care of his feet and avoid local trauma.
• He should reduce his cholesterol intake by following a low-cholesterol diet. If a lipid profile check 3 months later does not show improvement lipid-lowering agents will be started. There is some evidence that a statin should be

commenced in individuals with symptomatic lower limb arterial disease, irrespective of the lipid level.

A.5 He now has rest pain: the blood supply to the limb has deteriorated to such an extent that the leg's viability is threatened. You must take action:
• Repeat your physical examination.
• Repeat the Doppler studies.
• Reinforce your advice on the need to stop smoking.
• Make the patient aware of the high risk of losing his limb (or part of it).
• Arrange for the patient to be seen by a vascular surgeon, who will:
  – arrange imaging studies
  – suggest some form of intervention to try and improve blood supply to his foot.

A.6 Both a non-subtracted and subtracted angiogram are shown to assist with vessel orientation. The angiogram demonstrates normal aortoiliac arteries. The common femoral and profunda femoris vessels are also widely patent. Both superficial femoral arteries (SFA) (from groin to adductor canal) are extensively diseased, with a 7–8 cm long occlusion of the right SFA being shown. Collateral vessels via the profunda femoris arteries fill the popliteal arteries.

As a result of the more severe occlusive disease on the right side, the contrast filling the popliteal and proximal tibial vessels on this side is reduced, resulting in reduced opacification of the vessels.

A.7 As this patient has rest pain, revascularization should be undertaken, assuming his co-morbidities do not preclude intervention.

Approximately 30–60% of patients with disabling claudication or critical limb

Answers *cont.*

ischaemia (see Revision points) are suitable for percutaneous intervention (angioplasty, stent, thrombolysis or combinations of these techniques).

Many patients require bypass surgery, either owing to the length of the stenotic lesion/occlusion or as a result of the quality of the vessels above and below the lesion.

Revision Points

Chronic Lower Limb Ischaemia

Incidence
Approximately 5 : 1000 population/year in developed countries.

Aetiology
- Atherosclerosis (>90% of cases).
- Thromboangitis obliterans (Buerger's disease).
- Vasculitis.
- Arterial trauma.
- Rare causes: cystic adventitial disease of the popliteal artery, popliteal artery entrapment.

Differential Diagnoses
- Spinal canal disease.
- Sciatica.
- Peripheral neuropathy.

Note: presence of pulses, ankle–branchial index (ABI) or exercise ABI should allow differentiation between claudication and neurological cause of pain.

Risk Factors for Atherosclerosis
- Smoking.
- Diabetes.
- Hypertension.
- Genetic.
- Hyperlipidaemia.

Classification
See Table 23.1.

Natural History
Claudication
- Approximately 5–10% require lower limb intervention within 5 years for disabling claudication or deterioration to critical limb ischaemia.
- Limb loss in 2% during lifetime: majority of patients managed conservatively.
- Mortality 30% at 5 years (predominantly MI, CVA).

Critical limb ischaemia (rest pain or tissue loss)
- Revascularization attempted in 40–80%.
- Limb loss in 40% at 1 year.
- Mortality 20–30 % at 1 year (mainly cardiovascular).

Management
Claudication
- Conservative.
- Aggressive risk factor control.
- Only consider intervention if symptoms disabling.

Table 23.1 Classification of lower limb ischaemia		
Classification	**Doppler Ankle–Brachial Index (ABI) Approximate**	**Fontaine Stage**
Claudication	0.6–0.9	II
Critical limb ischaemia:		
• rest pain	0.3–0.6	III
• ulceration and/or gangrene	<0.4	IV

Revision Points *cont.*

Critical limb ischaemia
- Angiography with a view to revascularization.
- Stenting may be possible with durable results obtained in aortoiliac segments, less successful long-term results below the inguinal ligament.
- Selected centres rely on duplex ultrasound for planning revascularization.
- Lower limb bypass using autogenous vein is frequently required for limb salvage.

Issues to Consider

- How successful are conservative measures in the prevention of progression of occlusive vascular disease?
- What is neurogenic claudication and how does it differ from vascular claudication?
- What measures may help this man give up smoking?

Further Information

www.scvir.org *Home page of the American Society of Cardiovascular and Interventional Radiology. Interesting information and links about peripheral vascular diseases and the role of endovascular therapies.*

Norgen L, Hiatt WR, Dormandy JA, et al., TASC II Working Group, 2007. Inter-Society Consensus for the Management of Peripheral Arterial Disease (TASC II). Journal of Vascular Surgery 45, S1–S67.

Acute leg pain in a 73-year-old man

Robert Fitridge

You are relaxing in a comfortable chair in the doctors' mess, looking at the clock ticking towards the end of your shift when your thoughts are interrupted by a call from the ward.

The nurse would like you to see a 73-year-old man who is complaining of sudden-onset acute severe pain in his left leg. Two days earlier he had been admitted to hospital with an anterior myocardial infarction.

Q.1 What diagnoses go through your head as you head for the ward?

When you see the patient, you find him distressed with pain. He tells you the pain in his left leg came on abruptly about 40 minutes ago. The leg now feels numb and he cannot move it. He gives no prior history of claudication.

His blood pressure is 130/80 mmHg and his pulse rate 100 (irregularly irregular). Examination of the chest is unremarkable. There are no abnormalities in his abdomen. His femoral pulses are of good volume, the pulses in his right leg can all be felt. There are no pulses to be felt below the groin on the left side. The left leg is not swollen, but pale and cool to the touch.

Q.2 What do you think has happened? What further information would you like?

You are handed his in-patient notes. He had presented with 7 hours of chest pain. Work-up showed an acute anterior myocardial infarction. As his pain had subsided and he had developed Q waves in the anterior leads, he was not given any thrombolytic therapy.

He was immediately given oral aspirin and betablockers before being transferred for close monitoring in the coronary care unit. He remained there for 2 days before moving to the general ward. Now, 4 days since his admission, he has been slowly mobilizing. He was initially prescribed subcutaneous low molecular weight heparin, but you note on the drug chart that this was not continued on the ward since returning from coronary care.

His myocardial infarction was complicated by atrial fibrillation, with a rapid ventricular response rate on day 1. He had no ventricular arrhythmias and was treated with digoxin resulting in good rate control. He does not have any other significant past medical history.

Q.3 What would you like to do now?

An investigation is performed. One of the results is shown in Figure 24.1.

Figure 24.1

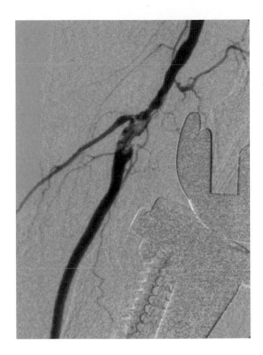

Q.4 What is this investigation? What does it show?

Q.5 What would you like to do now?

The patient underwent thrombolysis of the embolus radiologically using the 'pulse-spray' technique that often results in rapid clot lysis. Standard thrombolytic techniques would take 4–20 hours to achieve clot dissolution, and it was thought this patient's leg was unlikely to be viable if revascularization took this length of time. The 'pulse-spray' technique is much more rapid. After 1 hour of urokinase pulsing, the angiogram was repeated (Figures 24.2 and 24.3).

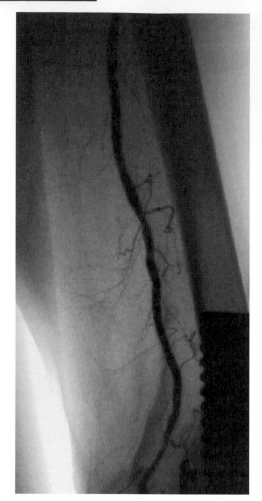

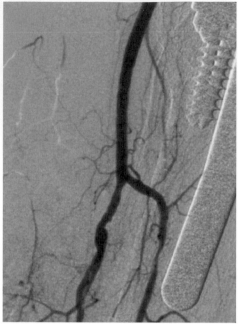

Figure 24.3

Figure 24.2

Q.6 What do these new angiograms show?

The patient was anticoagulated with heparin and plans were made to continue anticoagulation on oral warfarin for at least 6 months, or possibly indefinitely depending on his atrial rhythm.

Answers

A.1 There are few possible causes of an acute severely painful leg. The most likely diagnosis is one of arterial embolus to the left leg. Other less likely possibilities include thrombosis of a pre-existing arterial atherosclerotic plaque, an extensive deep vein thrombosis of the left leg or an aortic dissection extending into the left leg

Answers *cont.*

arteries. A muscle haematoma if on thrombolytic or anticoagulant therapy is also a possibility.

A.2 He has acute ischaemic limb. His leg is pale, pulseless, painful and 'perishing' with cold. In addition he may have paraesthesia and paralysis of the affected limb – the classic six Ps.

The presence of a femoral pulse on the left indicates that the occlusion is likely to be in the superficial femoral or popliteal artery.

The sudden onset, lack of previous history and recent myocardial infarction all suggest that this is an embolic phenomenon. He has most probably thrown off an embolus from the heart which has lodged in the femoral artery. Such an embolus would have arisen from a mural thrombus at the site of infarction (in the left ventricle) or dislodged from clot in an atrium that is fibrillating. A less likely cause in this instance would be acute thrombosis of an atherosclerotic lesion in the femoral or popliteal artery.

After your initial assessment you will want to examine the notes looking for information about his post-myocardial infarction course, the timing and duration of arrhythmias and whether or not he has been anticoagulated.

A.3 You should contact the vascular surgeons immediately. Emergency arteriography or CT angiography will be required to define the site and extent of obstruction.

Unless angiography can be performed without delay, you should consider anticoagulating the patient with unfractionated intravenous heparin. Baseline coagulation studies (APTT) must be performed before starting the heparin.

Heparin is dosed by weight and must be adjusted to maintain the APTT in the therapeutic range. A standard loading dose for an adult would be 5000 units, followed by an infusion of 1000 units/hour. Blood should also be collected for a complete blood picture, electrolytes and type and cross-matching. This patient is not a good candidate for general anaesthesia, but embolectomy or radiological intervention can be performed under local anaesthetic.

A.4 This is a digital subtraction angiogram, which demonstrates a filling defect in the left popliteal artery above the knee. At the level of the obstruction, there is a large collateral seen filling the distal popliteal vessel. This is consistent with a popliteal embolus. The proximal vessels are normal.

A.5 This patient has a threatened ischaemic leg requiring revascularization within 4 hours (see Revision points at end of chapter).

Management options include:
- Surgical removal of the embolus which could be done under local anaesthetic in some cases.
- Thrombolytic therapy. Possibilities include a rapid clot thrombolysis technique ('pulse-spray') or suction thrombectomy as a percutaneous radiological procedure. Urokinase and heparin can be 'pulsed' directly into the clot via a catheter traversing the thrombus.

A.6 The angiograms performed after 1 hour of thrombolysis demonstrated a good radiological result. The clot had lysed and there is satisfactory revascularization of the distal vessels. The filling defect was no longer visible.

Revision Points

Acute Lower Limb Ischaemia

Incidence
Approximately 2 : 10 000 population per year.

Aetiology
- Embolus – almost always due to mural thrombus post myocardial infarction or secondary to arrhythmia (occasionally can be from valvular heart disease or proximal aortic disease, e.g. aneurysm).
- Acute thrombosis of diseased artery.
- Bypass graft thrombosis.
- Trauma (e.g. knee dislocation, tibial plateau fracture).

Classification
Table 24.1 outlines classification criteria.

Investigations
- Following examination for pulses and assessment of severity of ischaemia, vascular surgeons should be consulted, and ECG, bloods, group and match performed. Doppler pressures (ankle–brachial index) may be performed. Anticoagulation should be commenced unless angiogram can be performed promptly.
- Also search for other sites of embolization (common sites include other leg, arms, brain and gut).
- Vascular imaging (ultrasound, CT angiography or angiography) will demonstrate the level of occlusion and may clarify the aetiology of acute ischaemia.

Management
Therapy will depend on aetiology, severity of ischaemia and patient co-morbidities.
   Options:
- Surgical thrombectomy under local, spinal or general anaesthetic (usually performed under local anaesthetic in the situation discussed).
- Thrombolysis performed radiologically (using urokinase or ± tissue plasminogen activator: TPA). Advanced catheter techniques such as suction thrombectomy or pulse-spray thrombolysis may be used in selected cases and decrease time taken to re-perfuse the lower limb (particularly in cases of profound ischaemia – category IIb).
- Bypass graft thrombectomy, thrombolysis or replacement for occluded (usually prosthetic) grafts.
- Surgical repair of artery ± bone fixation (for trauma).
- Immediate amputation for unsalvageable limb may be required.
- Occasionally palliative care is appropriate in selected cases.
   Note: fasciotomy of lower limb muscle compartments may need to be considered if ischaemia is profound and of lengthy duration prior to revascularization.

Table 24.1 Classification of severity in limb ischaemia

	Sensation (Calf/Foot)	Power (Foot Movement)	Calf Tenderness
1 Viable (urgent revascularization not required)	Normal	Normal	Nil
2 Threatened			
a) Needs revascularization (4–8 hours)	Slightly reduced	Normal	Nil
b) Needs urgent revascularization (<4 hours)	Reduced	Decreased	Often tender
3 Unsalvageable	Numb	Decreased/nil	Very tender (or paralysed)

Revision Points *cont.*

Outcomes
- Depend on severity and duration of ischaemia, and co-morbidities.

- Mortality rates are still 15–30%.
- Amputation rates in survivors 20–30%.

Issues to Consider

- What are the risks of surgery after a myocardial infarction?
- What are the other short- and long-term vascular complications of myocardial infarction? How may this patient's risk have been minimized?

Further Information

Norgen, L., Hiatt, W.R., Dormandy, J.A., et al., TASC II Working Group, 2007. Inter-Society

Consensus for the Management of Peripheral Arterial Disease (TASC II). Journal of Vascular Surgery 45, S1–S67.

Ouriel, K., 2002. Thrombolytic therapy for acute arterial occlusion. Journal of the American College of Surgeons 194, S32–S39.

A 68-year-old woman with a leg ulcer

Robert Fitridge

A 68-year-old woman attends the outpatient department with an ulcer on her left leg. She tells you it has been present for 2 months. She remembers knocking her leg on the end of her bed. The ulcer on her leg has become fairly painful over the last week. She has had a similar ulcer on her leg in the past which was treated by 'bandaging'.

What other information would you like from the history to ascertain the cause of the ulcer?

She is not a diabetic, but does take tablets for her blood pressure. She is not sure what these are. She is on no other medications. She has had no other illnesses of note, but has had varicose veins ever since the birth of her children. On further questioning, she reveals that the left leg was very swollen for 2 or 3 months after her third pregnancy but she never had any tests to see why. This has been her 'bad leg' ever since. Her leg ulcer is shown in Figure 25.1.

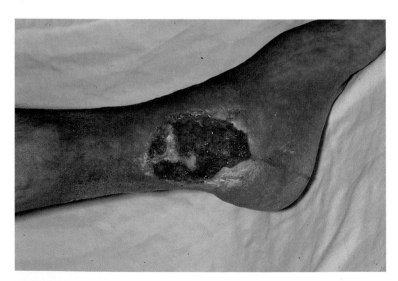

Figure 25.1

Q.2 | Describe what you see.

In addition to what is shown in the photograph, both legs show evidence of chronic venous insufficiency. There is loss of subcutaneous fat, and this atrophy has caused an 'inverted champagne bottle appearance'. There is pigmentation above each ankle. There are no ulcers on the feet or toes.

Q.3 | What else are you going to look for before you complete your examination of her legs?

On general examination she is mildly obese and has a blood pressure of 160/110 mmHg. The rest of the cardiorespiratory and abdominal examination is unremarkable. Her left leg shows varicosities in the distribution of the long saphenous vein. The right leg is similarly affected with varicosities and changes of chronic venous insufficiency in the lower third of the calf. You note the skin around the ulcer is mildly inflamed and tender and you think the ulcer is infected. The peripheral pulses and neurological exam of the lower limbs are normal.

Q.4 | What is your diagnosis now? What, if any, investigations should be performed? What is your initial management?

Answers

A.1 You would like to know if there is a history of:

- Varicose veins or deep venous thrombosis.
- Previous surgery on this leg.
- Pain in the lesion.
- Problems with her legs suggestive of arterial insufficiency, e.g. claudication, rest pain.
- Diabetes mellitus.
- Rheumatoid arthritis or other vasculitic process.

You also want to know the patient's general state of health, and occasionally their place of origin (tropical ulcers). You would also want to know about other medical problems like cardiovascular disease, renal disease, what medication she takes (e.g. steroids) and use of tobacco and alcohol.

A.2 There is an extensive ulcerated area over and above the medial malleolus approximately 8 × 5 cm. There is slough on the ulcer but with considerable healthy granulation tissue. The surrounding skin is discoloured, scaly and indurated. There are areas of haemosiderin deposition. This appearance is characteristic of venous ulceration secondary to chronic venous congestion.

A.3 On examination you need to ensure that pulses are present in the limbs (i.e.

Answers *cont.*

palpable femoral, popliteal and at least one of the dorsalis pedis or posterior tibial pulses). It is also important to exclude neuropathy by performing a screening neurological examination of the lower limbs.

A.4 The diagnosis is a venous ulcer. In the presence of cellulitis, take a swab and start antibiotics to cover *Staphylococcus aureus*, streptococcus and Gram-negative bacilli including *E. coli* and *Klebsiella*.

A venous incompetence duplex scan is not essential in this setting but will confirm underlying incompetence of the deep veins (usually secondary to a previous DVT) in approximately 40–50% of cases, or of the superficial veins (long or short saphenous ± perforating veins) in a further 40–50% of cases. Some individuals may have incompetence of both deep and superficial venous systems.

Initial management is based on compression therapy. You may delay commencing this for a few days until the cellulitis has settled. Most frequently, a four-layered compression bandaging system is applied on a weekly basis until the ulcer is healed. Smaller ulcers can be managed with occlusive dressings and class III (30–40 mmHg) compression stockings. Most clinicians use knee-high rather than full-leg stockings because of higher patient compliance levels. Many clinicians use class II (20–30 mmHg) knee-high compression stockings in elderly patients as compliance is better with these stockings.

Once healed, compression is maintained using knee-high stockings to reduce recurrence. Patients with isolated venous incompetence of the superficial systems (e.g. long saphenous vein ± perforator incompetence, with normal deep veins) should be considered for surgery or endovenous ablation of incompetent superficial veins to reduce the risk of recurrent ulceration. Skin grafting is infrequently required in venous ulcers.

In this patient healing will take many weeks. Therefore, she will require visits from a nurse who is experienced in wound care and assistance in the activities of daily living.

Revision Points

Assessment of Leg and Foot Ulcers

Table 25.1 describes the assessment of these ulcers. Note:

- Vasculitic ulcers: exclude above causes, may need biopsy.
- Malignant ulcers: biopsy suspicious ulcers and those not responding as expected.
- Combination of above aetiologies common.

Revision Points *cont.*

Table 25.1 Assessment of leg and foot ulcers

	Venous	Arterial	Neuropathic
Location	Lower calf area	Pressure areas – toes, 1st–5th MTP joints, heel, malleoli	Pressure areas
Swelling	Yes	Not usually	No
Pain	Usually not (or not severe)	Yes – except if also neuropathic	No
History	Often history of DVT/ varicose veins likely	May have claudication	Diabetes, alcohol, spinal pathology
Associated features	Venous skin change/ lipodermatosclerosis		
Presence of pulses	Yes, but may be difficult to palpate	No	Yes
Investigations	Nil initially required Venous incompetence duplex scan	Ankle–brachial index (usually <0.7)	Exclude arterial contribution to ulceration
Management	Compression Fix isolated superficial incompetence in selected cases	Revascularize if necessary	Pressure relief/ podiatry/orthotics

Issues to Consider

- What advice can be given to diabetics with neuropathy to avoid lower limb ulceration?
- What is the cause of tropical ulceration?
- What are the features of the various dressings available to specialist teams to manage lower limb ulceration?
- Why do varicose veins form and what are the associated complications?
- Do varicose veins predispose to deep vein thrombosis?
- How can chronic venous insufficiency be treated surgically?

Further Information

London, N.J.M., Donnelly, R., 2000. ABC of arterial and venous disease: ulcerated lower limb. British Medical Journal 320, 1589–1591. www.bmj.com *A superb overview of the subject.*

www.thediabeticfoot.net *An interesting resource about diabetic foot care.*

A 41-year-old man involved in a car crash

Andrew W. Perry

A 41-year-old man is brought in by ambulance to the emergency department of a tertiary hospital with trauma facilities from the scene of a car crash. The paramedic crew provides a history. The patient was a restrained driver in a sedan vehicle that had a head-on collision with another car whose occupant was pronounced dead at the scene. The car was not fitted with either driver or curtain airbags. There was significant intrusion of the engine block into the driver's compartment and the patient was trapped for about 30 minutes before extraction, with full cervical spine immobilization, by the emergency services. The patient is uncertain about whether he lost consciousness or not, but ambulance officers report he seems a little confused with poor recollection of events and has an obvious contusion to his right temple. Ambulance officers also report the smell of alcohol on the patient's breath.

During the ambulance journey from the scene of the crash the patient complained of shortness of breath and pain in the left side of his chest. He has been cardiovascularly stable throughout. The patient has been given oxygen by mask, one large-bore intravenous access has been obtained and 500 mL of crystalloid has been infused.

Q.1 Describe your initial assessment (history and examination) of this patient? What elements of the history are particularly important?

Your examination reveals the following:

Airway (with cervical spine control): the patient's airway is patent, he is speaking to you and has no evidence of facial trauma or airway foreign body. His cervical spine is immobilized with a hard collar.

Breathing: he has a respiratory rate of 30 bpm and his pattern of breathing is shallow. He is not centrally cyanosed. Examination of his chest reveals superficial abrasions and contusion to his left anterior hemithorax and shoulder. There is no evidence of paradoxical chest movement or open wound. He is tender over the anterior aspects of the left 6th–9th ribs and crepitus is present. There is a paucity of breath sounds on the left side and the percussion note is increased on that side. His trachea is central. Pulse oximetry measurement reveals his oxygen saturation is 99% on 15 litres of O_2 by non-rebreather mask.

Circulation: he has a pulse rate of 130/min and a blood pressure of 105/85 mmHg. His jugular venous pressure is not elevated and he has a peripheral capillary return time of 3–4 seconds. He has no obvious external haemorrhage or major long bone fractures. The examination of his abdomen reveals bruising consistent with a seatbelt injury and generalized tenderness of both upper quadrants, maximally on the left, with marked guarding.

Disability: a rapid skeletal and neurological survey shows that the patient has no obvious deformity or tenderness of his limbs, has normal power in all limbs and has normal sensation and reflexes.

His Glasgow Coma Scale score (GCS) is 14/15, with his verbal score being confused (4/5). His pupils are equal and react normally to light. You also note the odour of alcohol. Breath alcohol analyser shows a breath alcohol level (BAL) of 0.210 g/dL. He has no neck pain or midline cervical tenderness.

Exposure/environmental control: the patient's temperature is 36.1°C. In order to facilitate examination and X-rays his shirt and trousers' are cut off. He complains that he is cold in the resuscitation room.

Q.2 Describe your approach to the management of this patient in light of the above findings. What are your priorities? What investigations would you request during the initial management?

A second wide-bore intravenous cannula is inserted into a peripheral vein and 1 L of a crystalloid solution administered rapidly. Blood samples are collected for cross-matching, complete blood picture and biochemistry. In addition forensic blood alcohol samples are obtained. The chest X-ray is shown in Figure 26.1.

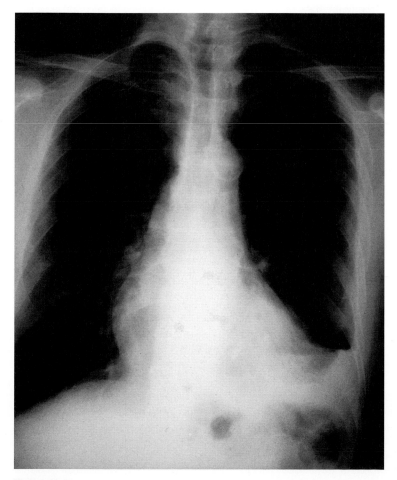

Figure 26.1

Q.3 Describe the abnormalities shown in this chest X-ray. In what ways may this condition be complicated?

The chest X-ray confirms your clinical suspicion of a haemopneumothorax. A chest drain is inserted successfully and connected to an underwater seal. Air and approximately 500 mL blood drain out. The patient confirms that his breathing is much improved.

A log roll and inspection of the patient's back is subsequently performed which is unremarkable. FAST scan done on arrival is equivocal.

The initial laboratory results are also unremarkable and his haemoglobin is 131 g/L.

One hour after admission and initial resuscitation you reassess the patient and note that although he has received a total of 2 L intravenous fluid and his pain is adequately controlled with parenteral opiates, his pulse has risen to 145/min and his blood pressure is 90/75 mmHg. His JVP is not visible. His airway and breathing are stable. Examination of his chest shows reasonable air entry to all areas, but there is still dullness at the left base. There is a further 100 mL fresh blood in the chest drainage bottle. His abdomen is markedly tender in the left upper quadrant.

Q.4 What is the probable cause of this change and what needs to be done now?

A further haemoglobin estimation is performed. It is now 102 g/L. He is rapidly transfused 2 units blood and a further 1 L crystalloid. His urine dipstick is negative for blood and a urinary catheter is inserted with hourly urine output monitored. His blood pressure stabilizes at 105/80 mmHg with a pulse of 120 bpm.

A CT scan of his head, cervical spine, chest, abdomen and pelvis is performed. A slice from the upper abdomen is shown in Figure 26.2.

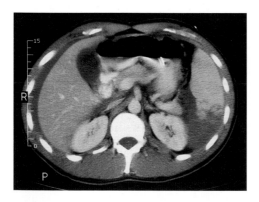

Figure 26.2

Q.5 What does the CT image show and how should this be managed?

The patient is transfused a further 2 units of blood. He remains stable, his tachycardia settles and so it is decided to trial treating his splenic injuries conservatively.

He is admitted to an intensive care unit where he is monitored closely and has an uneventful course. His chest drain is removed at day 5. His splenic injury is monitored with a further CT, which showed gradual reabsorption of the haematoma. He is discharged home 2 weeks after the accident and advised to avoid strenuous exertion for a further month.

Answers

A.1 This patient has been involved in a high-speed crash and is likely to be suffering from multiple traumatic injuries. In order to avoid overlooking significant injuries and to treat the most life-threatening conditions first it is wise to take a structured approach. Advanced Trauma Life Support® (also known as Early Management of Severe Trauma®) is one such system. This system relies on:

Airway (with cervical spine control).

Breathing and ventilation.

Circulation with haemorrhage control.

Disability (neurological evaluation).

Exposure/environmental control.

The mechanism of injury is especially important. You should establish the speed and type of vehicle and the mode of impact, i.e. direction and whether the car hit a mobile or immovable object. Also, the condition of the vehicle after the accident, the provision and use of safety features, the position of the patient, the ability to self-extricate or the time taken to release trapped victims are all important features and may give valuable information as to the likely nature and severity of injuries. Head injuries and alcohol intoxication may result in an altered mental state which may preclude the patient from being able to give a precise history or report pain, e.g. from a cervical vertebrae fracture.

A.2 As always in any resuscitation your priorities are **A**irway, **B**reathing and **C**irculation, with **D**isability and **E**xposure/environmental control of additional importance in trauma.

The assessment of this patient reveals no imminent problems with **A** and the cervical spine is being appropriately managed with hard collar immobilization. Further investigation of the cervical spine beginning with cross-table lateral X-ray should be arranged.

The assessment of **B** demonstrates problems that need to be addressed rapidly. The chest wall shows obvious signs of trauma with probable rib fractures of at least three ribs, the underlying lung is probably damaged and the increase in percussion note on the left side suggests a pneumothorax. The patient does not appear to be deteriorating rapidly, and the pneumothorax does not appear to be under tension. Therefore it is reasonable, in this case, to proceed to imaging of the chest to rule out diaphragmatic rupture and intrathoracic abdominal contents before proceeding to chest drain insertion. Whilst the X-ray is performed you ask for a chest drain set and underwater seal to be prepared and you proceed to assess C.

C: this is a relatively young patient who will have a good cardiovascular reserve. This means that even when bleeding and shocked, he can initially maintain his blood pressure and central perfusion. As he has a marked tachycardia and is diverting his blood from his peripheries (prolonging his capillary return), restoration of his circulating volume should be started immediately. Two large-bore peripheral cannulae should be adequate at this stage. After determining a baseline haemoglobin via a point-of-care haemoglobin analyser, blood samples should be sent for haematology, biochemistry and urgent six-unit cross-match. Coagulation studies may be of benefit if massive transfusion (the loss of one blood volume in 24 hours or 50% of blood volume in 3 hours) is thought likely. Many jurisdictions require all patients involved in motor vehicle accidents to have forensic blood alcohol samples taken. A large volume (1–3 L) of intravenous crystalloid (e.g. normal saline) should be

Answers *cont.*

infused over the first hour, titrated to physiologic response.

The history of injury to the left side of the torso must raise the possibility of damage to the rib cage and the abdominal wall, and the contents in the immediate vicinity. Any trauma of sufficient force to break ribs, particularly if associated with shock, may well have produced substantial internal injury.

Disability: a rapid skeletal and neurological survey shows that the patient has no obvious deformity or tenderness of his limbs and has normal sensation. Assessment of D may not show any immediate acute problems, but should be repeated later.

Exposure/environmental control: it is important to adequately and rapidly expose the patient so as to not miss injuries or other examination findings and to allow full access for investigations and interventions. This must be tempered with ensuring the patient is not allowed to become hypothermic so use of passive warming devices, e.g. blankets, or active warming, e.g. warm intravenous fluids, may need consideration.

Apart from X-rays of the chest and cervical spine, a pelvic X-ray should be performed, especially in view of his haemodynamic instability. An ECG should also be performed to look for evidence of cardiac contusion. Provided it can be arranged without compromising immediate patient care, a CT scan of the neck, chest and abdomen (including pelvis) will yield more information than plain radiology.

A.3 The X-ray shows collapse of the upper part of the left lung with air in the pleural space from the mid-zone to the apex. There is blunting and flattening of the left costophrenic angle, suggesting a

haemopneumothorax. There are fractures of the 6th–8th ribs.

In this situation the following potential complications must be remembered:

Tension Pneumothorax

With a rapidly developing pneumothorax a one-way valve may be created in the lung or chest wall and air enters the pleural cavity with each breath. This is known as a tension pneumothorax. These are dangerous because the accumulating air cannot only collapse the lung, but will push the mediastinum to the opposite side and increase intrathoracic pressure, preventing venous return and hence cardiac output. Features suggestive of a tension pneumothorax include rapidly worsening respiratory function, haemodynamic instability and hypotension, together with engorgement of neck vessels and tracheal deviation. A tension pneumothorax is an emergency and must be dealt with immediately, prior to any imaging. Needle thoracocentesis must be immediately performed whereby a large-bore cannula should be inserted in the 2nd intercostal space in the mid-clavicular line overlying the affected lung, prior to definitive insertion of a chest drain.

Haemothorax

Extensive damage to the intercostal vessels can lead to a rapidly enlarging haemothorax. With this condition the breath sounds on the affected side are diminished, and the percussion note is markedly dull, as is vocal resonance. A large-gauge chest drain should be inserted and the blood drained.

Flail Segment

Multiple ribs fractured in more than one place prevent that section of the chest moving normally. The affected section of

Answers *cont.*

the chest moves paradoxically and can limit normal ventilation. It is not this that causes hypoxia, but the associated severe contusion to the underlying lung. Contused pulmonary tissue is very sensitive to both under- and over-perfusion. Very careful fluid balance is needed in these cases. A short period of assisted ventilation (which may be non-invasive or invasive) may be required to optimize ventilation and perfusion of the affected lung.

A.4 Despite your initial resuscitation this patient has become hypotensive and this is likely to be due to hypovolaemia. While other causes of hypotension must be considered, in this setting the cause of the problem is almost certainly blood loss. The patient requires:

• Prompt resuscitation (with blood transfusion).
• A careful assessment made for the site of blood loss. This is likely to be either into the left chest, the abdominal cavity or both.

Apart from a further clinical examination, imaging studies must be considered. The two main imaging methods used in these circumstances are CT scan and ultrasound.

If available, ultrasound examination in the emergency department (FAST scan – focused assessment with sonography of trauma) by the emergency physician or trauma surgeon is useful in the unstable patient, and can be performed in the resuscitation cubicle. It is particularly useful for rapidly detecting free fluid (e.g.

haemorrhage) in the abdomen and has largely replaced the more invasive diagnostic peritoneal lavage.

A CT scan with intravenous contrast is the imaging investigation of choice, and will aid in defining internal injuries including splenic injury. A CT scan showing a contained splenic bleed with acceptable patient haemodynamics may allow non-operative management and spleen preservation. This might include splenic embolization. If the patient is significantly haemodynamically unstable moving the patient out of the emergency department or resuscitation area for an imaging investigation may be dangerous. In this case a diagnosis of ruptured internal organ may be made solely on clinical grounds and the patient moved straight to theatre from the emergency department.

When scanning this patient it is likely that he would receive a 'full body scan', i.e. a scan of his head to look for cerebral contusions or bleeds, of the cervical spine to clear his neck (see Issues to Consider), of the chest to look at the extent of chest injury, and of the abdomen and pelvis to assess for intra-abdominal injury.

A.5 This is a section through the upper abdomen. Free blood can be seen between the right lobe of the liver and the abdominal wall. There is a large haematoma within the spleen, particularly involving the lower pole. The laceration goes towards the splenic hilum and most of the splenic capsule appears to be intact.

Revision Points

Care of the Trauma Patient

Multiple and major trauma requires a structured and organized approach. A team approach is essential. Many of the steps discussed will happen simultaneously, but must be coordinated by one individual, usually the emergency medicine physician. Involvement of multiple specialties such as anaesthetists, surgeons and radiologists is frequently essential.

The first hour following major trauma is the most important. Rapid assessment, diagnosis and intervention during this period are essential for favourable outcome.

Many hospitals have dedicated trauma teams and some are designated trauma centres where this approach to trauma care is highly rehearsed and senior staff from all required specialties are on site. Outcomes in these hospitals are significantly better than in hospitals without them.

A structured approach such as that provided by EMST® or ATLS® is pivotal:
- **A**irway (with cervical spine control).
- **B**reathing and ventilation.
- **C**irculation with haemorrhage control.
- **D**isability (neurological evaluation).
- **E**xposure/environmental control.

Any change in the condition of the patient should make you go back to the beginning and start again.

Issues to Consider

- What are the indications for applying cervical immobilization? How do you clear a cervical spine as being free of bony injury? Does alcohol intoxication affect cervical spine management?
- What is the role of ultrasound in trauma? What other organs can be visualized using portable ultrasonographs?
- What are the indications for splenectomy in abdominal trauma and what measures need to be taken after an emergency splenectomy has been performed to protect the patient from future infection?
- Discuss the different forms of shock. How is haemorrhagic shock classified?

Further Information

Stiell, I.G., Clement, C., McKnight, R.D., et al., 2003. The Canadian C-spine rule vs the NEXUS low-risk criteria in patients with trauma. New England Journal of Medicine 349, 2510–2518.

Wahl, W.L., Ahrns, K.S., Chen, S., et al., 2004. Blunt splenic injury: operation versus angiographic embolization. Surgery 136 (4), 891–899.

www.trauma.org/ *An independent, non-profit organization providing global education, information and communication resources for professionals in trauma and critical care.*

Management of acute coronary syndrome

Matthew Pincus

A 67-year-old man presents to the emergency department with chest pain.

Q.1 What questions would you ask the patient about the pain?

The pain has been present for 2 hours, is a retrosternal 'heaviness' graded at 6 out of 10 and radiates to both arms. It began while the patient was sitting watching television. He has not made specific attempts to relieve the pain and does not think changes in posture or inspiration alter the intensity. The only accompanying symptom is mild dyspnoea but this is much less prominent than the pain. On questioning, the man says he experienced a similar discomfort while walking quickly uphill a week ago, but it had resolved after a few minutes of rest.

Q.2 What aspects of the past medical history are particularly important?

The patient has never been diagnosed with, or been investigated for, coronary artery disease.

He has a 20 pack-year smoking history and quit about 20 years ago. He also has hypertension. He has been tested for hypercholesterolaemia and diabetes and not been diagnosed with either of these conditions.

Current medication is perindopril 10 mg daily for hypertension.

Q.3 What components of the physical examination are particularly important?

The patient is mildly hypertensive at 150/90 mmHg in both arms, has a regular heart rate of 90/min, oxygen saturation of 96% on room air, two heart sounds with no murmur, gallop or rub, non-elevated JVP and a clear chest to auscultation.

Q.4 What is the likely diagnosis?

Q.5 What is the most important initial investigation and what would you look for in it?

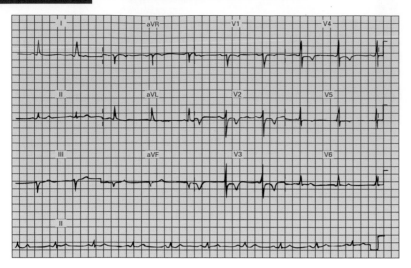

Figure 27.1

Q.6 What does the ECG show?

You interpret the ECG (Figure 27.1), and your consultant asks you your opinion.

Q.7 What can be said about the patient's diagnosis at this point?

Q.8 Could the patient be having a non-ST elevation myocardial infarction (NSTEMI)?

You have made your diagnosis, now you need to decide what to do about it.

Q.9 What treatment should the patient be given?

You institute urgent therapy, as per guidelines. Five minutes after administration of the GTN the chest pain has improved but not resolved, and he is given 10 mg IV morphine which results in complete resolution. He is admitted to the coronary care unit for continuous ECG monitoring.

Thirty minutes later the troponin-I comes back at 1.8 µg/L (normal range <0.04 µg/L).

Q.10 What implications does this have for the patient's diagnosis and management?

Q.11 Should the patient be given an intravenous glycoprotein IIb/IIIa inhibitor?

Q.12 Should the patient have a coronary angiogram? If so, how urgently?

The day after presentation the patient is taken to the cardiac catheterization laboratory where a coronary angiogram is performed (Figure 27.2). It shows a severe stenosis of the left anterior descending coronary artery and this is treated with percutaneous coronary intervention (PCI) with the use of a bare metal stent. A left ventriculogram is also performed and shows normal left ventricular systolic function. No heparin is required after a PCI, so the heparin infusion is stopped.

The day after the PCI (48 hours after admission), the patient is asymptomatic, has no abnormalities on cardiovascular examination and ECG monitoring has shown no arrhythmias.

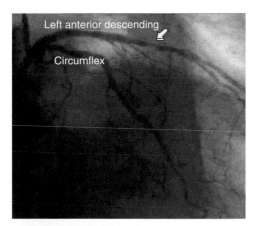

Left anterior descending

Circumflex

Figure 27.2

Q.13 When can the patient be discharged?

Q.14 What medications should the patient be discharged on?

Q.15 What other aspects of long-term management need to be addressed?

He is discharged the day after the PCI, with no complications. You see him in clinic after 6 weeks, and he is actively participating in the cardiac rehabilitation programme at your hospital. You advise him that he is doing well, and to continue his current medications.

Answers

A.1

- The duration of the pain.
- The severity and nature of the pain.
- The location of the pain and whether it radiates from the chest.
- What he was doing when the pain began.
- What, if any, attempts the patient has made to relieve the pain and whether they have been effective.

  Whether inspiration or changes in posture change the severity of the pain.

- Whether the pain is associated with other symptoms including dyspnoea, cough, haemoptysis, palpitations, gastrointestinal symptoms.
- Whether there is a recent history of chest pain related to exertion or emotional stress.

A.2

- Whether there has previously been a diagnosis of, or investigations for, coronary artery disease, and if so, whether there has been any coronary revascularization (coronary artery bypass graft surgery or percutaneous coronary intervention).
- Risk factors for coronary artery disease: smoking, hypercholesterolaemia, hypertension, diabetes, family history of premature coronary artery disease.
- What regular medications the patient is taking.

A.3

- Haemodynamic status (blood pressure and heart rate).
- On cardiac auscultation the presence of a gallop rhythm or murmur.
- Signs of congestive cardiac failure – gallop rhythm, elevated JVP, lung crackles.

- Findings suggesting a non-coronary cause of pain, for example aortic dissection, pericarditis, pulmonary disease.

A.4 An acute coronary syndrome (ACS).

This patient has symptoms which have been shown to be predictive of coronary artery disease (CAD), namely retrosternal location of pain, radiation to the arms, recent discomfort on physical exertion with relief from rest. He also has two well-established risk factors for CAD. Unlike some other causes of chest pain, CAD often has relapsing symptoms, so that patients presenting with chest pain will often have a history of investigation or treatment for CAD and this will often have included revascularization either surgically or percutaneously.

A.5 Current guidelines recommend that a patient presenting with symptoms that potentially represent an acute coronary syndrome should have an ECG within 10 minutes of presentation. The most important task on examining the ECG is to find or exclude ST segment elevation in a pattern consistent with an ST elevation myocardial infarction (STEMI) or find a new left bundle branch block (LBBB), because these patients are given a diagnosis of STEMI and require emergency reperfusion therapy (either thrombolysis or percutaneous coronary intervention). Crucially, *no other* investigation is required to make this diagnosis and institute reperfusion therapy.

Other investigations performed at presentation include a chest X-ray, cardiac biomarkers (troponin), electrolytes and creatinine, full blood count and blood glucose level.

Answers *cont.*

A.6 Sinus rhythm, normal axis and anterior T wave inversion.

A.7 The patient is having a non-ST elevation acute coronary syndrome (NSTEACS) (a syndrome being a collection of signs and symptoms).

All acute coronary syndromes can be put into one of two categories: (1) STEMI or (2) non-ST elevation ACS (NSTEACS). We have diagnosed this patient with an ACS and he does not have ST segment elevation, so we must diagnose a NSTEACS at this point.

A.8 It is certainly possible, but we cannot make that diagnosis until the cardiac biomarker result is available. A NSTEMI is diagnosed when a patient has symptoms consistent with an acute coronary syndrome *accompanied by* cardiac biomarkers above the upper limit of normal. No matter what abnormalities are present on the ECG, a NSTEMI cannot be diagnosed unless the cardiac biomarkers are elevated, and we do not know that yet.

A.9 The patient should be placed on electrocardiographic monitoring and given guideline-based treatment for a NSTEACS:

1. Chest pain relief:
   Sublingual glyceryl trinitrate (GTN), followed by intravenous morphine if the GTN does not result in resolution of the pain. The purpose of these agents is symptom relief. Neither has been shown to reduce death or myocardial infarction.
2. Oral antiplatelet agents:
   Oral aspirin 300 mg loading dose followed by 75–150 mg daily. Aspirin has been shown to improve survival in clinical trials in ACS.
   plus

Oral clopidogrel 300 mg loading dose followed by 75 mg daily. When added to aspirin, clopidogrel has been shown to reduce recurrent myocardial infarction in ACS.
3. Anticoagulation:
   Intravenous unfractionated heparin (UFH) has been shown to reduce the combined endpoint of death or MI. A loading dose and infusion should be used, targeted to an APTT 1.5–2.5 times the upper limit of normal. The anticoagulation should be continued for at least 48 hours or until coronary angiography.
   or
   Subcutaneous enoxaparin (a low molecular weight heparin). Clinical trials have shown this to be an acceptable alternative to UFH. Caution must be used in patients with renal impairment because of an increased risk of bleeding.
   or
   Alternative agents for anticoagulation are bivalirudin and fondaparinux.
4. Beta blockers:
   Oral metoprolol or atenolol. These agents reduce death and MI after an ACS, but should be avoided in patients who are in heart failure or haemodynamically unstable.

A.10 The biomarker elevation enables us to now diagnose a NSTEMI – i.e. a myocardial infarction.

Patients with a NSTEACS have a variable short-term risk of death or myocardial infarction depending on how many high-risk features are present. The best known of these features are cardiac biomarker elevation (troponin) and ischaemic ECG changes. But other variables have also been shown to be important for risk

Answers *cont.*

stratification including age, congestive cardiac failure, haemodynamic compromise, ventricular arrhythmias, previous known coronary disease and diabetes. Summation of high-risk features can be performed to produce a risk score, the TIMI and GRACE scores being the best known examples.

The elevated troponin level (*NSTEMI*) in our patient immediately puts him in a high-risk category. However, it is important to note from the risk variables mentioned in the previous paragraph that it is possible to be high risk without biomarker elevation.

A.11 Probably not at this point. Although trials have shown that these agents reduce myocardial infarction in high-risk NSTEACS patients, recent trials have shown no coronary benefit and an increased risk of bleeding from their routine use in these patients prior to coronary angiography. Their use can be left to the discretion of the interventional cardiologist at the time of angiography.

A.12 Yes. Patients with a high-risk NSTEACS benefit from early coronary angiography to guide coronary revascularization during their initial hospitalization. Guidelines recommend angiography be performed within 48–72 hours in high-risk patients if they remain pain free and haemodynamically stable. The revascularization can be performed by percutaneous coronary intervention (PCI) or by coronary artery bypass grafting (CABG), depending on the distribution of coronary disease. Generally, the more widespread the coronary disease, the more suitable the patient is for CABG rather than PCI.

A.13 The day after the PCI in the absence of a complication. Patients with a NSTEACS treated with PCI are at low risk

of developing recurrent ischaemia or life-threatening arrhythmias more than 24 hours after the onset of chest pain. They are generally monitored electrocardiographically for a total of 48 hours and are able to be discharged 24 hours after the PCI provided they are stable and the PCI was performed without complication.

A.14 Discharge medications include the following combination:

- Aspirin 75–150 mg daily indefinitely.
- Clopidogrel 75 mg daily for 12 months.
- A beta blocker.
- A statin. This drug class has been shown to reduce recurrent ischaemia after ACS and should be used irrespective of the lipid levels.
- The preadmission ACE inhibitor should be continued. Whether an ACE inhibitor should be routinely started after NSTEACS in a patient who does not have hypertension or left ventricular systolic dysfunction is more controversial.
- Sublingual GTN for chest pain.

A.15 Treatment of the hypertension should continue with a target blood pressure of <130/80 mmHg, as is recommended for patients with established coronary disease.

The patient should be advised to call an ambulance if he has chest pain that has not resolved 10 minutes after GTN.

He should attend a cardiac rehabilitation service for advice on physical activity, nutrition, exercise and alcohol consumption. Trial evidence supports this recommendation.

He should consume about 1000 mg of omega-3 polyunsaturated fatty acids per day, through a combination of oily fish and

Answers *cont.*

fish oil capsules or liquid. Trial evidence supports this recommendation.

You should advise him about the legality of driving, and consult your local guidelines.

This is important, and often overlooked. Providing him with a copy of the driving guidelines may be helpful.

Revision Points

- Acute coronary syndromes can be divided into ST elevation myocardial infarctions (STEMI) and non-ST elevation acute coronary syndromes (NSTEACS).
- In a patient with a presentation consistent with an acute coronary syndrome, an ECG is the only investigation required to diagnose a STEMI.
- The major distinction between the management of patients with STEMI and those with a NSTEACS is that STEMI patients should be treated with emergency reperfusion therapy with either thrombolysis or emergency percutaneous coronary intervention (PCI).
- The management of patients with a NSTEACS is dependent on an assessment of their short-term risk of death or myocardial infarction.
- The most well known high-risk features in NSTEACS are an elevated cardiac

biomarker (most commonly troponin) and ischaemic ECG changes. It is necessary for a biomarker to be elevated to diagnose a non-ST elevation myocardial infarction (NSTEMI). However, it is possible to have a high-risk NSTEACS without biomarker elevation.
- Patients with a high-risk NSTEACS benefit from the routine administration of aspirin, clopidogrel, anticoagulation, beta blockade, a statin and coronary angiography with revascularization as appropriate (CABG or PCI). A glycoprotein IIb/IIIa inhibitor may also be beneficial in the highest risk cases.
- After a NSTEACS, there are pharmacological and non-pharmacological aspects to reducing the likelihood of further cardiovascular events and death.

Issues to Consider

- How do you use the TIMI risk score in NSTEMI?
- What are the complications of NSTEMI, and of the medications used to treat it (aspirin, thienopyridines, IIb/IIIa inhibitors)?

Further Information

http://circ.ahajournals.org/cgi/reprint/ CIRCULATIONAHA.107.185752 *ACC/AHA NSTEACS guidelines.*

http://www.escardio.org/guidelines-surveys/ esc-guidelines/GuidelinesDocuments/ guidelines-NSTE-ACS-FT.pdf *European Society of Cardiology NSTEACS guidelines.*

http://content.nejm.org/cgi/content/ full/360/21/2237 *Very short review of NSTEACS management.*

Breathlessness in a young woman

David Platts

A 28-year-old woman presented to the emergency department following and 3-day history of a dry cough, ankle swelling and progressively worsening shortness of breath. At presentation, the patient was severely breathless at rest. She had had an acute viral-like upper respiratory tract infection 6 weeks earlier.

On examination, she looks unwell and is in respiratory distress. Her heart rate was 110 bpm in sinus tachycardia, blood pressure 100/60 mmHg, respiratory rate 24 and oxygen saturations 92%. The jugular venous pressure was elevated at 8 cm. Praecordial examination revealed a displaced, volume loaded apex beat, a soft S1, normal S2 and an S3 with a 3/6 pansystolic murmur. Respiratory examination revealed reduced breath sounds in the left base with fine inspiratory crackles to the mid zones. There was mild pitting oedema in the ankles. You think she has acute heart failure.

Q.1   What further questions should be asked to help obtain a diagnosis?

There is no other medical or surgical past history. The patient is a non-smoker and non-drinker. She has not been pregnant recently. There is no family history of cardiac problems. She was not taking any medications. For the last 2 nights, the patient has been unable to sleep due to respiratory distress whenever she lay flat. The patient has also been nauseous and anorexic for 24 hours. There have been no palpitations or episodes of presyncope or syncope.

Q.2   What other examination findings are important?

The patient was not peripherally or centrally cyanotic. The peripheries were cool to touch. There was no fever. Abdominal examination was unremarkable other than mild hepatic tenderness. There was no clinical evidence of anaemia. The peripheral pulses were palpable and mildly reduced in intensity.

Q.3   What investigations would you initially order to help assess this patient?

The full blood count is normal. U&Es show a Na$^+$ of 131, K$^+$ of 3.8, creatinine of 97 and urea of 5. Liver function tests reveal a total protein=55, albumin=23, ALP=235, GGT=187, ALT=23, bilirubin=12. INR=1.3. BNP=2187. Cardiac enzymes are normal.

A 12-lead ECG showed a sinus tachycardia, normal axis, normal intervals and no ST-T wave changes.

The chest X-ray showed an increased cardiothoracic ratio, a small left pleural effusion and interstitial and alveolar oedema.

Q.4 What is the likely diagnosis?

Q.5 What is the next investigation that should be ordered?

A transthoracic echocardiogram was performed at the bedside in the emergency department, which showed a dilated and severely globally impaired left ventricle with a left ventricular ejection fraction (LVEF) of 20%. The right ventricle was also dilated and severely impaired. There was moderate mitral regurgitation, moderate tricuspid regurgitation and no pulmonary hypertension.

Q.6 What is the initial management of this patient in the emergency department?

This patient had acute cardiogenic pulmonary oedema due to a recent onset of a viral dilated cardiomyopathy. As the patient was hypoxic, she should be given oxygen and be sitting upright. A bolus dose of 40 mg of intravenous furosemide was given, followed by an infusion of glyceryl trinitrate (GTN).

Q.7 What further treatment should be commenced when the patient is more stable on the ward?

The patient's breathlessness improved and she was transferred to the coronary care unit on telemetry. She was commenced on an ACE inhibitor (tritace 2.5 mg bd), regular oral furosemide (40 mg daily) and a heart failure beta blocker (carvedilol, initially starting at 3.125 mg bd). Over the next 5 days, the patient's condition stabilized. Contact was made with the hospital multidisciplinary heart failure team (consisting of a heart failure cardiologist, heart failure nurse, pharmacist and physiotherapist) and they coordinated the patient's ongoing inpatient and outpatient care, in consultation with the patient's usual general practitioner. The patient was discharged on day 7 on ramipril 5 mg bd, carvedilol 6.25 mg bd, and furosemide 40 mg daily.

Q.8 What sort of follow-up should be arranged after discharge?

The patient had close follow-up through the heart failure outpatient service, which included outpatient visits to the heart failure cardiologist and heart failure nurse, telephone contact and monitoring by her general practitioner. A follow-up CXR showed cardiomegaly, no pleural effusions and clear lung fields. A repeat transthoracic echocardiogram at 3 months showed a moderately dilated left ventricle, a LVEF of 25%, mildly impaired right ventricular function and mild tricuspid regurgitation and mild mitral regurgitation only.

Q.9 What options are available if the patient severely deteriorates?

The patient re-presented to the emergency department 6 months later with severe acute cardiogenic shock, with a heart rate of 130 and a blood pressure of 70/40 mmHg. This did not respond to conventional therapy and after extensive consultation with the cardiac transplant team, the intensive care unit and cardiothoracic surgery, a left ventricular assist device was inserted. This was used as a bridge to transplantation and the patient underwent a successful heart transplantation 4 months later. The patient was discharged 2 weeks after her transplant, with no episodes of rejection, and is now back at work.

Answers

A.1

- The history of a recent viral illness should alert to the possibility of a viral respiratory infection, a postviral pneumonia or even a virally induced cardiomyopathy.
- A history of recent pregnancy or childbirth is also important due to the possibility of this being a peripartum cardiomyopathy. It is important that family history is obtained as some cardiomyopathies are familial in aetiology.
- Conventional medical history-taking will also provide clues as to other possible causes (such as diabetes, haemochromatosis, hypertension, thyroid disorders, drugs or medications, alcohol or rheumatic heart disease).
- The history of being unable to lie flat due to breathlessness (orthopnoea) or waking up during the night breathless (paroxysmal nocturnal dyspnoea) is a very important feature as this is usually due to heart failure.
- The nausea and anorexia may be due to several causes but in this case, liver congestion due to congestive heart failure is the likely cause. It is important to ask whether there have been any palpitations or dizzy turns as these may indicate the presence of an associated arrhythmia (such as ventricular tachycardia or atrial fibrillation).

A.2 When examining an acutely unwell patient, both the severity of the cardiac dysfunction and the end organ consequences of reduced perfusion must be assessed. Starting at the peripheries: is there evidence of reduced perfusion (cool or warm peripheries) or cyanosis (although cyanosis is usually a manifestation of severe cardiorespiratory failure)? Are the peripheral pulses palpable? What is the cardiac rhythm (is there a sinus tachycardia, atrial fibrillation or a relative bradycardic state)? What is the blood pressure (this may be so low that it is not detectable unless via invasive means)? Is the jugular venous pressure (JVP) elevated? Palpation of the praecordium may reveal an altered apex beat (is it displaced, indicating a dilated heart)? Listen carefully to each component of the heart sounds in turn; it may help to say to yourself 'I am listening to S1, to

Answers *cont.*

systole, to S2, to diastole, to any added sounds'. Ask yourself about the intensity of the heart sounds (is there a soft S1, which occurs in severe mitral regurgitation?). Are there any added heart sounds (either an S3/S4 or gallop rhythm)? Are there any murmurs (such as mitral regurgitation, aortic regurgitation, aortic stenosis or a ventricular septal defect)? Listening to the chest, is there evidence of pulmonary oedema or a pleural effusion? In severe cases of pulmonary oedema, there may be just severely reduced breath sounds or a wheeze.

It may not be possible to lay the patient flat in severe pulmonary oedema to examine the abdomen adequately. In congestive heart failure there may be evidence of tender hepatomegaly (due to congestion) or a pulsatile liver (due to severe functional tricuspid regurgitation). There may be evidence of ascites if there is significant right heart involvement. There may also be peripheral oedema.

Reduced perfusion from cardiac dysfunction can have significant consequences on other organ systems. The patient may be agitated or delirious due to reduced cerebral perfusion. The respiratory distress associated with pulmonary oedema can result in respiratory fatigue and exhaustion which may require management with mechanical ventilation. Reduced perfusion of the kidneys can result in pre-renal failure and a reduced urine output. Liver dysfunction can also occur from prolonged hypotension (although this is difficult to detect clinically).

A.3 The investigations required for heart failure are important because they will help establish a diagnosis, determine the severity of the illness, point toward an aetiology,

find precipitating or exacerbating factors and help in guiding therapy.

The initial investigations in the emergency department should be an ECG, CXR and blood tests (full blood count, urea, creatinine and electrolytes, liver function tests, thyroid function tests and BNP). Investigations performed later include those that aim to determine the aetiology of the heart failure, and those that help establish severity and prognosis. These tests include assessing for coronary artery disease (such as a nuclear perfusion scan, stress echocardiogram, cardiac MRI, coronary CT angiogram, or invasive coronary angiogram), haemodynamic assessment with a right heart catheter, 6-minute walk test, cardiopulmonary exercise test, myocardial viability assessment and a cardiomyopathy blood screen (such as iron studies for haemachromatosis, autoantibody screen for disorder such as lupus, serum and urine electrophoresis for amyloidosis, and a viral screen).

A.4 By integrating the history, examination findings and initial investigations, the likely diagnosis is heart failure due to a dilated cardiomyopathy. This may have been caused or precipitated by a recent viral infection. It is important to recognize that heart failure is a *syndrome* and not a diagnosis. There is a three-stage process to assessing this patient. Firstly, establish the presence of a heart failure syndrome has been determined. Secondly, determine the type of cardiac dysfunction that is causing the heart failure. The third step is to determine the underlying aetiology of the cardiac dysfunction.

Not all heart failure is due to left ventricular systolic dysfunction (although this is the most common cause). Other important causes include diastolic heart

Answers *cont.*

failure (or heart failure with normal ejection fraction: HFNEF), right heart failure (without left heart involvement) or non-myocardial heart failure (such as pericardial disease, valvular disorders or a cardiac mass/tumour).

Once the cardiac mechanism has been identified, the cause of this dysfunction has to be determined. In this case, the heart failure due to a dilated cardiomyopathy is most likely due to the preceding viral illness. A viral aetiology is a common cause of a dilated cardiomyopathy and common aetiological agents include Coxsackie virus, enterovirus and adenovirus.

The other common causes of heart failure in Western countries are coronary artery disease, hypertension, valvular heart disease (such as untreated aortic stenosis or mitral regurgitation), toxicity from alcohol or chemotherapy, and other disorders affecting the myocardium – such as viral infections, infiltration (sarcoid and amyloid), metabolic abnormalities (such as thyroid dysfunction or haemochromatosis) or genetic disorders such as hypertrophic cardiomyopathy.

A.5 The next investigation that should be ordered is a transthoracic echocardiogram. This is a fundamentally important investigation in heart failure and should be performed in all patients that are suspected of having heart failure. It provides an accurate, safe, non-invasive, time-efficient evaluation of cardiac structure and function, valvular function, and assessment of cardiac haemodynamics and presence of pulmonary hypertension or intra-cardiac thrombus.

A.6 Acute pulmonary oedema is a medical emergency. The initial management requires oxygen, diuretics and a nitrate vasodilator. The oxygen is to correct the hypoxia and may be given via a face mask, or in more severe cases, positive pressure ventilation. Mechanical ventilation may be required for those in significant respiratory distress. Intravenous loop diuretics (such as furosemide) are required to increase sodium and water excretion (and furosemide also has an immediate venodilator effect). This may be given as either a bolus (such as 40–80 mg) or an infusion (starting as 5 mg/hour). Nitrates are also important as they are predominantly a venodilator and have very rapid onset of action. They are particularly useful in heart failure due to myocardial ischaemia as they also dilate the coronary arteries. The nitrate is usually given as a continuous intravenous infusion. If IV access cannot be immediately obtained, the nitrate can be given as a topical patch as a temporary measure.

If these measures do not result in improvement of the patient's condition, other options need to be considered. These include non-invasive assisted ventilation, intubation and ventilation, inotropic therapy and finally mechanical support (such as an intra-aortic balloon pump or ventricular assist device).

A.7 Once the patient is more stable on the ward, the treatment for heart failure is both increased and broadened. Treatment centres around ACE inhibition and beta blockade. All patients with LV systolic dysfunction (irrespective of functional class) should be commenced on an ACE inhibitor, with the dose up-titrated to maximal dose or that which is tolerated. ACE inhibitors have been shown to improve survival, improve symptom class, reduce hospitalizations and increase left ventricular ejection fraction.

Answers *cont.*

Beta blockers are also fundamental in the management of chronic heart failure. They help to inhibit the chronic activation of sympathetic nervous system (which in the long term is toxic to the myocardium). Beta blockers have also been shown to improve survival (both by reducing sudden arrhythmic cardiac death, and by reducing progressive heart failure). Beta blockers also improve symptom class and left ventricular ejection fraction. Beta blockers should not be commenced until the patient has recovered from the acute pulmonary oedema and are generally better tolerated when the patient is euvolaemic. To reduce the likelihood of beta blocker side-effects (such as hypotension, fatigue, worsening heart failure), they should be started at a low dose and gradually increased.

Diuretics in the chronic situation may be required to maintain euvolaemia and control symptoms. However, they do not confer a survival benefit in isolation. Additional pharmacological therapy that may be required, depending upon response and severity of heart failure, includes aldosterone antagonists (spironolactone and eplerenone), digoxin, angiotensin 2 receptor blockers, nitrates and hydralazine. Some patients may also require long-term anticoagulation, usually with warfarin.

A.8 When the patient is discharged, it is important that they are linked into a heart failure programme and closely monitored in conjunction with their general practitioner. Heart failure management is a dynamic process with alterations in treatment and dosing a common occurrence. Further up-titration of heart failure medications is continued in an outpatient setting. Patient education is important. This includes fluid intake control, daily weighing, exercise programmes and good lines of communication with their GP and heart failure programme.

Patient compliance with prescribed therapy is important and poor compliance is a common cause for re-presentation with worsening heart failure. Other precipitants for heart failure include arrhythmias, infection, myocardial ischaemia, anaemia, alcohol excess, thyroid disorders, pregnancy, medications (such as steroids or NSAIDs) and pulmonary embolism.

A.9 If the patient does not respond to conventional medical therapy, there are other important options to consider. These include device therapy and surgical treatment. In some patients who do not respond to appropriate medical therapy, biventricular pacing (cardiac resynchronization therapy – CRT) may be of benefit. In this form of pacing, both ventricles are paced to try and induce mechanical synchrony between the two ventricles. The right heart is paced via a right ventricular lead and the left heart is paced via a lead passing through the coronary sinus and into a cardiac vein, usually on the lateral aspect of the left ventricle. In this way, the left ventricle can be paced via access from the venous system. Some patients, whose LVEF remains below 35%, may also be candidates for insertion of an implantable cardiac defibrillator (ICD).

Surgical options are also important to consider in the refractory heart failure patient. Ventricular assist devices (VADs) are small mechanical pumps that provide circulatory support and can be either implanted within the thoracic cavity or abdomen, or be extra-corporeal and sit outside the chest or abdominal wall. There are various types of pumps available which

Answers *cont.*

can provide either pulsatile or continuous rotary blood flow support.

In the more chronic setting, cardiac surgery may be needed to correct the cause of the heart failure. Common examples include surgical revascularization for heart failure due to coronary artery disease, or an aortic valve replacement for severe aortic stenosis or severe aortic regurgitation.

The final management option is cardiac transplantation. There are strict criteria as to who is eligible for heart transplantation and this form of therapy is only offered to a select group of patients who have undergone an extensive screening process and for whom no other form of therapy is available. This is due to a shortage of donor organs and the complexity of the procedure and resources required to maintain a cardiac transplant programme. Following cardiac transplantation, 1-year survival is approximately 85% and 5-year survival 65%. Early complications include acute cellular rejection and infection, while more long-term complications include coronary artery vasculopathy (CAV – a form of chronic rejection), malignancy, hypertension and renal dysfunction. However, this therapy is both a lifesaver and provides the opportunity to have an excellent quality of life, neither of which would occur in the non-transplanted state.

Revision Points

Heart failure is one of the commonest reasons for admission to hospital and is likely to increase with the ageing population.

Heart failure is not a diagnosis, but a syndrome; therefore a specific cause has to be found in each case. In Western communities, the two common causes are coronary artery disease and hypertension. However, there is an extensive list of alternative aetiologies.

Treatment options for heart failure include the following:
- Non-pharmacological (such as fluid intake control, exercise programmes and other lifestyle modifications).
- Pharmacological (such as ACE inhibitors and beta blockers).
- Devices (such a biventricular pacemakers and implantable defibrillators).
- Surgical therapy (such as coronary artery bypass surgery, mechanical support and cardiac transplantation).

Issues to Consider

- What are the most common causes of heart failure in your country?
- What services are available for heart failure patients at your institution? Where is your nearest advanced heart failure/transplant unit?
- Is echocardiography or cardiac MRI available in your institution? Ask to watch a study being performed and reported.

- What is the average survival after cardiac transplantation?

Further Information

Heart Foundation of Australia and the Cardiac Society of Australia and New Zealand, 2006. Guidelines for the prevention, detection and management of chronic heart failure in Australia, 2006. http://www.heartfoundation.org.au/

Professional_Information/Clinical_Practice/CHF/Pages/default.aspx.

Hunt, S.A., Abraham, W.T., Chin, M.H., et al., 2009. 2009 Focused update incorporated into the ACC/AHA 2005 Guidelines for the diagnosis and management of heart failure in adults. Journal of the American College of Cardiology 53, e1–e90. http://content.onlinejacc.org/cgi/content/full/j.jacc.2008.11.009.

Task Force for Diagnosis and Treatment of Acute and Chronic Heart Failure 2008 of European Society of Cardiology, Dickstein, K., Cohen-Solal, A., Filippatos, G., et al., 2008. Guidelines for the diagnosis and treatment of acute and chronic heart failure. European Heart Journal 29, 2388–2442. http://www.escardio.org/guidelines-surveys/esc-guidelines/Pages/acute-chronic-heart-failure.aspx.

A 25-year-old woman with chest pain and breathlessness

Fiona Kermeen

You are currently working in the emergency department on an evening shift. A 25-year-old woman has come to you for urgent assessment tonight with difficulty breathing and right-sided chest pain. The pain began suddenly 1 week ago. She describes it as sharp and worse on breathing in. It is now constant and has increased in severity. She has also become progressively more breathless on exertion over the last few days and is now unable to perform activities such as showering without feeling 'out of puff'.

You ask her more history – she has not had a fever, cough or wheeze and she has never previously suffered any respiratory complaints. The woman has polycystic ovarian syndrome and has been using the oral contraceptive pill to help regulate her menses in the last couple of years. Her health has otherwise been good. She is an active smoker, averaging 10 cigarettes per day for the last 7 years.

You examine her – she is obese with a weight of 110 kg. She is sweaty and looking unwell. She is taking short shallow breaths and her respiratory rate is 30 breaths/minute. Her temperature is 37.5°C, her pulse is 120 beats/minute and feels regular. Her blood pressure is 125/60 mmHg with oximetry showing oxygen saturation on room air of 88%. Her jugular venous pressure is visualised at 5 cm. Both heart sounds are present with no murmurs or pericardial rub audible. There are reduced breath sounds at both lung bases. No crackles, wheeze or pleural rub are heard. You note that there is tenderness behind her left calf but no associated leg swelling. Her admission CXR is reported as having mild basal atelectasis, but as being otherwise normal.

> **Q.1** What are the most likely diagnoses? What further history would help?

On further questioning, the patient reports having had left calf pain for 1 month but she thought it was a 'cramp'. She has had no episodes of haemoptysis or syncope. She has not had recent surgery. There is no known family history of heart or lung problems. She is compliant with her oral contraceptive pill and she is not pregnant. She has not embarked on any recent long distance travel. She has had a recent papsmear which was negative for malignancy.

> **Q.2** What further investigations are you going to organize now?

Complete blood picture and baseline electrolytes are normal.

Investigation 29.1 Arterial blood gas analysis			
pO_2	65 mmHg	pCO_2	28 mmHg
pH	7.48	Calculated bicarbonate	29 mmol/L
O_2 saturation (calc.)	90%		

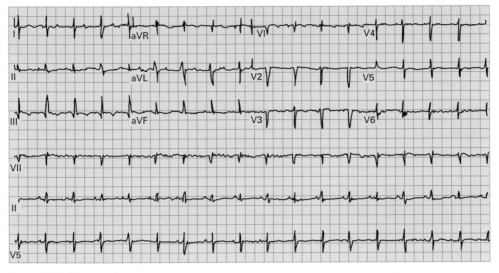

Figure 29.1 Electrocardiograph.

Q.3 What do the above investigations show?

An imaging study is undertaken and two images from the sequence are shown (Figure 29.2). Her left Doppler showed an extensive clot into proximal femoral veins.

Figure 29.2

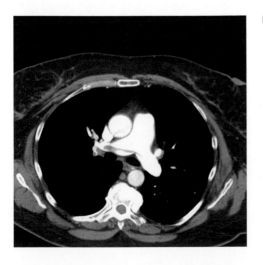

What do these images show? What clinical signs may reflect the underlying severity of the condition?

The nurse asks you to review the patient again because she is concerned that her BP is now 85/60 mmHg. Her pulse has increased to 128 beats/min with no central or peripheral cyanosis. She appears distressed and her oxygen saturations are 90% on 2 L/min O_2 with use of nasal prong. In addition to her raised JVP, you palpate a left parasternal heave. A third heart sound is now heard (gallop rhythm). You order an urgent bedside echocardiogram and the sonographer tells you the right ventricle is moderately dilated with moderate RV dysfunction and RVSP of 40 mmHg.

Q.5 What actions do you take now?

Intravenous unfractionated heparin loading dose is given calculated to your institution's weight-based protocol. O_2 is increased to 10 L with non-rebreather mask. The patient is taken to ICU. Thrombolysis is given with alteplase. Within 4 hours the patient is normotensive, pulse rate 82 and O_2 requirements have reduced and her JVP is not visible. The next day the patient is transferred to your ward with IV heparin running.

Q.6 How do you manage her ongoing anticoagulation?

Oral warfarin is commenced early, while on IV heparin. Once her INR has been within the therapeutic range for 2 days, the IV heparin is ceased. An echocardiogram is repeated and shows normalization of right ventricular size and function. Prior to discharge, her thrombophilic screen of tests is reported as showing no abnormalities.

Advice is provided about her condition and taking warfarin tablets. The hospital's outpatient warfarin clinic is going to monitor her INR, and an alert bracelet is arranged for her to wear oral contraceptive pill is ceased and referal to gynaecologist regarding progestrone only contraception.

Q.7 What advice would you give her before discharge?

The woman returns to see you in the outpatient clinic after 3 months. She has been well and no longer experiences chest pain or breathlessness on exertion. Her INR has been well maintained within the therapeutic range. She has quit smoking.

Q.8 How long should she be on warfarin, and are any tests required before stopping it?

Answers

A.1 This young lady has pleuritic chest pain, dyspnoea and hypoxia (based on pulse oximetry) unexplained by her chest X-ray.

- Pulmonary embolism (PE) is the most likely and important diagnosis to consider as it carries a significant mortality risk when untreated:
  - her risk factors for PE are: obesity, smoking and use of the oral contraceptive pill
  - the left calf tenderness on examination raises the possibility of deep vein thrombosis (DVT) which is found in 70% of patients with confirmed PE.
- Spontaneous pneumothorax has been excluded in this case with the chest X-ray.
- Inflammatory pleurisy from pneumonia is less likely because more infective symptoms would be expected a week after onset (sputum production and constitutional symptoms) along with definite features of consolidation on chest X-ray and/or on clinical examination (bronchial breath sounds).
- Pericarditis is another condition that sometimes mimics pleurisy but does not usually cause hypoxia, unless associated with acutely decompensated heart failure.

Further specific questions should be asked to determine her pre-test probability of DVT/PE:

- Recently abdominal/pelvic/orthopaedic surgery?
- Major trauma or lower limb fractures requiring casts?
- Pregnant or recently given birth?
- History of DVT or PE?
- History or family history of thrombophilia?
- Prolonged immobility such as long-haul air travel?
- History of any malignancy, (especially breast cancer in this case)?

A.2 The following investigations must be undertaken:

- Arterial blood gas analysis (to determine degree of hypoxia).
- ECG (looking for right-heart strain pattern).
- Complete blood picture (anaemia, leucocytosis).
- Biochemistry (baseline electrolytes).
- Specific imaging. The standard imaging studies used for the detection and assessment of PE are:
  - Isotope ventilation–perfusion scan ('V/Q scan'). The ventilation component of the scan is obtained when the patient breathes a radioactive gas (e.g. Xenon 133) and the perfusion scan obtained by injecting the patient with a gamma-emitting radionuclide (e.g. technetium-99m). A pulmonary embolus is detected through the identification of a 'mismatch' between ventilation (normal) and perfusion (reduced). This is the better investigation for detection of small peripheral embolic lesions. There are no concerns about contrast allergies, but it is of limited value in the presence of other forms of lung disease which can include atelectasis, pneumonia, COPD or pleural effusions.
  - CT-pulmonary angiography (CTPA). This is the better tool if there is co-existent lung disease. These high-definition scans are capable of detecting small pieces of blood clot in the major pulmonary vessels. Some patients may be allergic to the contrast and there can be concerns about the contrast load in patients with renal impairment, particularly the elderly.
  - Venous leg Doppler ultrasound (to exclude extensive venous thrombosis, which may require IVC filter).

Answers *cont.*

A D-dimer blood test is *not* appropriate in this case as it is only useful in excluding a diagnosis of PE when there is a low pre-test clinical probability. This lady has known risk factors for and a clinical picture consistent with PE; therefore, specific imaging should be performed. A CTPA should be chosen in this setting because there is atelectasis on her chest X-ray which makes a V/Q scan difficult to interpret.

A.3   The arterial blood gases show the following:

- Hypoxia (low oxygen tension).
- Hypocapnia (low carbon dioxide tension).
- Respiratory alkalosis.
- Calculated A-a gradient of 55.

This is type 1 respiratory failure, and suggests an acute event, causing hypoxia. The patient then hyperventilates to compensate, and releases carbon dioxide leading to hypocapnia and an alkalosis. A similar pattern may be seen in acute asthma, pneumothorax and pulmonary oedema.

This ECG shows the classically quoted changes seen with PE of S-wave in lead I with a Q-wave and T-wave inversion in lead III (S1Q3T3). However, this is a rare occurrence and the most common abnormality seen is sinus tachycardia. More extensive emboli often result in new-onset atrial fibrillation.

A.4   This high-definition image confirms the diagnosis of PE showing clot at the bifurcation of the pulmonary artery into its right and left main branches (saddle PE).

The signs of PE will generally depend on the size of the embolus and underlying co-morbidities. Large, haemodynamically significant PE, as in this case, can be associated with:

- Tachycardia.
- Raised JVP.
- Left parasternal heave (consistent with right ventricular enlargement).
- Gallop rhythm (consistent with right ventricular third heart sound).
- Leg and sacral oedema (consistent with right heart failure).
- Cardiogenic shock with systemic hypotension.
- Cyanosis.
- Sudden cardiac arrest into pulseless electrical activity (PEA).

A.5   This patient requires emergency resuscitation. You need to increase the oxygen requirements, anticoagulate the patient with IV heparin and call for help from senior colleagues. Blood should be sent for thrombophilic screen to detect underlying abnormalities of coagulation prior to commencing heparin. These include:

Testing for Prothrombotic Disorders

- Factor V Leiden (activated protein C resistance).
- Protein C and S levels.
- Prothrombin gene mutation (20210A).
- Autoantibodies (ANA, ENA, anticardiolipin/ lupus inhibitor).
- Homocystein MTHFR mutation.
- Plasminogen level.
- Fibrinogen levels.
- Factor XII (for deficiency).
- Factor VIII (for level >150%).
- CRP.

Immediate anticoagulation is the usual treatment for PE. In this case, unfractionated IV heparin should be given to achieve rapid anticoagulation.

Thrombolyis is indicated for life threatening PE when associated with one or more of the following features:

Answers *cont.*

- Cardiogenic shock with systemic hypotension (<90 mmHg systolic or drop >40 mmHg from usual value).
- Circulatory collapse (including syncope or need for cardiopulmonary resuscitation).
- Echocardiographic findings indicating significant right ventricular systolic dysfunction.
- Severe, unresponsive hypoxia.

Thrombolysis should be performed in consultation with a major centre experienced in PE management.

This young woman is in impending cardiogenic shock (as defined above). Provided there are no contraindications, IV thrombolysis should be given and the patient should be transferred to HDU/ICU. Rarer treatment options that are only available in highly specialized centres include surgical embolectomy (where the clot is surgically removed) and catheter fragmentation (where the clot is broken up into smaller pieces with a special device) in patients with contraindications to thrombolysis.

Contraindications to Thrombolysis
Absolute
- Recent major trauma, major operation or non-compressible.
- Vascular puncture (within 10 days).
- Recent stroke (within 2 months) or any history of haemorrhagic stroke.
- Active internal bleeding.
- Significant bleeding diathesis.

Relative
- Prolonged cardiopulmonary resuscitation.
- Pregnancy.
- Diabetic proliferative retinopathy.

ANA, antinuclear antigen; CRP, C reactive protein; ENA, extractable nuclear antigen; MTHFR, methylenetetrahydrofolate reductase.

A.6 Intravenous (systemic) alteplase was chosen for thrombolysis as this has been shown in clinical trials to be effective in treatment of acute massive PE with right ventricular dysfunction.

Baseline coagulation studies are important (INR and APTT). A prolonged APTT prior to heparin is a common presentation of a lupus anticoagulant, and may indicate an underlying thrombophilic disorder. Thrombophlia is a very important diagnosis as it will mean the APTT cannot be used to monitor the heparin therapy if unfractionated heparin is to be used.

She requires ongoing anticoagulation both in the short and long terms.

- Unfractionated heparin (UFH) has the advantage of being rapidly reversible when given intravenously (by stopping the intravenous infusion and, if necessary, giving protamine). It can also be used in patients with renal impairment or obesity, and should be first-line therapy in massive PE. The disadvantages of UFH are need for more frequent APTT monitoring dose, and risks of both under-anticoagulation (under-treating the patient) versus over-anticoagulation (increasing the chance of haemorrhage).
- Low molecular weight heparins (LWMH such as enoxaparin) are convenient as they are dosed by weight and are administered subcutaneously. LWMH are well validated for use in acute coronary syndromes. However, there are significant disadvantages in the treatment of acute PE. Firstly, LWMH cannot be reversed if haemorrhage occur after thrombolysis. Also LWMH has been poorly studied in obese patients and there are concerns about efficacy, especially considering that PE is a life-threatening event.

Answers cont.

• Warfarin (oral vitamin K antagnonist) should be commenced early. It should be given at the same time each day, usually in the evening. Hospitals have set guidelines as to warfarin loading and monitoring and you need to familiarize yourself with these. Heparin should not be stopped until a minimum of 48 hours (i.e. 2 consecutive days of overlap) have elapsed with the INR greater than 2.0. Plans must be made for close monitoring of the INR and specialized warfarin clinics exist to assist patient with this. In addition, any doctor involved in the patient's care must be made aware that the patient is anticoagulated with warfarin, and a Medi-alert bracelet is advised.

A.7 The patient should be issued with an information card about warfarin, a medical alert bracelet, and advised not to commence any new medications without first talking to a doctor. She must understand that warfarin can interact with many drugs. Alcohol, antibiotics, and non-steroidal anti-inflammatory drugs (NSAIDs) are common culprits in these instances. Also, contraception while on warfarin is essential as it is teratogenic in the first trimester. The oral contraceptive pill has been associated with increased risk of venous thrombosis, and expert opinion of alternative contraception methods should be sought (e.g. intra-uterine device, barrier methods, etc. depending on patient preference).

The patient should also be encouraged to lose weight through regular exercise and a good diet. She should have regular breast examinations and pap smears to ensure that an underlying malignancy does not become apparent. Furthermore, she should be helped to stop smoking.

A.8 The minimum treatment duration of warfarin therapy is 3 months which is appropriate in situations where there has been a short-lived risk factor such as recent surgery or orthopaedic injury.

A V/Q should be performed between 3 and 6 months after acute PE to reassure you that there has been resolution of thrombus as evidenced by normalization of perfusion.

A proportion of patients with life threatening PE go on to develop high blood pressure in the pulmonary circulation, known as chronic thromboembolic pulmonary hypertension (CTEPH). This is a rare but serious complication that can occur after acute PE and is often missed. CTEPH should be considered in patients who present with progressive breathlessness who have a distant history of PE or DVT. CTEPH is life-threatening but potentially curable with surgery called pulmonary thromboarterectomy.

Revision Points

Pulmonary Embolism
Definition
Venous thrombus which embolizes to the pulmonary circulation. Most arise from thromboses in the deep venous system of the legs and it follows that risk factors for pulmonary emboli are identical to those for deep vein thromboses.

Risk Factors
Divided into three groups as first described in Virchow's triad:

Revision Points *cont.*

Stasis: e.g. bed rest, immobility.

Endothelial damage: e.g. surgery, trauma.

Abnormalities of coagulation: e.g. inherited thrombophilia versus acquired (malignancy including myeloproliferative disorders, pregnancy, oral contraceptive pill, nephrotic syndrome, heparin-induced thrombocytopaenia, thrombotic thrombocytopaenic purpura).

Clinical Presentation

Varies greatly – from mild dyspnoea to sudden cardiovascular collapse and death – depending upon thrombus burden within the pulmonary circulation. The classic presentation includes sudden onset of shortness of breath and pleuritic chest pain. PE will have a greater impact on those with poor cardiovascular reserve (e.g. chronic obstructive pulmonary disease, congestive cardiac failure), and a sudden deterioration in breathing of such patients should raise suspicions of a PE.

Treatment

Long-term anticoagulation as outlined in Answer 6.

Patients with underlying malignancy have a high risk of developing thromboembolism, and unexplained DVT or pulmonary embolus in a previously well patient may be the first suggestion of occult malignancy. In patients with unexplained DVT/pulmonary embolus, a family history and personal history for previous episodes of clotting is very important in establishing whether they may have an inherited or acquired thrombophilia.

Chronic thromboembolic pulmonary hypertension (CTEPH) is a rare but important complication to recognize. It can occur in the years following an acute PE resulting in breathlessness again. It is identified by an incomplete normalization of a V/Q scan with ongoing right ventricular systolic dysfunction and pulmonary hypertension on echocardiogram.

Issues to Consider

- What is the role of echocardiography in the management of PE?
- In what situations would you prefer unfractionated over low molecular weight heparin?
- Are you familiar with your local guidelines for heparin and warfarin?

Further Information

Task Force for the Diagnosis and Management of Acute Pulmonary Embolism of the European

Society of Cardiology (ESC), 2008. Guidelines on the diagnosis and management of acute pulmonary embolism. European Heart Journal 29, 2276–2315.

Hamilton-Craig, C.R., McNeil, K., Dunning, J.D., et al., 2008. Treatment options and strategies for acute severe pulmonary embolism. Internal Medicine Journal 38, 657–667.

McNeil, K., Dunning, J.D., 2007. Chronic thromboembolic pulmonary hypertension (CTEPH). Heart 93, 1152–1158.

Recurrent collapse in a 56-year-old truck driver

Jamie Layland

A 56-year-old truck driver presents to the emergency department with a 6-month history of recurrent episodes of loss of consciousness. He has had four episodes in total and his most recent event occurred while he was driving his vehicle. Luckily he was not seriously injured. You are the attending doctor in the emergency department and are assessing him.

Q.1 What specific questions would you ask the patient and what are the possible causes of syncope?

On further questioning you find out that the patient's episodes are unprovoked and come on at any time without warning. There is no postural element to the symptoms and they are not exertional. He denies any urinary or faecal incontinence during the attacks and makes a prompt recovery following events. His wife has witnessed the attacks and tells you that there are no associated seizure-like movements. Until now he has not injured himself as a result of the syncopal attacks. In between attacks he has been systemically well. He has not had any recent headaches or head injuries and denies any abdominal symptoms or unplanned weight loss. He denies any chest pain or shortness of breath and there is no history of sudden cardiac death within the family. He seldom drinks alcohol, does not smoke and denies any history of illicit drug use. He is not taking any regular medications.

Q.2 What would you look for on physical examination?

Physical examination is essentially unremarkable with no abnormal cardiovascular findings and a normal neurological exam. The only positive finding is that of centripetal obesity consistent with the patient's elevated body mass index. You request an ECG in light of the normal physical examination (Figure 30.1).

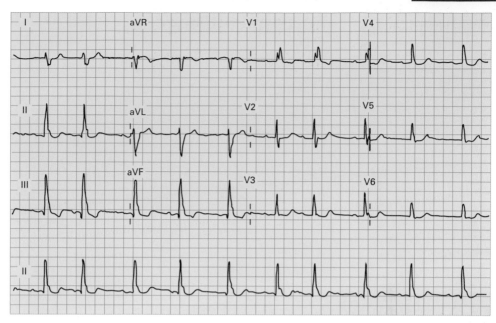

Figure 30.1

Q.3 What does it show and what else would you look for on the ECG? What further investigations would you consider requesting in a patient presenting with syncope?

Following a period of overnight cardiac monitoring that was essentially unremarkable our patient was discharged home for further outpatient evaluation.

Q.4 The results of initial investigations fail to provide a definitive cause for the syncope. What other investigations could you suggest?

The patient went on to have a 24-hour ambulatory cardiac monitor. He had several episodes of syncope during this time. Figure 30.2 shows the electrocardiogram during the events.

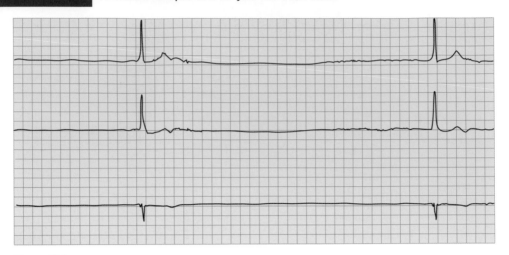

Figure 30.2

Q.5   What does the ECG strip show and what would you do now?

Based on this information, your patient is admitted to hospital and has a dual-chamber pacemaker inserted without complication and recovers well at home. Dual-chamber pacing is preferred over single-chamber left ventricular pacing as it is more physiological and associated with fewer long-term adverse sequelae. Another option, as the patient had sinus node disease, would have been to implant a single-chamber atrial lead. However, given the conduction system disease on his resting ECG it was felt that a ventricular lead should be inserted because of the risk of developing bradycardia due to atrioventricular node/His–Purkinje dysfunction in the future.

    An important consideration in any patient presenting with syncope is their suitability to drive a vehicle following the attack. These will vary depending on state or country and will also depend on the type of licence that the patient holds. Generally, patients with a commercial vehicle licence have more stringent regulations placed upon them than patients with a private licence.

    Your patient is discharged on the day after pacemaker insertion, with advice to observe the pocket site for infection, and follow-up pacemaker check in 3 months' time.

Answers

A.1   When approaching a patient presenting with loss of consciousness it is important to use the history to attempt to derive the most likely diagnosis. It may be appropriate to speak to a family member in order to obtain as much collateral history as possible since the patient may have difficulty recalling the situation.

Firstly, the patient's demographic provides an important clue in the diagnosis. Vasovagal syncope is more common in young patients although syncope in the elderly has a greater risk of adverse outcomes. Also, knowing the situation in which the syncopal event occurred is important. For example, if the patient has

Answers *cont.*

been standing for a long time in a hot environment prior to losing consciousness or has a syncopal event following (not during) exercise, again this is suspicious for a vasovagal episode.

Does the patient have a characteristic warning prior to the syncope? Patients with vasovagal syncope classically have a prodrome that consists of a lightheaded sensation, feeling nauseous and diaphoretic prior to the attack. An absence of a warning prior to the episode of loss of consciousness often indicates a more sinister aetiology such as a cardiac arrhythmia.

Syncope occurring soon after standing suggests orthostatic hypotension that may occur on its own or be a part of a systemic process such as autonomic neuropathy. It is worthwhile enquiring what medications the patient is taking as new medications such as diuretics and anti-hypertensives can augment the postural hypotensive response.

A history of headache prior to syncope should make you think of a subarachnoid haemorrhage as a potential cause. Diplopia and vertigo may suggest brainstem ischaemia from cerebrovascular disease; however, syncope is uncommon in anterior circulatory cerebral ischaemia.

It is also important to determine the recovery period following the syncopal episode. Prolonged recovery suggests a possible seizure whereas a more rapid recovery occurs more commonly in vasovagal syndromes and cardiac arrythmias.

A history of exertional syncope suggests hypertrophic cardiomyopathy or aortic stenosis. A family history of sudden cardiac death is a very important component of the history and may make you more suspicious of possible structural heart disease or an

acquired genetic disorder such as long QT syndrome. Shortness of breath and chest pain associated with syncope suggests a pulmonary embolism.

Causes of Syncope

- Neurally mediated.
- Vasovagal syncope:
  - carotid sinus syndrome
  - micturition/cough syncope.
- Orthostatic hypotension.
- Autonomic neuropathy:
  - hypovolaemia, e.g. dehydration, acute haemorrhage
  - medication related, e.g. diuretics
  - Addison's disease.
- Cardiac arrhythmias:
  - bradycardia – sinus node disease, atrioventricular conduction system disease
  - less commonly tachycardia – supra and ventricular tachycardia.
- Structural cardiac causes:
  - hypertrophic obstructive cardiomyopathy
  - severe aortic stenosis
  - cardiac tamponade
  - pulmonary embolism.
- Ischaemic heart disease:
  - significant coronary artery disease such as left main stem disease.
- Neurological:
  - brainstem ischaemia
  - seizures.
- Metabolic:
  - hypoglycaemia.
- Psychiatric.
- Unknown aetiology.

A.2 The physical examination is really aimed at trying to identify specific causes of syncope and so it is essentially a system-by-system exam considering possible diagnoses.

Answers *cont.*

General Appearance

Pallor or pale conjunctivae suggest anaemia and possible haemorrhage – particularly a large acute haemorrhage that may also be a cause of syncope.

Neurological System

Focal neurological deficit such as limb weakness, cranial nerve palsy on physical examination may indicate a transient ischaemic attack, stroke or subarachnoid haemorrhage as a potential cause.

Cardiovascular Examination

A heart murmur on physical examination raises the possibility of a structural heart defect such as hypertrophic cardiomyopathy or aortic stenosis. Bradycardia suggests underlying electrical conductive system disease. Tachycardia in the appropriate clinical context may be the only clinical sign of a pulmonary embolism. A significant postural drop in blood pressure suggests primary orthostatic hypotension as an aetiology but also could suggest hypovolaemia from causes that include haemorrhage or dehydration.

Respiratory Examination

Features of respiratory compromise such as hypoxia, tachypnoea and clinical signs of right heart strain such as an RV heave, a loud pulmonary component to the second heart sound and a raised JVP suggest pulmonary embolism as a possible cause.

Abdominal Examination

A mass in the abdomen could suggest an underlying malignancy that might lead to anaemia. Equally, the presence of an abdominal aortic aneurysm in the context of syncope should alert you to the possibility of a leak or rupture.

A.3   The ECG shows first-degree AV block, left posterior hemiblock and right bundle branch block that together constitute trifasicular block. Alternatively trifasicular block can occur with left axis deviation, right bundle branch block and first degree heart block.

Other specifics to look for on the ECG would be evidence of pre-excitation such as a delta wave and widened QRS that may predispose the patient to developing SVT; prolongation of the QT interval that would again predispose the patient to ventricular arrythmias; ischaemic ECG changes such as ST depression and T wave inversion may alert you to the fact that the patient may have underlying ischaemic heart disease; Evidence of prior AMI with pathological Q waves is also an important finding. ST elevation of aVR is particularly concerning for a proximal main vessel stenosis that may precipitate syncope. Features of right heart strain (RBBB, RAD, T wave inversion V1-V3, S1Q3 T3 is not specific) is also important to exclude.

Further investigations will be guided on your findings from history and examination but as a general rule any patient presenting with syncope should initially have a systematic work-up that includes an ECG and the following:

Blood tests: full blood count – the presence of anaemia should alert you to the possibility of an underlying haemorrhage; urea and electrolytes – might indicate underlying dehydration or suggest adrenal insufficiency. It is not necessary to perform cardiac enzymes on all patients presenting with syncope unless there are ECG changes consistent with ischaemia or the patient is experiencing chest pain. A blood sugar should be a routine part of a syncope evaluation.

Chest X-ray: increased cardiothoracic ratio may indicate an underlying

Answers *cont.*

cardiomyopathy or the presence of a pericardial effusion.

In our particular patient the history and ECG suggest that a cardiac cause is a likely diagnosis and in such patients a period of inpatient cardiac monitoring may be necessary. An assessment of left ventricular function with an echocardiogram is also an important test. Patients with systolic left ventricular dysfunction are at increased risk of developing ventricular arrhythmias. The echocardiogram can also determine the presence of any structural heart defects or valvular pathologies such as hypertrophic cardiomyopathy. It can also provide you with an assessment of right heart function, which may be abnormal in patients who have had a pulmonary embolism and in those rare patients with arrhythmogenic right ventricular dysplasia, a genetic disorder where patients can present with syncope. Whether this needs to be done as an inpatient or an outpatient will be determined by your underlying clinical suspicion. In our patient it is reasonable to perform an echocardiogram as an outpatient as we have no reason to suspect structural heart disease based on our history and examination.

A.4 The aim of further investigations is to obtain a recording of heart rhythm when the patient is symptomatic. This can be achieved in several ways and will depend upon the frequency of patient symptoms. If the patient experiences daily symptoms then a 24-hour ambulatory cardiac monitor can be organized. This involves the patient wearing surface ECG electrodes for 24 hours that are attached to a recording device. There is continuous ECG recording during this period. The patient records times when they experience symptoms and the corresponding rhythm recorded by the device is compared. If the patient experiences less frequent symptoms then an event recorder may be a more appropriate investigation. This is similar to the 24-hour ambulatory monitor but this time the patient has to press a button to store the ECG. These can be worn for a much longer period of time – typically 1–2 weeks, and often longer.

If ambulatory cardiac monitoring fails to elucidate the nature of the syncope then the next investigation available is a loop recorder. These are small devices, roughly the size of a USB flash drive that is placed subcutaneously in the left infraclavicular position. They are able to remain in situ for 2–3 years. Following a syncopal event the patient places an activator over the device and the ECG over that time period is stored. They are valuable devices in the management of recurrent syncope but their expense and invasive nature limit their blanket use and therefore they should only be used in patients with recurrent syncope in whom a cardiac cause is suspected.

Tilt table testing is a test that is useful in patients in whom you suspect underlying vasovagal syndrome, postural hypotension or autonomic neuropathy as a cause of their syncope. The patient is tilted from supine to 70° over a period of time and may be given medication such as isoprenaline to promote susceptibility to the test. However, up to 40% of patients with vasovagal syndrome may have a normal result and so a negative result is not conclusive. However, the test can be useful when positive at confirming the diagnosis with the replication of the patient's symptoms.

The final investigation available is an electrophysiology study (EPS). This is an invasive test performed via the right femoral vein with a small but significant morbidity

Answers *cont.*

associated. An EPS can detect sinus or atrioventricular nodal disease, bypass tracts and the readiness of a patient to develop ventricular arrhythmias. However, there is generally a low diagnostic yield if it is used in everybody presenting with syncope and indeed recent guidelines suggest only utilizing an EPS in patients with structural heart disease, an ECG that may be suggestive of an arrhythmic cause (e.g. LBBB) or in patients with a family history of sudden cardiac death.

A.5 The ECG shows sinus pauses of up to 5 seconds and these occurred during the day. It is considered normal to have sinus pauses at night of up to approximately 3 seconds due to increased vagal tone. However, in our patient the pauses were greater than 3 seconds and occurred during the day. He therefore meets current guideline indications for a pacemaker.

Revision Points

Current Guidelines for Pacing

Guidelines usually weight pacing indications depending on available literature into three levels, with class I evidence considered the highest achievable level. There are many different pacing indications with differing weights of evidence from class I (permanent pacing is definitely beneficial) to class III (pacing may be harmful) but it is worth knowing what the class I indications are.

Class I Indications for Permanent Cardiac Pacing
Sinus node disease
  – symptomatic sinus bradycardia
  – symptomatic chonotropic incompetence.

Atrioventricular node disease
  – symptomatic complete heart block
  – symptomatic Mobitz I or Mobitz II second-degree AV block
  – exercise-induced second- or third-degree AV block
  – Mobitz II second-degree AV block with widened QRS or bifasicular block.
Neurocardiogenic syncope.
Significant carotid sinus hypersensitivity following minimal carotid sinus massage.

Issues to Consider

- How does cardiac syncope classically differ from a neurological seizure?
- What are the indications for implantable cardiac defibrillators?
- What are the complications of pacemakers in the short and long term?
- What different types of pacing modes are available in different devices?

Further Information

Epstein A.E., DiMarco J.P., Ellenbogen K.A., et al., 2008. ACC/AHA/HRS 2008 Guidelines for device-based therapy of cardiac rhythm abnormalities. Journal of the American College of Cardiology 51, 1–62.

http://content.onlinejacc.org/cgi/content/full/51/21/2085

www.blackouts.edu.au

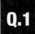

PROBLEM 31

A 68-year-old woman with breathlessness and yellow sputum

Hubertus P.A. Jersmann

You are working in the emergency department one winter evening. A 68-year-old woman is brought in by ambulance, acutely short of breath. The history is obtained mainly from the patient's daughter, because the patient is too breathless to talk, very tired and also a little drowsy. She says she has had difficulty with her breathing for many years and can now only walk at a slow pace for 100 metres and then has to stop due to breathlessness. She has had a smoker's cough for as long as she can remember and has produced phlegm on most days for many years. She has had a number of chest infections this winter despite repeated courses of antibiotics and as a result the local doctor started her on a purple inhaler. On this occasion the woman has been unwell for 1 week. During this time she has been producing thick yellow-green sputum which she has found difficult to cough up. She has been sitting up at night in a chair and has been unable to do anything due to her breathlessness and extreme fatigue. She has become nauseated and is eating very little.

She has not had a temperature or shivers or chest pain. She has not noticed any blood in her sputum and she has not had ankle swelling. The patient has been on antibiotic tablets for 5 days but there has been no improvement.

The woman suffered a myocardial infarction at the age of 60 and underwent coronary bypass surgery. She has not had recurrent angina since then and is not on any cardiac medication. She does not have hypertension or diabetes mellitus. She had experienced pain in the left calf on walking up until the last 6 months when she has been more troubled by breathlessness.

She is on a salbutamol puffer, 2 puffs 4-hourly, fluticasone/salmeterol 250 mg/25 mg 2 puffs bd and amoxicillin 500 mg three times a day for the past 3 days. She currently smokes 5 cigarettes a day, but until 3 months ago smoked 30–60 a day and had done so since the age of 17. She claims she finds benefit from the smoking as it seems to aid the clearing of her sputum.

Q.1 What is the likely diagnosis? What factors may have precipitated her recent deterioration?

You ponder the differentials, and move on to examining the patient.

Q.2 Describe the key components of the examination.

The woman is agitated and looks exhausted and cyanosed. She sits up on the examination couch, in obvious respiratory distress. She is tachypnoeic at 30 breaths/minute. She has prolonged expiration with an audible wheeze, and is coughing frequently, producing thick yellow-green sputum. She has a ruddy complexion, and appears moderately dehydrated.

Her temperature is 38°C, her pulse 140 bpm, regular and bounding, and her blood pressure is 150/100 mmHg with a paradox of 25 mmHg. The patient has a barrel chest with markedly reduced chest expansion and a tracheal tug with use of her sternocleidomastoid muscles and intercostal recession. Precordial dullness is lost. There is no finger clubbing or flap.

Her jugular venous pulse is raised 4 cm. Her apex is not palpable and her heart sounds are inaudible. Her chest is hyper-resonant with globally reduced breath sounds, a prolonged expiratory phase and a loud wheeze. There is no cervical lymphadenopathy and the abdomen is not examined formally due to the patient's distress. There is mild ankle oedema. She is unable to perform simple spirometry due to the severity of her breathlessness.

Q.3   What investigations would you like at this stage?

The following result is obtained:

Investigation 31.1 Arterial blood gas analysis on air	
pO_2	41 mmHg
pCO_2	75 mmHg
pH	7.25
HCO_3	32 mmol/L

Q.4   What does this investigation show?

The patient is placed on 3 L/min oxygen via nasal cannulae. The arterial blood gas estimation is then repeated after 30 minutes. Biochemical analysis, complete blood picture, blood cultures, sputum cultures, CXR and an ECG are also obtained.

Investigation 31.2 Arterial blood gas analysis on 3 L/min O_2	
pO_2	58 mmHg
pCO_2	89 mmHg
pH	7.21
HCO_3	32 mmol/L

Investigation 31.3 Complete blood picture			
Haemoglobin	181 g/L	White cell count	14.3×10^9/L
Platelets	259×10^9/L	Neutrophils 86%	12.3×10^9/L

The electrolytes are normal other than bicarbonate.

The chest X-ray is shown in Figure 31.1.

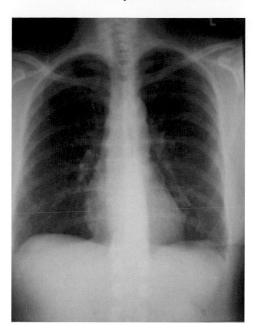

Figure 31.1

An ECG shows a sinus tachycardia with a right axis deviation and a prominent R wave in lead V1.

Q.5 | What do these results indicate?

Q.6 | How are you going to manage this patient?

The patient is managed in the specialist respiratory ward. Her blood gases are maintained within a satisfactory range using low-flow nasal cannulae at 1 L/min oxygen. Salbutamol nebulizers are given hourly.

After blood cultures have been taken, she is started on oral amoxicillin/clavulanic acid and intravenous clarithromycin. Oral steroids are given starting at 50 mg prednisolone.

Q.7 | If her respiratory failure had continued to worsen, what options would have been open to you?

Twenty-four hours later you are called to see the patient because she has an obvious tremor and a temperature of 37.6°C. Her pulse is 140 bpm and her blood pressure is 140/90 mmHg.

Q.8 | What are the possible explanations for her deterioration? What should you do?

Her chest findings are unchanged and abdominal examination is unremarkable. A repeat chest X-ray shows no change and an ECG shows a sinus tachycardia with a rate of 146 bpm.

Her nebulized salbutamol is decreased to 4 hourly and the tachycardia slowly improves. The prednisolone dose is decreased and then ceased over 7 days. Tiotropium is instituted as a once-daily inhaler.

Seven days after admission she has improved to the extent where she can walk slowly around the ward. Formal pulmonary function tests are done prior to discharge. The results are as follows:

Investigation 31.4 Forced expiratory volumes			
	Pre-bronchodilator	Post-bronchodilator	Predicted
FEV_1	0.81 (28%)	1.37 (48%)	(2.89)
FVC	2.84 (78%)	3.71 (102%)	(3.62)
FEV_1/FVC	29%	37%	(80%)
Single Breath Diffusing Capacity			
DLCO corrected for haemoglobin (mL/min/mmHg)		Observed	Predicted
		10.2 (42%)	24.5

Investigation 31.5 Arterial blood gases on air	
pO_2	50 mmHg
pCO_2	61 mmHg
pH	7.40
HCO_3	34 mmol/L

The patient is told firmly that she must stop smoking immediately.

Q.9 **What do these results tell you? How will you manage the patient before discharge and in the future?**

The patient ignores your advice on smoking. She qualifies for home oxygen but is not issued the treatment due to her current smoking. She survived another 18 months, dying of another episode of acute on chronic respiratory failure.

Answers

 A.1 She has at least a 100 pack/year history of smoking and chronic obstructive pulmonary disease (COPD) secondary to cigarette smoking is the most likely underlying diagnosis. This includes chronic bronchitis and emphysema and there may also be an element of reversible airways obstruction, i.e. asthma. Infection of the tracheobronchial tree causing an increase in airway inflammation and volume and viscosity of sputum is the most common precipitant of deterioration in these patients.

Cardiac failure, either diastolic failure secondary to ischaemia or decompensation of cor pulmonale secondary to increasing pulmonary artery pressures, are important

Answers *cont.*

factors to consider as precipitants or as confounders.

Other factors contributing to deterioration may include increased tobacco use, non-compliance with medication, use of sedative drugs, intercurrent pneumonia, left ventricular failure, pneumothorax, thromboembolism and development of a bronchogenic carcinoma or development of anaemia.

The differential diagnosis includes adult-onset asthma and bronchiectasis, and heart failure.

The occupational history is important as the woman may have pneumoconiosis in addition to her smoking-related disease. Exposure may be indirect, such as having laundered her husband's clothes contaminated with asbestos material etc. Occupational history including exposure related to hobbies must always be asked about, even with an obvious smoking history. A history of childhood respiratory problems including exposure to pulmonary tuberculosis may also be relevant.

A.2 During the examination of this patient you will focus on:
- Disturbance of the mental state, e.g. agitation or drowsiness, suggesting underlying hypoxia or hypercapnia.
- Cyanosis and polycythaemia.
- Clubbing (which suggests an underlying lung carcinoma).
- Metabolic flap (hypercapnia).
- Fever (suggests systemic infection).
- Tachycardia and arrhythmia (e.g. sudden-onset atrial fibrillation could contribute to decompensation of cor pulmonale).
- Blood pressure including pulsus paradoxus.
- Pursed lips respiration.
- Use of accessory muscles and intercostal recession.

- Chest signs of over-inflation (loss of precordial dullness, increased resonance, reduced breath sounds) and airways obstruction (wheeze). Also evidence of pneumothorax (reduced breath sounds) or consolidation (bronchial breath sounds).
- Evidence of right heart failure (cor pulmonale).
- Evidence of primary and metastatic malignancy (e.g. cachexia, pleural effusion, supraclavicular lymphadenopathy, hepatomegaly).
- Sputum.

A.3 Initial investigations (and reasons why):
- Spirometry (if available).
- Arterial blood gas analysis (an objective measure of the degree of derangement of lung function and to detect respiratory failure).
- Chest X-ray (evidence of emphysema, consolidation, airways thickening, pneumothorax, cor pulmonale and primary lung malignancy).
- ECG (arrhythmia, right ventricular hypertrophy or hypoxia-induced ischaemia/infarction).
- Complete blood picture (anaemia or polycythaemia, leucocytosis).
- Biochemistry (baseline electrolytes).
- Sputum culture and cytology (bacterial pathogens by Gram stain and culture, malignant cells).
- Blood serology (raised titres of antibodies against bacteria, e.g. *Legionella* and *Bordetella pertussis*).
- Blood cultures (septicaemia).

A.4 The initial blood gas indicates acute on chronic respiratory failure. The bicarbonate is halfway between what is expected in acute respiratory acidosis

Answers *cont.*

(lower bicarbonate) and chronic respiratory acidosis (higher bicarbonate). This suggests renal (metabolic) compensation for chronic hypercapnia and acidosis by bicarbonate retention. This would normalize the pH in the chronic state. With an acute deterioration this compensation cannot occur, resulting in a moderate acidosis.

A.5 With the application of 3 L/min of oxygen there has been improvement in oxygenation but also further CO_2 retention and exacerbation of the acidosis.

The patient has a raised haemoglobin, which is likely to reflect a secondary polycythaemia induced by chronic hypoxia. She has a neutrophilic leucocytosis, which indicates bacterial infection.

The chest X-ray reveals a cardiac size within normal limits and prominent pulmonary arteries. The lung fields are grossly inflated and there is some scarring at the lung apices. There is no evidence of consolidation. This suggests chronic obstructive pulmonary disease (COPD) with pulmonary hypertension. This diagnosis is supported by the ECG changes of right ventricular strain (right axis deviation and a prominent R wave in V1).

Overall, the clinical picture indicates that the patient has COPD with probable cor pulmonale. There has been an acute deterioration precipitated by infection but there is no evidence of pneumonia.

A.6 Oxygenation is the key. Patients need oxygen if they are hypoxic, but excessive supplemental oxygen can result in dangerous hypercapnia with mental stupor or coma and respiratory arrest. A compromise is needed. Improvement of the pO_2 towards 50–60 mmHg should be attempted using the smallest amount of oxygen possible. At this level pulmonary

vasodilatation is achieved. This is when Venturi masks are useful: low-dose oxygen via 24% Venturi mask improves oxygen without causing dangerous respiratory depression. If these cannot be tolerated, nasal cannulae can be substituted at 1 L/min. A modest rise in pCO_2 is acceptable provided that the patient remains alert. If a 24% Venturi mask is tolerated, particularly if the patient improves, a 28% mask (or nasal cannulae at 1.5–2 L/min) may be tried. The blood gases will need to be checked to exclude deterioration in ventilation.

In addition to oxygen, the treatment of any reversible airways obstruction by removing secretions and treating infection will help. If these measures to improve ventilation and ventilation–perfusion mismatch fail non-invasive ventilation (NIV) will have to be considered, including with continuous positive airways pressure (CPAP) or bi-level positive airway pressure (BiPAP). Usually endotracheal intubation and mechanical ventilation would be regarded as the last resort.

The patient may only have a small component of reversible airways obstruction but attempted bronchodilatation by frequent salbutamol nebulizers is accepted practice. Salbutamol intravenous infusion is hardly ever used.

Steroids are used in acute exacerbations of chronic airways obstruction, although they are more important in asthma, and their effectiveness in the management of COPD is not uniform. A similar dose is often used during the acute phase of the illness, but unless there is a significant component of bronchospasm in the obstruction, the chronic use of steroids is not recommended.

Clearance of airway secretions in this patient is important. In the acute stage she would not tolerate routine chest physiotherapy, but regular encouragement of coughing and possibly nasotracheal suction should be performed.

Although the patient has no consolidation she has a fever and a severe deterioration associated with purulent sputum; intravenous antibiotics such as amoxicillin (or amoxicillin/clavulanic acid), doxycycline or clarithromycin should be added. It must be remembered that the macrolide antibiotics (erythromycin, roxithromycin, clarithromycin) interact with many medications including warfarin, anticonvulsants, oral contraceptives and any drugs metabolized by hepatic cytochrome P450. Intravenous erythromycin is now avoided wherever possible, as it can be associated with a highly irritant superficial thrombophlebitis.

This patient is critically ill with respiratory failure, and should be admitted to a dedicated respiratory speciality ward or if that is not available to a high dependency unit. If repeated gas measurements are necessary, an arterial line can be considered.

A.7 She would need some form of respiratory support. This would probably be non-invasive in the form of non-invasive ventilation such as BiPAP, or CPAP. Both these forms of ventilatory support are supplied via well-fitting face or nasal masks. If her respiratory failure worsened further or her conscious level decreased then she would need endotracheal intubation.

A.8 The most likely explanation for the tachycardia is the combination of fever and the frequent administration of salbutamol. Potassium levels may have changed, especially if diuresis has occurred. In addition, she may have cor pulmonale which makes her prone to atrial

tachyarrhythmias, further exacerbated by hypoxaemia. You should arrange an ECG to rule out ischaemia, given her history, repeat electrolytes and a chest X-ray.

A.9 Her lung function tests show an obstructive pattern with significant reversibility to salbutamol. According to GOLD criteria this lady has severe COPD with respiratory failure, stage IV. The reduced DLCO demonstrates markedly impaired gas exchange and is typical of severe emphysema.

Her gases show a return to her chronic state. She is no longer acidotic and her bicarbonate has risen back to its chronically elevated level.

In the short term she should finish her course of antibiotics and tail off her steroids over the following week.

She should have an assessment of her inhaler technique and if required receive more education on device use. She should be discharged with inhalers of tiotropium and a corticosteroid/long-acting beta agonist combination as well as salbutamol if needed.

She must stop smoking. Tobacco smoke inhibits mucociliary function and hence clearance of airway secretions. Smoking also stimulates increased airway mucus production so cessation of smoking will decrease sputum production and bronchospasm. In addition home oxygen cannot be prescribed if the patient continues to smoke, because of the fire hazard.

This patient should have the pneumococcal vaccine every 5 years and an annual influenza vaccine. Compliance with medication should be ensured and inhaler technique should be checked regularly. Infective exacerbations should be treated early with oral antibiotics,

Answers *cont.*

and intensive chest physiotherapy. If manifestations of cor pulmonale (such as ankle swelling) worsen, they may have to be treated with diuretics.

Referral to a respiratory rehabilitation programme is helpful, and provision of home improvements may improve the

ability of the chronically breathless person to cope. This patient would fit the criteria for home oxygen provided she can become an established non-smoker and that there is reversal of hypoxaemia with domiciliary oxygen without progressive hypercapnia.

Revision Points

Chronic Obstructive Pulmonary Disease (COPD)

Cigarette smoking is by far the most important aetiological factor in this disease. Smoking cessation slows the progression of the disease and there may be improvement in airway obstruction. Marijuana smoking has been largely undervalued as a risk factor and it is estimated that one marijuana cigarette may be as damaging as 8–15 cigarettes.

Diagnosis

- Clinical examination is a good tool to rule out alternative diagnoses, but notoriously poor to rule in COPD. In addition, patients often deny symptoms or symptoms become manifest only when the disease is quite advanced.
- Thus, suspicion based on history (including smoking status) should lead to early use of spirometry.
- Spirometry shows a reduction in the forced expiratory flow rate (FEV_1).
- A low FEV_1/FVC ratio will confirm obstruction.
- More complex pulmonary function tests include measurement of the gas diffusion coefficient (DLCO), static lung volumes and lung elastic recoil or compliance.
- Lung function testing provides the data needed to assess the severity of COPD

according to GOLD criteria (Global Initiative for Chronic Obstructive Lung Disease – http://www.GOLDCOPD.com).
- Cor pulmonale is a bad prognostic indicator.
- Blood gas analysis in the acute setting must be interpreted in the light of the patient's chronic status. The renal bicarbonate compensation for chronic hypercapnia will usually cause the pH to be within the normal range. This means that a patient with acidosis has usually had a major decompensation.

Treatment

- Smoking cessation is the only intervention in COPD which has been shown to reduce the rate of decline in lung function.
- There are two inhaled therapies for COPD authorized by the PBS, which reduce exacerbations and, hospitalizations and improve quality of life:
  - tiotropium (Spiriva), indicated for all stages of COPD (New England Journal of Medicine 2008;359:1543–1554. 'UPLIFT')
  - fluticasone/salmeterol (Seretide) indicated for moderately severe and severe COPD, predominantly patients with frequent exacerbations (New England Journal of Medicine 2007;356:775–789. 'TORCH').

Revision Points *cont.*

- When used in combination patients derived an even greater benefit than from treatment with either drug alone (Annals of Internal Medicine 2007;146:545–555. 'OPTIMAL').
- The evidence for benefit from inhaled corticosteroids (ICS) alone is less convincing.
- Short-acting bronchodilator drugs such as salbutamol are useful for symptomatic improvement.
- Oral steroids are indicated in acute airflow obstruction exacerbations. They have no role in the long-term treatment of COPD.
- Vaccination against pneumococcus and influenza virus is advisable and early treatment of chest infections is important.
- If the PaO_2 is below 55 mmHg long-term oxygen therapy >16 h per day or longer prolongs survival as well as improves the quality of life in COPD.

Issues to Consider

- How do you clinically measure pulsus paradoxus?
- What disorders, other than smoking, can cause chronic respiratory failure?
- How are patients assessed to qualify for home oxygen therapy?

Further Information

www.COPDX.org.au *The COPD-X Plan, Australian and New Zealand guidelines for the management of chronic obstructive pulmonary disease.*

www.GOLDCOPD.com *GOLD – Global Initiative for Chronic Obstructive Lung Disease.*

www.lungfoundation.com.au *The Australian Lung Foundation is a key agent of change in Australia for promoting the understanding, management and relief of lung disease.*

Persistent cough in a young woman

Richard A. Stapledon

A 37-year-old woman of Caucasian origin presents with an irritating cough of 3 months' duration and recent episodes of small amounts of blood-stained sputum. She is a non-smoker. She has consulted her family doctor twice during this period and has had only a modest response to successive courses of antibiotics. She has also noticed some lethargy and more recently occasional night sweats.

On examination she appears mildly unwell, has evidence of recent weight loss and a temperature of 38.2°C. No other abnormal findings were elicited.

Q.1 What further history should be obtained?

You question the patient further. Five years ago she spent 2 years as a volunteer teacher in Malawi. When she returned she underwent TB screening and had a 'positive' tuberculin skin test and a normal chest X-ray. At the time, the clinic placed her on a 6-month course of isoniazid preventive therapy, which she had apparently completed.

You arrange a chest X-ray. The PA and lateral views are shown in Figures 32.1 and 32.2.

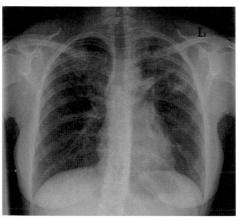

Figure 32.1   Figure 32.2

Q.2 What does the chest X-ray show? What might the findings suggest? Would any other imaging be of help?

Q.3 What simple investigation would you request urgently? Are there any other investigations that may assist in making the diagnosis?

Your suspicions have been aroused, and you admit her to an isolation ward for investigation and treatment. Later, your lunch is interrupted by a call from the microbiology laboratory advising that the smear from her sputum is heavily positive for acid-fast bacilli (AFBs).

Q.4 Why does this result necessitate an urgent call? What should you do now? What additional investigations are indicated?

Q.5 What treatment would you recommend initially and why? What are the main treatment concerns?

Q.6 Are there any other issues that you need to address promptly?

Your patient is surprised and concerned that she is sick, and wants to know if this could have been prevented.

Q.7 Could this illness have been prevented?

Answers

A.1 A careful history in a patient with persistent cough and haemoptysis may provide clues about a possible diagnosis before any definitive investigations are undertaken.

Causes include:

- Lung abscess/pneumonia.
- Bronchiectasis.
- Active tuberculosis (TB).
- Mycetoma.
- Lung cancer (e.g. carcinoid).
- Chronic bronchitis.
- A-V malformation.
- No cause is found in up to 30% of cases.

This patient's fever and night sweats strongly imply an infective cause. The more chronic nature of her history suggests that tuberculosis must be excluded. Disease caused by a non-tuberculous mycobacterium can present a similar clinical picture to TB but in this instance is considered less likely to be the causative agent. Lung abscess or malignancy would also seem less likely. You need to specifically enquire about any TB risk factors:

- Known close contact with a TB case (especially family).
- Past residence or visits to a high-risk country for an extended period, including

223

Answers *cont.*

India, Asia, Africa and Aboriginal and Torres Strait Islander people(s).

- History of previous treatment for TB disease or 'preventive' treatment for latent TB infection.
- Causes of immunosuppression such as HIV infection, immunosuppressive medications particularly TNF agents and steroids.

A.2 The chest X-ray shows a cavitating lesion in the left upper lobe, with some air space opacity in slightly contracted upper lobes.

These chest X-ray findings are highly suspicious of post-primary TB disease, especially in this clinical context. However, no chest X-ray pattern is absolutely diagnostic. Lung malignancies need to be considered and may also co-exist.

TB disease that follows primary infection can produce lower zone infiltrates, hilar or mediastinal lymph node enlargement or pleural effusions. More varied and less specific features can be seen in up to a third of cases, particularly the elderly and immunosuppressed. This can include those of primary disease, a miliary pattern, solitary or multiple nodules or even 'normal' chest films. Remember, TB is the 'great mimicker'.

The radiological changes seen so far are highly suspicious of pulmonary tuberculosis and a CT scan is unlikely to provide any more definitive information. The CT scan is more sensitive than the standard chest X-ray in the examination of the lung parenchyma, mediastinum and pleura. It may be useful in those patients with less obvious or atypical features, or suspicion of other diagnoses such as cancer.

A.3 An urgent sputum sample is required to screen for acid-fast bacilli (AFBs). Collection of the specimen should be in a well-ventilated area, and the patient placed in isolation. A further two morning specimens on consecutive days must also be requested. One specimen alone will fail to detect about 20% of smear-positive cases and about 50% of culture-positive cases. For the patient unable to produce sputum, inhalation of nebulized hypertonic saline should be undertaken. Otherwise bronchoscopy and lavage has a good yield and would also be indicated in the sputum smear-negative case with these symptoms and chest X-ray findings.

An elevated ESR, normocytic anaemia and depressed sodium are non-specific findings which may be present.

The tuberculin skin test or interferon gamma release assay (IGRA) are *rarely* indicated. These tests cannot distinguish latent TB infection from active disease and false-negative results occur in as many as 20% of active cases. Similarly, false-positive results are an issue for those from high-prevalence regions as high rates of reactivity in these populations can be expected.

Nucleic acid amplification tests (NAAT) have been recently developed, making it possible to detect *Mycobacterium tuberculosis* complex from a smear positive specimen and a proportion of smear negative specimens in 24 hours. Due to the urgent treatment and public health implications, nucleic acid amplification could be requested if your clinical suspicion of TB is high but other results are less certain. NAAT are not alternative to conventional methods, as culture is essential for drug-resistance testing. Some NAAT systems are able to detect rifampicin resistance simultaneously which is a marker of multidrug-resistant TB and etc. may be useful in overseas born patients from high burden TB settings.

A.4 TB is the likely diagnosis, requiring the following measures:

Answers *cont.*

- Isolation, in a room with negative pressure ventilation if available, and treatment.
- Strict infection control measures need to be followed. Those with smear-positive cavitary disease who cough frequently as in this case represent the most infectious cases.
- Sputum culture will provide a definitive answer and importantly allow for drug susceptibility testing.
- Urine should be tested for AFBs as a positive urine culture is not an uncommon finding in pulmonary TB cases.
- Screening for HIV infection is important, given the history of residence in an endemic area. HIV associated TB continues to have a substantial impact on TB control in many high burden countries.
- The possibility of undiagnosed diabetes also should not be overlooked. Checking for evidence of impaired renal or hepatic function and a baseline ophthalmology review are important with respect to treatment choices.

A.5 Standard drug treatment for drug susceptible TB is a 4 drug combination of isoniazid, rifampicin, pyrazinamide and ethambutol for an initial 2 months followed by isoniazid and rifampicin for a further 4 months (the initial 4 drug combination also covers for possible isoniazid resistance, the

most likely in a TB endemic area). Pyridoxine is often recommended as a supplement to isoniazid to prevent peripheral neuropathy especially in pregnant women or those with diabetes, renal disease, HIV infection or nutritional deficiency.

Important treatment principles need to be followed to prevent disease relapse and acquired drug resistance:

- Always use combination treatment to which the organism is fully susceptible.
- Treatment adherence is essential and direct observation (directly observed therapy – DOT) should be considered in all patients especially in the initial 2-month intensive phase.
- Never add one drug alone to a failing regimen.
- Duration needs to be for a minimum of 6 months (dependent on drug susceptibility, tolerance and extent/site of disease).
- Correct application of these rules results in a failure rate of less than 2–5%.
- Adverse drug reactions are relatively frequent but severe forms uncommon (Table 32.1).
- Discharge of this patient can occur when there is evidence of good clinical improvement, cough reduction or absence, the quantity of AFBs on smear microscopy is substantially reduced and treatment is assured. Regular follow-up is required to

Table 32.1 Important side-effects and drug interactions

Drug	Side-Effect	Interaction
Isoniazid	Peripheral neuropathy, hepatitis, rash	Anticonvulsants (increased level)
Rifampicin	Hepatitis, rash, flu-like syndrome, thrombocytopenia	Warfarin, oral contraceptives, oral hypoglycaemics, anticonvulsants (reduced level)
Pyrazinamide	Hepatitis, rash, arthralgia, gout	
Ethambutol*	Optic neuritis	

*Use three times weekly or avoid in those with renal impairment or avoid in those with renal impairment.

Answers *cont.*

monitor disease response, check for side-effects and assess compliance.

A.6 Prompt notification to the relevant public health authority is required for surveillance purposes and to facilitate contact investigation. The infectious risk of this person is potentially high, based on her clinical presentation (persistent cough and cavity on chest X-ray) and positive sputum smear result. It is important to promptly identify close contacts, particularly children less than 5 years old and the immunosuppressed; the risk of progression to disease if infected is greatest in these latter groups.

Contact tracing for notifiable diseases should be performed by a specialized service as there is a delicate balance between preservation of patient confidentiality and protecting public health.

A.7 You suspect that this woman became infected during her 2-year stay in Africa. The doctor correctly assumed the tuberculin result reflected TB exposure (no evidence of disease) and advised isoniazid 'preventive' treatment. Isoniazid for 6 months (minimum) is generally recommended, but 9 months is optimal and preferred for children and the HIV-infected. If resistance to isoniazid is strongly suspected or known then rifampicin alone for 4 months is the recommended option. Failure to prevent disease may have reflected poor compliance or an isoniazid-resistant strain.

This case also highlights the need to 'think TB' particularly in individuals from high-prevalence populations or with a history of close TB contact.

Revision Points

Pulmonary Tuberculosis

Causative Organism
- Mycobacterium tuberculosis Complex.

Mode of Transmission
- Inhalation of airborne droplet nuclei.

Incidence
- Uncommon in industrialized countries: rates >5–10 : 100000.
- 90% of cases occur in resource-poor countries: rates >50–100 : 100000.

Risk Groups
- People from endemic areas.
- Recent close contacts of infectious cases.
- The socially disadvantaged.
- The elderly, particularly those with medical co-morbidities or who are on immunosuppressants.
- HIV co-infected patients.

Pathology
- Primary TB infection is usually asymptomatic.
- Risk of progression is about 5% within the first 2 years; average lifetime disease risk of 10–15% dependent on age and immune status.
- If HIV co-infected the risk of developing active TB is 10% per year.
- Most disease in low endemic countries is pulmonary from reactivation of latent infection (post primary or secondary).
- Extrapulmonary disease occurs in 15–20% but is more frequent with increasing immune suppression. The more common sites include lymph nodes, pleura, bone and kidney.
- The classic histological feature is necrotizing epithelioid granuloma.

Revision Points *cont.*

Immunopathology

- Immune responses in TB are complex and mediated mainly by T cells. They cause either a necrotic hypersensitivity or immune protective reaction but the factors responsible for these responses are not well understood.

Clinical

- Classic presentation of pulmonary disease is not always the case. Atypical presentations are frequent in the elderly and immunosuppressed, and TB should always be in the back of the mind as a differential diagnosis.

Diagnosis

- Chest X-ray abnormalities can be consistent with active pulmonary TB but are not diagnostic. Atypical features will be present in up to 30% of cases and CT scan may assist.
- The tuberculin skin test or IGRA blood test cannot distinguish active TB from latent infection.
- Sputum smear microscopy is rapid but insensitive for detection of AFBs, i.e. may miss cases, but should be positive in 40–60% of pulmonary cases.
- Culture remains the gold standard but confirmation takes 7–21 days in smear-positive specimens and 3–6 weeks in smear-negative specimens. Drug

susceptibility testing (DST) requires a further 10–15 days.

Treatment

- Multi-drug treatment is essential to cover resistance, and directly observed therapy strongly recommended at least in the initial 2 month phase.

Public Health

- Notification is usually a legislative requirement and allows for contact investigation.

Prevention

- Treatment of those recently infected/ exposed (no active disease) is up to 90% effective.
- Patients who become immunosuppressed and who also have a clear history of prior exposure to TB should be considered for anti-TB medication as a secondary preventive measure.
- BCG vaccination in the uninfected has protective benefit in neonates and young children but its value to adults remains unclear. It is considered in TST- or IGRA-negative health workers who are at high risk of exposure to MDRTB cases. This is because of the unproven benefit of preventive therapy if infected with an MDR strain.

Issues to Consider

- What would you do if a patient with infectious TB refused treatment?
- What is the role of screening programmes in the detection of tuberculosis?
- Why has TB not been eliminated in high income countries and why should we remain vigilant?

Further Information

www.nlm.nih.gov/medlineplus/tuberculosis.html *A National Library of Medicine website. Comprehensive coverage of tuberculosis with links to a wide variety of sites dealing with many aspects of this disease.*

www.who.int/gtb *A superb web resource from the World Health Organization dealing with the global fight against tuberculosis infection.*

Cough, dyspnoea and fever in a 55-year-old man

Narin Bak

A 55-year-old man presents with 3 days of anorexia, headache, general weakness, aches and pains all over his body. He thought he had the flu and has been treating himself with paracetamol.

However, in the last 24 hours he has become very unwell, with a high fever, irritating dry cough, breathlessness and diarrhoea and he has vomited a number of times. He has no pleuritic pain but has a dull generalized ache in his abdomen. There is no significant past medical history. He has no pets, animal contacts or recent holiday travel but likes gardening. He smokes about 20 cigarettes a day and consumes 30–50 g of alcohol daily. He is not on any regular medications and has no known allergies.

On examination he looks unwell and flushed. He is orientated but agitated and easily distracted. He has a temperature of 39.5°C. The patient is not cyanosed, clubbed, jaundiced or anaemic. He has dry mucous membranes and a coated tongue. His pulse rate is 105 bpm and regular, his blood pressure is 120/75 mmHg and his oxygen–haemoglobin saturation is 90%. His cardiovascular system is otherwise normal. His respiratory rate is 30 breaths per minute and he has a hacking cough productive of small amounts of mucoid sputum. His chest is resonant and the breath sounds vesicular. There are scattered inspiratory crepitations throughout the right lung only. His abdomen is soft and non-tender. There is no neck stiffness and there are no focal neurological signs.

Q.1 What is the most likely diagnosis?

Q.2 What initial diagnostic investigations would you perform and why?

You review the chest X-ray Figure 33.1 and the results of your other tests can be seen in Investigation 33.1.

Q.3 What do the results show ? How would you interpret them?

Figure 33.1

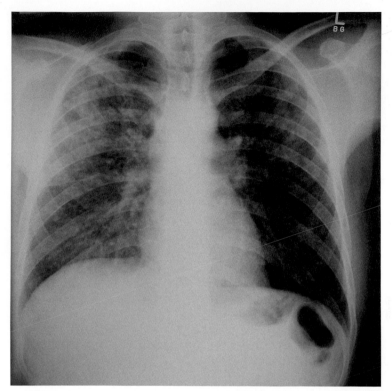

Investigation 33.1 Summary of results

Haemoglobin	161 g/L	White cell count	12.2×10^9/L
RBC	4.39×10^{12}/L	Neutrophils 50%	6.1×10^9/L
PCV	0.53	Lymphocytes 38%	4.6×10^9/L
MCV	86.9 fL	Monocytes 7%	0.9×10^9/L
MCH	29.5 pg	Eosinophils 2%	0.2×10^9/L
MCHC	340 g/L	Basophils 3%	0.4×10^9/L
Platelets	278×10^9/L		
Sodium	128 mmol/L	Calcium	2.16 mmol/L
Potassium	3.1 mmol/L	Phosphate	1.15 mmol/L
Chloride	106 mmol/L	Total protein	66 g/L
Bicarbonate	25 mmol/L	Albumin	39 g/L
Urea	10.1 mmol/L	Globulins	27 g/L
Creatinine	0.19 mmol/L	Bilirubin	16 µmol/L
Uric acid	0.24 mmol/L	ALT	62 U/L
Glucose	4.9 mmol/L	AST	75 U/L
Cholesterol	3.5 mmol/L	GGT	80 U/L
LDH	212 U/L	ALP	131 U/L
INR	1.0	APTT	35 sec
Arterial blood gases on room air			
pO$_2$	61 mmHg	pCO$_2$	32 mmHg
pH	7.50	Calculated bicarbonate	25 mmol/L

Urinalysis: 1+(0.3 g/L) protein, 1+(5–10 red cells/µL) blood – no active sediment

> **Q.4** What organisms are likely to have caused this man's illness? How would you expect the clinical signs to differ with different pathogens?

> **Q.5** How do you assess severity of pneumonia and level of risk to patient?

You assess him as having moderately severe pneumonia. His age, his mental state and the multi-lobar involvement are high-risk characteristics requiring admission to hospital, and you arrange a bed in the respiratory unit.

> **Q.6** How are you going to manage this patient?

The patient is placed on oxygen via nasal cannula at 4 L/min. An intravenous line is inserted and 1 L isotonic saline is set up running over 2 hours to rehydrate the patient. You check with the patient and his family to ensure he is not allergic to penicillin.

The nurse is kindly drawing up the antibiotics, and your IV fluids are running. His family have started asking you some questions.

> **Q.7** What complications may be expected to occur?

The patient was commenced on erythromycin 1 g 6-hourly and ceftriaxone 1 g intravenously. He was rehydrated using isotonic saline so as not to exacerbate the hyponatraemia. The hypokalaemia was corrected.

Sputum culture on special medium was positive for *Legionella pneumophila* after 3 days. Urine was positive for legionella antigen (specific for *L. pneumophila* 1). Blood cultures were negative. His respiratory status was closely monitored with the assistance of oximetry and serial blood gases. Initial serology for *Legionella* species by indirect fluorescent antibody was <1:4. At 16 days the *L. pneumophila* titre was 1:1024. Intravenous erythromycin was continued for 7 days and an oral dose of clarithromycin 500 mg 12-hourly was given for a further 2 weeks.

He improved after 72 hours and made a slow recovery over the following 10 days. The disease was notified to the Department of Health and *L. pneumophila* was subsequently isolated from a sprinkler system in the patient's greenhouses. The water system was decontaminated. The patient was told that his cigarette smoking and alcohol intake had put him at increased risk of contracting this illness. He was advised to stop smoking and was given options to assist with this process.

Answers

A.1 The presentation of this case strongly suggests community-acquired pneumonia. The patient has fever, cough, dyspnoea and abnormal respiratory signs but no hard clinical signs of consolidation. His respiratory rate is markedly increased, which is an important sign of respiratory compromise. Gastrointestinal symptoms (vomiting and diarrhoea) are not uncommon in pneumonia and may be misleading features for site of infection. Audible crackles on respiratory examination is a

Answers *cont.*

frequent and an important sign not to miss. Signs of consolidation is present in only about 30% of patients.

However, some patients can present with fever without localizing symptoms.

Pneumonia can also be referred to anatomically as in right lower lobe pneumonia or on the basis of aetiology such as pneumococcal pneumonia.

Differential diagnoses include pulmonary embolism, pulmonary vasculitis, malignacy, and hypersensitivity pneumonitis.

A.2 The following investigations are required to confirm diagnosis, assess severity and investigate for causative organism:

- Complete blood examination, serum chemistry and coagulation studies to assess severity of illness and assist diagnosis.
- Arterial blood gas analysis on air to ascertain the degree of respiratory impairment that is present, and oximetry performed for ongoing assessment.
- Chest X-ray to confirm diagnosis, and may provide clue to severity.
  To identify aetiology:
- Blood cultures (*prior* to any antibiotics).
- Sputum collection for Gram and acid-fast stains and for culture (including for *Legionella*, mycobacteria).
- Urinary pneumococcal and legionella antigen.
- Nasopharyngeal swabs for the respiratory viruses (influenza, parainfluenza, respiratory syncytial virus, adenovirus).
- Serology (acute and convalescent) for respiratory pathogens including:
  – viral
  – *Mycoplasma pneumoniae*
  – *Chlamydia pneumoniae*.

A.3 There is only a mild leucocytosis (much lower than would be expected for

pneumococcal pneumonia). The patient has hyponatraemia, which is not uncommon with some pneumonias. It may be the result of pulmonary production of ADH-like substances. A hyponatraemia of less than 130 mmol/L can be associated with legionella pneumonia, but is not diagnostic. There is mild renal impairment, which may be due to dehydration or the underlying illness. There is a hypokalaemia which needs correction.

- The liver enzymes are abnormal. This is often a feature in pneumonias caused by 'atypical' organisms such as *Legionella* and *Mycoplasma*.
- The urinalysis is abnormal, highlighting the systemic illness.
- The coagulation studies are normal and this excludes disseminated intravascular coagulation.
- The arterial blood gas shows moderate hypoxaemia with hyperventilation and respiratory alkalosis.

These findings are in keeping with a moderately severe pneumonia with systemic sepsis. They would be consistent with legionellosis but could still represent pneumonia caused by other pathogens.

The chest X-ray shows significant bilateral pulmonary infiltrate, consistent with a clinical diagnosis of pneumonia. The right lung is extensively involved, particularly the upper lobe with consolidation and atelectasis. The appearances suggest bronchopneumonic change without major lobar volume loss. There is also patchy infiltrate in the left mid and upper zones. The heart size is normal.

A.4 Community-acquired pneumonia in the immunocompetent host can be caused by a broad range of pathogens which differ from those seen in hospital-acquired pneumonias and pneumonias in immunocompromised hosts (Table 33.1).

231

Answers *cont.*

Table 33.1 Aetiology of community-acquired pneumonia

Causative Oragnism	Percentages
Streptococcus pneumoniae	42
Mycoplasma pneumoniae	9
Legionella species	3
Chlamydia species	2
Gram-negative	3
Haemophilus influenzae	5
Staph. aureus	1
Respiratory viruses	14
Other or unknown	21

Table 33.2 Treatment of community-acquired pneumonia

Mild (Low-Risk) Pneumonia	Moderate Severity Pneumonia	Severe (High-Risk) Pneumonia
Outpatient treatment	Hospital admission	Hospital admission – consider intensive care assessment/admission
Oral amoxicillin plus doxycycline or	IV benzyl penicillin and gentamicin plus oral doxycycline or macrolide	IV ceftriaxone or Tazocin plus IV azithromycin
Oral macrolide (clarithromycin or roxithromycin, azithromycin)	or	
	IV ceftriaxone plus IV erythomycin/azithromycin	

A.5 You should always assess the severity of pneumonia in every patient. It predicts the risk and prognosis, and determines admission and the types of recommended empiric antibiotics (see Table 33.2). The 30-day mortality for low-risk or mild pneumonia is less than 1%, while the 30-day mortality for severe (high-risk) pneumonia is approximately 27%.

The severity of pneumonia can be graded and scored and is based on the following factors:
- Age >50 years.
- Co-existing illness (e.g. diabetes, renal disease, cardiac failure, splenectomy).
- Abnormal physical signs on examination (confused, pulse >125 bpm, respiratory rate >35 per minute, systolic blood pressure <90 mmHg, or temperature <35°C or >40°C).
- Abnormal investigations (pH<7.35, PaO_2<60 mmHg on air, extensive CXR changes).

A.6 The initial antibiotic selection should be empirical as clinical and chest X-ray findings are not sufficiently specific for causal organism. The antibiotic choice should cover both pneumococcus and other less common organisms such as *Legionella*, *Mycoplasma* and *Chlamydia* pneumonias (see Table 33.2).

In severe pneumonia, IV vancomycin may need to be added to the empiric regimen as community-acquired methicillin-resistant *Staphylococcus aureus* is a rare but emerging pathogen. In some tropical

Answers *cont.*

regions, empiric treatment for severe pneumonia in patients with diabetes or chronic renal failure may need to also cover *Burkholderia pseudomallei* and *Acinetobacter baumanii*.

A.7 Most patients respond well to treatment but complications can occur. If patients are not improving, consider the following:

- The diagnosis is incorrect (e.g. pulmonary malignancy or pulmonary oedema).

- The antibiotic does not cover the pathogen (e.g. *Mycobacterium tuberculosis* or methicillin-resistant *Staphylococcus aureus*, or HIV-associated *Pneumocystis* pneumonia).
- Parapneumonic effusion (common).
- Empyema or lung abscesses.
- Sputum plug causing lobar collapse.
- Development of pulmonary embolism.
- Development of ARDS or multi-organ failure.
- Drug fever.

Revision Points

Community-Acquired Pneumonia

Aims of Management at Presentation

- Assess severity and risk. Severe cases need admission to hospital.
- Identify aetiologic agent. This can guide subsequent antibiotic choice and duration.
- Remember that underlying illnesses that impair the patient's immune system will extend the spectrum of possible infecting agents (so-called opportunistic infection).
- Exclude other diagnoses.
- Initiate treatment appropriately:
  - high-flow oxygen
  - intravenous rehydration and monitoring of fluid balance and renal function

  - antibiotic therapy (*after* blood cultures taken) as guided by local policy and microbiology results; the initial antibiotic choice depends on assessment of severity
  - severe cases require early admission to an intensive care unit for ventilatory support.
- Remember to consider the patient's fitness. For the elderly, those with serious co-morbid conditions such as diabetes, COPD or cardiac failure or those with immune compromise, pneumonia may be rapidly life-threatening and may require specialized management.

Issues to Consider

- What are the implications of the widespread use of parenteral cephalosporins in the management of community-acquired pneumonia?
- What other respiratory disorders can be transmitted from environmental exposure?

Further Information

www.brit-thoracic.org.uk *The website of the British Thoracic Society, with access to the*

excellent guidelines for the management of community-acquired pneumonia.

www.legionella.org *Public access website from the USA with plenty of information on this organism and the public health issues related to it.*

Breathlessness and weight loss in a 58-year-old man

Hubertus P.A. Jersmann

A 58-year-old accountant presents with 3 months of progressive breathlessness on exertion. He has no associated chest pain or wheeze but has had a smoker's cough for years. He has lost 5 kg over the last 3 months but says that his appetite is normal. He complains of a 'frog in his throat' for the last 6 weeks, which he has put down to his smoking. His breathlessness has progressed to such an extent that he has been unable to work for the last few days and was only able to walk up the one flight of stairs to your clinic with difficulty. Apart from feeling generally lethargic, he reports no other symptoms.

He has a history of hypertension for which he takes ramipril. He smokes 20–30 cigarettes a day; his alcohol consumption is regular and has never exceeded an average of 20 g a day. He is in his second marriage and has two young children aged 9 and 14.

> **Q.1** What other information would you like from the history? What will you look for on examination?

On examination he is slightly plethoric and has signs of recent weight loss. He has a hoarse voice. His pulse is 80 bpm, his blood pressure is 155/95 mmHg and he is afebrile. He is tachypnoeic with a respiratory rate of 25 breaths per minute and appears to be centrally cyanosed. Cardiovascular examination is normal.

His trachea is in the midline and the chest is not obviously over-inflated. The percussion note is dull in the lower zone of the right chest. The breath sounds are reduced in this area and there is an associated increased vocal resonance. There is a widespread polyphonic wheeze throughout both lung fields. There are no other clinical signs on full examination.

> **Q.2** What are the possible diagnoses?

The man looks unwell and dyspnoeic and you decide to admit him to hospital for further management.

> **Q.3** What investigations will you order?

You receive the results shown in Investigation 34.1.

234

Investigation 34.1 Summary of results			
Haemoglobin	175 g/L	White cell count	18.5×10^9/L
Platelets	500×10^9/L	Neutrophils 80%	$14.8 \times ts\}10^9$/L
Sodium	123 mmol/L	Calcium	2.85 mmol/L
Potassium	4.2 mmol/L	Phosphate	0.65 mmol/L
Chloride	106 mmol/L	Total protein	59 g/L
Bicarbonate	27 mmol/L	Albumin	32 g/L
Urea	5.1 mmol/L	Globulins	27 g/L
Creatinine	0.076 mmol/L	Bilirubin	12 μmol/L
Uric acid	0.24 mmol/L	ALT	22 U/L
Glucose	4.4 mmol/L	AST	32 U/L
Cholesterol	3.5 mmol/L	GGT	17 U/L
LDH	212 U/L	ALP	230 U/L
Arterial blood gases on room air			
pO_2	52 mmHg	pCO_2	50 mmHg
pH	7.38	Base excess	–2.5

Q.4 What do these results tell you?

A chest X-ray is shown in Figure 34.1.

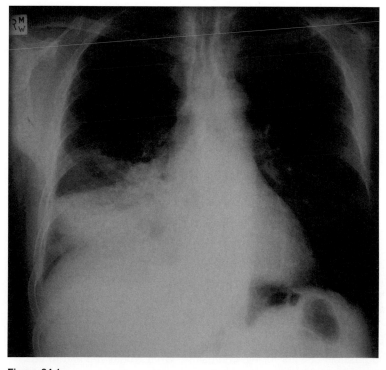

Figure 34.1

Q.5 What does the chest X-ray show? How are you going to manage this patient?

Q.6 What further investigations should now be considered?

A further radiological investigation is performed. Two representative films are shown (Figures 34.2 and 34.3).

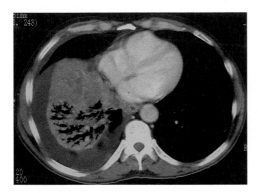

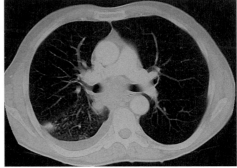

Figure 34.2   **Figure 34.3**

Q.7 What do these CT scans show?

A bronchoscopy is performed. The right vocal cord is adducted and does not move. A tumour is found obstructing the right main bronchus. The right middle lobe and the right lower lobe bronchi could not be entered. Biopsy of this tumour reveals a poorly differentiated adenocarcinoma.

Q.8 What treatment options are open to you at this stage? What will you tell the patient?

Five days after admission you are called to see him on the ward. He has become confused over the past 24 hours. A decision has been made not to proceed with chemotherapy or radiotherapy. The nurses report that he has not opened his bowels for 4 days.

On examination he is mildly confused with a GCS of 13. Despite his humidified oxygen he has dry mucous membranes and has decreased skin turgor. He is afebrile. The examination is otherwise unchanged since admission.

Q.9 What are the possible causes for his confusion? What would you like to do?

Some serum biochemistry had been performed earlier that day. The results are shown in Investigation 34.2.

Investigation 34.2 Summary of results

Sodium	130 mmol/L	Calcium	3.8 mmol/L
Potassium	4.4 mmol/L	Phosphate	0.16 mmol/L
Chloride	102 mmol/L	Total protein	57 g/L
Bicarbonate	27 mmol/L	Albumin	30 g/L
Urea	15.6 mmol/L	Globulins	27 g/L
Creatinine	0.28 mmol/L	Bilirubin	16 μmol/L
Uric acid	0.24 mmol/L	ALT	28 U/L
Glucose	4.4 mmol/L	AST	40 U/L
Cholesterol	3.5 mmol/L	GGT	17 U/L
LDH	212 U/L	ALP	354 U/L

Q.10 What is the problem and what would you like to do now?

He received rehydration and a single dose of pamidronate. This was associated with clearing of his confusion and after discussion with his wife he elected to be transferred to inpatient hospice care. His hypercalcaemia rapidly recurred and he died peacefully surrounded by his family 3 weeks after his initial presentation.

Answers

A.1 Find out the following:

- The nature and severity of his shortness of breath. After how much exertion does he get short of breath? How rapidly did this develop? Does it occur at rest, during the night or when he lies flat? How many pillows does he sleep with?
- The nature of his cough. Has it changed? Is it productive and if so is it purulent? Has he coughed up any blood?
- Has he had any other symptoms to explain his weight loss? Has he had fevers or night sweats?
- Enquire further about his smoking history. How long has he smoked? Express the smoking history in 'pack-years' where 20 cigarettes a day for 1 year is 1 pack-year.

Thus a comparative figure can be derived for overall consumption of tobacco measured in terms of the total number of pack-years.

- Are there any other risk factors for lung disease such as industrial exposure to asbestos in the past? Does he keep birds? Has he had any recent foreign travel? Is there a family history of pulmonary disease? Has he had previous cancers or is there a family history of cancers such as colon cancer? Has he had any previous blood clots?

On examination you should look for signs or evidence of the following:

- Respiratory distress, e.g. tachypnoea, cyanosis and the use of accessory respiratory muscles.

Answers *cont.*

- Chronic lung disease, wheeze and hyperinflated lungs.
- Pneumonia, e.g. fever and lobar consolidation.
- Malignant lung disease, e.g. clubbing, pleural effusions, lymphadenopathy, hepatomegaly and ascites.
- Anaemia.
- Cardiac disease, e.g. cardiomegaly, raised jugular venous pressure, atrial fibrillation or peripheral oedema.

In addition you should measure oxygen saturation via pulse oximetry and perform spirometry.

A.2 His smoking history makes it likely that he is suffering from a degree of chronic obstructive pulmonary disease (COPD). Patients with severe COPD often suffer from weight loss and become cachectic but this is usually in the context of a reduced intake due to severe dyspnoea at rest.

He may be suffering from an infective process but the length of the history makes it unlikely that this is bacterial in nature. The presence of weight loss raises the possibility of tuberculosis and you should ask about risk factors.

Other intrinsic lung diseases such as fibrosing alveolitis are possibilities but the presence of weight loss, the problems with his voice and his smoking history all make this a less likely diagnosis.

Cardiac failure leading to weight loss (cardiac cachexia) is unlikely in the absence of paroxysmal nocturnal dyspnoea or orthopnoea.

Anaemia may explain his shortness of breath, lethargy and, depending on the cause, his weight loss.

By far the most likely diagnosis in this man, who is a heavy smoker, has experienced recent weight loss and shortness of breath and has localizing pulmonary signs, is lung cancer. The hoarseness of his voice is an extremely sinister symptom and may be due to malignant infiltration of the recurrent laryngeal nerve by a hilar tumour causing a vocal cord paralysis.

A.3 Perform these investigations:
- Complete blood picture: look for evidence of anaemia or infection (leucocytosis).
- Urea, electrolytes, creatinine, calcium, liver function tests.
- Chest X-ray.
- Arterial blood gases, looking for evidence of respiratory failure.
- Sputum collection for microscopy, culture, AFB and cytology.

A.4 He is likely to have polycythaemia secondary to his long history of smoking (you would like to see his haematocrit). He has a neutrophilia which raises the possibility of an underlying infective process but this may be a nonspecific finding in any inflammatory condition. His mild thrombocytosis also supports an inflammatory process.

He has a moderately severe hyponatraemia in the context of otherwise normal renal function and in the absence of any culpable drugs. This may well be the syndrome of inappropriate ADH (SIADH) seen in many pulmonary conditions and particularly in bronchogenic adenocarcinoma. Paired serum and urine osmolalities would help to confirm this. If SIADH is present you would expect to see inappropriately concentrated urine in the presence of dilute or normal serum.

He has a raised alkaline phosphatase which may be due to liver infiltration with metastatic carcinoma (expect to see a raised GGT in addition) or due to bony involvement. The mild hypoalbuminaemia is

Answers *cont.*

likely to be due to his chronic illness or, if there is liver involvement, synthetic liver dysfunction. It is highly unlikely to be due to nutritional deficiency despite his recent weight loss.

He has a mild hypercalcaemia. This may be due to production of a parathormone-like peptide by a lung adenocarcinoma. Alternatively, in conjunction with the raised ALP, bony involvement is a distinct possibility.

His blood gases show that he has type 2 respiratory failure with both hypoxia and hypercapnia. The normal pH implies that this is a relatively well compensated and, therefore, a chronic process.

A.5 The "chest X-ray" is reported as follows:

There is partial collapse and consolidation in the right middle lobe. There is also an abnormal convexity to the posterior aspect of the right hilum and the appearances are suspicious of a right hilar mass resulting in the collapse and consolidation of the right middle lobe. There is some increased opacity in the subcarinal region and lymphadenopathy in this region is suspected. The left lung and pleural reflection appear clear.

He is in respiratory failure. You should administer oxygen by Venturi mask to correct his hypoxia. Repeat his blood gas analysis in 30 minutes to ensure he does not decompensate due to carbon dioxide retention.

In view of the X-ray appearances and the leucocytosis, the administration of antibiotics would be appropriate. An intravenous penicillin and oral macrolide would be suitable until the results of microbiological culture are known.

Remember that although the history and investigations so far point towards an advanced lung cancer, this has not yet been proven. He should be managed in a respiratory unit and intensive care support requested should he deteriorate.

If he is suffering from SIADH then fluid restriction may be appropriate. However, in the presence of hypercalcaemia, fluid restriction may lead to profound dehydration. It would be wise not to restrict his fluid intake and, if he is unable to drink, to provide the patient with maintenance intravenous fluids using isotonic saline. Daily checks on his electrolytes and calcium will help you adapt his fluid and electrolyte regimens accordingly.

A.6 Once he is stabilized he will need:
• A CT scan of his chest to further define the hilar and mediastinal abnormalities.
• A fibreoptic bronchoscopy to look for a bronchial tumour and to obtain histological samples for diagnosis. The lymph nodes should be sampled via transbronchial needle aspiration (TBNA) or with endobronchial ultrasound (EBUS) guidance. These techniques are safe and not only enhance the chance of securing tissue diagnosis in one procedure but often also deliver important staging information at the same time as initial diagnosis. This saves time and unnecessary mediastinoscopies.
• If the bronchoscopy is inconclusive, a slightly more risky CT-guided fine needle biopsy may be necessary. (This particular patient would be too unwell for a mediastinoscopy.)

A.7 The "CT scans" are reported as follows:

There is a large soft tissue mass in the subcarinal region of the mediastinum consistent with lymphadenopathy. This is associated with soft tissue enlargement

Answers *cont.*

with surrounding of the right pulmonary artery by the soft tissue mass lesion. The appearances are consistent with bronchogenic carcinoma with involvement of the mediastinum. There is distal consolidation and partial collapse of the lung within the right middle and lower lobes. The left lung shows no evidence of any sinister parenchymal lesion. There is a right pleural effusion. The appearances are consistent with a bronchogenic carcinoma involving the right hilum.

A.8 This man is highly likely to have advanced (stage IV) lung cancer with respiratory failure, hypercalcaemia, SIADH and probable liver and/or bone involvement. Any treatments that you offer him at this stage are palliative.

The presence of mediastinal involvement, respiratory failure and probable metastatic disease rule out the possibility of surgery. Surgery remains the only real option for cure in non-small cell lung carcinoma but is only effective in stage I and II disease and in patients with good lung function and performance status. Surgery is now being performed in some centres for more advanced disease (IIIA), often in conjunction with either chemotherapy or radiotherapy.

Radiotherapy alone has resulted in 'cure' in a small number of reported cases with lower-stage disease but inoperable on general grounds, but it is largely used for palliation.

Chemotherapy for non-small cell tumours has also produced disappointing results. Aggressive regimens involving the taxanes and platinum-based drugs have been shown to be useful as palliation in selected patients. This man's respiratory failure and metabolic upset make him poorly suited for any such treatment.

His outlook is poor. When breaking bad news it is important to be in possession of all the facts and prepared for questions. If possible, the most senior member of your team should be present when bad news is broken. It is important that you speak to him in a quiet, private environment in the presence, if he wishes, of friends and family. Allow good time, as he is likely to have many questions. Be honest and frank but avoid medical jargon and do not remove all hope. It is important to avoid phrases such as 'there is nothing we can do' as, although there is no chance of a cure, there are many interventions which can relieve symptoms and improve his quality of life in his final days. The main fear of many patients told they have a terminal disease is that they will die in pain or without dignity. With modern palliative care, this should not be the case. He has a young family and the devastating effects of his diagnosis on them must not be forgotten. The involvement of palliative care professionals at an early stage is important.

A.9 There are several possible causes for confusion in this man:
- Hyponatraemia: his sodium was low on presentation; this may have worsened.
- Hypercalcaemia: he may have worsening hypercalcaemia.
- Respiratory failure: he may have become more hypoxic or/and have increasing hypercapnia.
- Sepsis: keep in mind common causes of confusion. Is there any sign of sepsis?
- Cerebral metastases: he has widespread disease. The presence of cerebral metastases with attendant cerebral oedema needs to be considered.
- Alcohol withdrawal: the patient stated when first seen that he 'drinks regularly', and you must remember that most

Answers *cont.*

patients will underestimate their alcohol consumption.
- You should check his electrolytes, calcium and blood gases. If it looks likely that there are no metabolic causes for his symptoms then you could consider a CT scan to identify metastases.

It is important to identify easily treatable causes of his deterioration if such treatment will result in improved symptomatology and quality of life. However, in the setting of palliative care, investigations and interventions should only be carried out if they are likely to lead to such improvements. If not then treatments should aim for symptom control and comfort. Always involve his relatives, particularly his next of kin. Palliative care professionals can also be very helpful.

A.10 He has hypercalcaemia with associated dehydration and renal failure.

Fluid restriction instituted at first for his hyponatraemia may have exacerbated this situation.

Hypercalcaemia of malignancy often occurs in the presence of bone metastases but may also be mediated by the production of a parathormone-like peptide from malignant cells; a so-called paraneoplastic syndrome. It often produces a dramatic clinical picture and should be treated in all but the most terminal of cases.

Treatment involves initial rehydration with isotonic saline. This man is likely to need 3–4 litres over the next 24 hours. Bear in mind that this may exacerbate his hyponatraemia.

A bisphosphonate such as pamidronate can be added to palliate the hypercalcaemia if this were thought appropriate. These drugs work by inhibiting the mobilization of calcium from the skeleton.

Revision Points

Lung Cancer

Epidemiology
- The most common form of cancer in men and now, in most developed countries, in women.
- Causes more deaths in the USA than breast, prostate and bowel cancer combined.
- On the increase, especially in women due to a dramatic rise in female smoking. Also increasing in developing societies.
- Almost all forms of lung cancer are a direct result of tobacco smoking, making it one the West's biggest preventable health problems.

Presentation
- Always suspect in smokers with unexplained deterioration in health and/or weight loss.
- May have no pulmonary symptoms. The presence of shortness of breath, pain and haemoptysis often imply advanced disease. Hoarseness of voice if recurrent laryngeal nerve involvement.
- Sometimes picked up incidentally in medical assessments.

Types
Two major groups
- Small cell lung cancer
  - accounts for 10–15% of total number of cases

Revision Points *cont.*

– tumours tend to be rapidly progressive
– responds to high-dose chemotherapy regimens ± radiotherapy but have a very high recurrence rate following treatment. Metastatic disease is common.
• Non-small cell lung cancer (NSCLC). Three subtypes:
– adenocarcinoma
– squamous cell carcinoma
– large cell carcinoma.

Diagnosis

New bronchoscopic techniques, in particular transbronchial needle aspiration with endobronchial ultrasound (EBUS), often allow not only tissue diagnosis but also hilar and mediastinal staging with a single procedure. This often saves valuable time and resources by avoiding readmission and mediastinoscopy. The state-of-the-art method for staging for distal disease is positron emission tomography (PET) using radioactive 18F-fluorodeoxyglucose. An additional CT brain is required because of the inability of PET to detect brain metastases due to the high glucose utilization of the cerebrum.

Treatment

Treatment depends on stage.
• Surgical resection ± adjuvant therapy are options for early-stage tumours (IA–IIB).
• For later-stage tumours, treatment is largely palliative. New high-dose chemotherapeutic regimens may improve quality and prolong length of life.
• Current research involves a variety of approaches, e.g. novel chemotherapy agents, photodynamic therapy and vaccine therapy.
• Palliative care measures and psychological support especially important in patients with advanced disease.

Prognosis

• Prognosis of NSCLC depends on stage at presentation. IA (small volume local disease with no nodes or metastases) has a 5-year survival of up to 70%. Only 1% of patients with stage IV disease (presence of metastases) will be alive at 5 years.
• Overall, prevention by not smoking is the most important approach for this disease. Advising patients and their relatives not to smoke should be the responsibility of all healthcare professionals.

Issues to Consider

• What are the factors that influence the incidence of smoking in various countries? Are there any effective measures that might be used to treat nicotine addiction and thus reduce the incidence of cigarette smoking?
• What other paraneoplastic phenomena occur in advanced lung cancer? How can they best be treated?
• What palliative care options exist for the treatment of respiratory distress in this situation?

Further Information

http://en.wikipedia.org/wiki/Non-small_cell_lung_carcinoma_staging *Summarizes the latest revision to the NSCLC staging system (January 2009).*

www.cancerresearchuk.org *Website of the Cancer Research Campaign in the UK with lots of information and links for lung and other tumours.*

www.lungcancer.org *Excellent website with links and information for patients and health-care professionals alike.*

A 35-year-old woman vomiting blood

Jonathan Mitchell

It is 7 p.m. on a busy Saturday night. You are called urgently to the emergency department. A 35-year-old woman has been brought in by her husband. She has vomited bright red blood on three occasions over the last 2 hours. The last episode was on arrival in the resuscitation room. The nurses say it was around 500 mL. She is pale but conscious with a GCS of 15. Her pulse is 120 and her blood pressure is 96/57 mmHg. She has an oxygen saturation of 94% on room air.

Q.1 What are your immediate priorities?

Q.2 What further elements of the history would you like from the woman and her partner?

Blood tests become available as follows:

Investigation 35.1 Summary of results
White cell count: 10.1×10^9/L
Haemoglobin: 11.8 g/dL
Platelets: 78×10^9/L
Prothrombin time 17.6 seconds
Sodium: 131 mmol/L
Potassium: 3.8 mmol/L
Bicarbonate: 12 mmol/L
Urea: 18.7 mmol/L
Creatinine: 54 mmol/L
Albumin: 32 g/L
ALP: 114 U/L
Bilirubin: 23 mmol/L
AST: 63 U/L
ALT: 47 U/L
GGT: 61 U/L

Q.3 What do these results tell you? What would you like to organize next?

A further detailed history reveals that the woman has never vomited blood before but did have one episode of black stools 3 weeks earlier which she put down to diet. She has had no indigestion and has not taken any non-steroidal anti-inflammatories. She has never had any operations. Her partner volunteers that, up until 3 years ago, she had had longstanding problems with alcohol excess and had seen a hospital specialist who had warned her that she would die if she continued to drink. They had made a decision to move across the country to start a new life and she had not had an alcoholic drink since.

Q.4 Does this information change your immediate management?

You organize an urgent endoscopy. The endoscopist finds a large amount of fresh and altered blood in the stomach. No bleeding source is identified in the stomach or the duodenum. Figure 35.1A, B shows the positive findings.

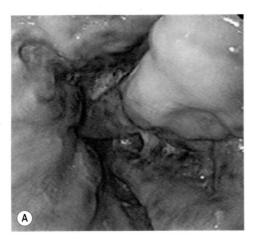

Figure 35.1A

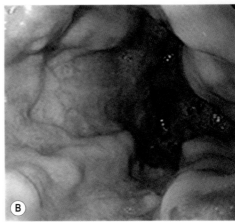

Figure 35.1B

Q.5 What abnormality do these images show? What options are available to the endoscopist?

The endoscopist places four bands on the varices, with apparent haemostasis. She returns to the ward. It is now 11 p.m.

Q.6 Is any other treatment appropriate at this stage?

At 5 a.m. you are called to the ward. The woman has had no further haematemesis. She has become confused and is trying to remove intravenous cannulae and get out of her bed. Her blood pressure is 120/79 mmHg, her pulse 90 and her SpO$_2$ 98% on room air. She has had 3 units of FFP. A fourth unit of packed cells is running.

Q.7 What may be happening and why? How can you manage the situation?

Shortly after your arrival, she has a further large haematemesis. Her GCS is 11. Her pulse has risen to 130 and her blood pressure fallen to 86/49 mmHg. She is sweaty and peripherally cool. The nurses and her husband are very concerned and look to you for answers.

Q.8 What are you going to do?

The woman is taken to the endoscopy suite once more. Copious fresh blood is seen in the oesophagus. Despite their best efforts, haemostasis cannot be achieved. A balloon tamponade tube is inserted with airway control. The patient is taken to the intensive care unit.

The following morning a definitive procedure is performed. An image taken from this procedure is shown (Figure 35.2).

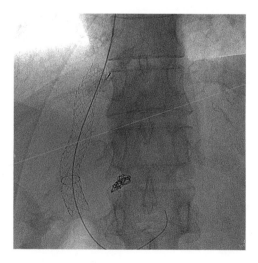

Figure 35.2

Q.9 What procedure has been performed? What are the potential risks of this procedure?

Three days later the woman is discharged. Two years later, she remains well. She works full time as a chef and has had no further bleeding.

Answers

A.1   The patient has had a significant upper GI bleed with a very large witnessed haematemesis. Despite her young age, she is already showing signs of shock with a tachycardia. Her airway may be at risk if she vomits further. High-flow oxygen should be administered. Intravenous access with two large-bore cannulae should be secured. Blood should be taken immediately for a 6 unit cross-match, full blood count, clotting, electrolytes and liver enzymes. Intravenous fluids can be used to restore circulating volumes although note cautions later. There are many debates about the best fluids to use (crystalloid vs colloid) but there is no doubt that the best of all in this situation is blood.

A.2   You will want to know any previous medical history including previous GI bleeding, peptic ulceration or liver disease. Has this happened before? Has it been accompanied by abdominal pain or dyspepsia, suggestive of a peptic cause? Did she have 'normal' vomitus before bringing up blood? This may suggest a Mallory–Weiss tear following trauma to the oesophageal mucosa. This can produce surprisingly brisk haemorrhage. Does she take any culpable medications including often short courses of non-steroidals or aspirin. Has she had melaena? The absence of melaena in the context of a large haematemesis normally implies an oesophageal source.

A.3   She has a very mild anaemia. This is often overtly reassuring but remember! In the acute stages of any form of bleeding the *haemoglobin concentration* is initially well maintained until haemodilution occurs. Haemoglobin concentration is not the same as total haemoglobin so do not be falsely reassured. Her platelet count is very low.

While there are many causes, it may signify hypersplenism and, therefore, portal hypertension and liver disease.

There is further evidence of this in her liver synthetic function. She has a slightly increased prothrombin time and a mildly depressed albumin. In addition she has minor abnormality of her liver enzymes.

The urea : creatinine ratio is helpful in ascertaining the source of any GI bleed. In this case, we know from her presentation that it is upper GI. However, in cases of melaena or passage of fresher blood rectally, this ratio can be helpful. The sudden appearance of a high protein load in the upper gut generates a high level of blood urea in upper GI blood loss. Later, this becomes relevant in this case.

The woman needs an endoscopy urgently. In view of the possibility of variceal haemorrhage, the patient is likely to need a general anaesthetic for airway protection. You may want to consider platelet transfusion.

A.4   This information makes the presence of significant liver disease and, therefore, a variceal bleed, all the more likely. Variceal bleeding is an endoscopic emergency. You may even want to consider giving a potent vasoconstrictor such as terlipressin if endoscopy is likely to be delayed. Get advice now. Antibiotics may need to be considered. Beware over-zealous volume resuscitation. (See later to find out why.)

A.5   These are endoscopic images of the lower oesophagus: four variceal cords are seen. There are several 'red spots' which are signs of high-risk bleeding points although no active bleeding is currently seen. The endoscopist rightly asserts that the bleeding has come from the varices and places bands on the varices

Answers *cont.*

endoscopically. There is good evidence that this technique is significantly superior to older 'injection' sclerotherapy.

A.6 In variceal bleeding, broad-spectrum antibiotics reduce septic complications and short-term mortality. If bleeding has not been reliably controlled, terlipressin may be required but this drug is a potent vasoconstrictor and can cause ischaemic complications if not used with care. She is now at risk of hepatic decompensation.

A.7 First consider the possible latent effects of sedative or anaesthetic agents especially in a patient with liver disease in whom these drugs are often metabolized extremely slowly. However, she has emptied a large 'high protein load' into her gut – i.e. blood. This provides a substrate for gut bacteria to produce ammonia.

Ammonia, and associated by-products of protein metabolism, may enter the systemic circulation via the portosystemic shunts, of which her varices are examples, which define portal hypertension. In addition, poor synthetic function means that ammonia entering the liver via the portal circulation

will not be adequately metabolized. This then causes hepatic encephalopathy.

Hepatic encephalopathy may have been precipitated by drugs, as above, or signify further bleeding. A patient in this situation is at risk of losing airway control. Further sedatives are not appropriate outside a high dependency/intensive care environment. Aperients such as lactulose may be useful later on.

A.8 The situation has deteriorated significantly and she is now in grave danger. She needs to be intubated and taken to ITU as soon as possible. If not already given, a vasoconstrictor such as terlipressin should be administered.

It is quite likely that *over-enthusiastic* fluid resuscitation has led to a rise in her portal pressure to provoke further bleeding. Once stabilized, she will need a further endoscopy.

A.9 This is a transjugular portosystemic shunt stent or TIPSS. The metallic stent is seen lying between the hepatic veins and portal vein in an artificially created channel. The radiologist has also inserted some metallic coils into one of the collateral vessels feeding her bleeding varices.

Revision Points

Management of Variceal Haemorrhage

Airway and Breathing

- Patients with variceal bleeding are at high risk of compromising their airway.
- Involve ITU early. **All** patients requiring endoscopy for actively bleeding varices will need to be intubated.

- Bleeding is often complicated by encephalopathy. Think aspiration!

Resuscitation

- Resuscitation is paramount.
- Two large-bore peripheral cannulae, blood for FBC, clotting and 6 unit cross-match.

Revision Points *cont.*

- Blood is the best colloid! Consider group-specific or O neg blood.
- **Avoid over-filling!** This raises portal pressure and can promote further bleeding. Aim for a systolic BP of 100, a pulse of <100 and a CVP of 6–10.
- Consider platelets if <50. There is no evidence that the use of FFP is beneficial. Conversely, its use may raise portal pressure and promote bleeding.

Vasoconstrictors

- In patients with active suspected variceal bleeding, give a 2 mg IV bolus of terlipressin.
- Post endoscopy, terlipressin should be continued at 1–2 mg IV qds for a maximum of 72 hours. This can be shortened further if adequate haemostasis is achieved at endoscopy.
- Watch out for ischaemic complications in long-term use.

Endoscopy

- Involve the on-call endoscopist early. Variceal haemorrhage is an endoscopic emergency.
- Endoscopic band ligation (EBL) is the treatment of choice but alternatives in skilled hands include tissue or 'super' glue sclerotherapy, especially in non-oesophageal varices where band ligation is not an option. Older sclerotherapeutic agents such as ethanolamine are no longer used.

Antibiotics

- All patients with a confirmed variceal haemorrhage must receive parenteral broad-spectrum antibiotics.
- There is excellent evidence that this prevents the late septic complications which lead to renal failure, hepatic decompensation and death. There is even evidence that sepsis, for example from spontaneous bacterial peritonitis in a patient with ascites, may be the trigger that leads to increased portal blood flow and bleeding in the first place.

Balloon Tamponade

- 'Sengstaken' or 'Minnesota' tubes (Figure 35.3) can be life-saving but in inexperienced hands may be extremely dangerous and should always be placed by experienced operators in an intubated patient.
- With improved access to endoscopy and improved endoscopic techniques as well as the availability of TIPSS, they are required less and less.

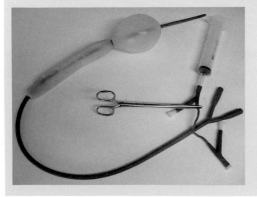

Figure 35.3

Revision Points *cont.*

Further Management

- The majority of patients will need to be managed on HDU/ITU immediately post endoscopy.
- The majority of deaths occur from the complications of bleeding including liver decompensation, encephalopathy, sepsis and renal failure.

- Stable patients normally require a repeat endoscopy within 48–72 hours. In those in whom endoscopy fails and in patients with non-oesophageal varices (e.g. gastric, duodenal), TIPSS is the treatment of choice and is being used earlier than ever before.

Issues to Consider

- Using the information above and your knowledge of physiology, what major complication might follow TIPSS insertion?
- What class of medication has been shown to reduce the risk of variceal haemorrhage in the long term and why is choice of drug important?
- What are the Blatchford and Rockall scores? Would they have been useful here?

Further Information

http://www.patient.co.uk/doctor/Upper-Gastrointestinal-Bleeding.htm *A decent article on upper GI bleeding with a useful 'calculator'.*

www.daveproject.org *An excellent online source of fascinating endoscopy videos.*

A young woman with jaundice

Usama Warshow

A 25-year-old woman presents with a 2-week history of general malaise. She had developed a sore throat and fever followed by nausea and diarrhoea. She has vomited and has been eating little. Yesterday, a friend noticed that her eyes had turned yellow. Her urine has turned dark brown but she has not noticed what colour her bowel motions are. She is thin, jaundiced and looks unwell. She has tattoos, puncture marks in her antecubital fossae and tracks along the lines of her veins in her forearms. She has no lymphadenopathy. Cardiovascular and respiratory examinations are normal. Her abdomen is soft without ascites. Her liver is palpable 4 cm below the costal margin and is smooth and tender. The spleen is not palpable. There are no stigmata of chronic liver disease. She is not encephalopathic. Her urine is positive for ketones and bilirubin.

Q.1 What extra questions would you like to ask this young woman?

She is admitted and admits that she has used intravenous drugs for 2 years. She claims that she has only ever shared needles with her current boyfriend of 4 months.

Q.2 What preliminary investigations would you perform on this patient?

The results of some initial investigations are as follows:

Investigation 36.1 Initial laboratory investigations

Haemoglobin	125 g/L	White cell count	6.2×10^9/L
Platelets	475×10^9/L	Lymphocytes	3.1×10^9/L
INR	1.2	Blood film: occasional atypical lymphocyte	
Sodium	145 mmol/L	Calcium	2.16 mmol/L
Potassium	4.4 mmol/L	Phosphate	1.15 mmol/L
Chloride	106 mmol/L	Total protein	67 g/L
Bicarbonate	27 mmol/L	Albumin	40 g/L
Urea	5.9 mmol/L	Globulins	27 g/L
Creatinine	0.12 mmol/L	Bilirubin	171 µmol/L
Uric acid	0.24 mmol/L	ALT	1563 U/L
Glucose	4.4 mmol/L	AST	1284 U/L
Cholesterol	3.5 mmol/L	GGT	75 U/L

Q.3 Interpret these blood results. What other investigations should be performed?

The following results become available:

Investigation 36.2 Ultrasound of liver

- Enlarged liver with heterogenous echotexture with normal contours.
- Thin-walled gallbladder with no gallstones seen.
- Normal calibre to common bile duct and intrahepatic ducts.
- Spleen at the upper limit of normal.

Investigation 36.3 Department of virology

Anti-hepatitis A IgM:	Negative
Hepatitis B surface antigen:	Positive
Anti-hepatitis B core IgM:	Positive
Anti-hepatitis C IgG:	Negative
Hepatitis C antibody:	Positive
Hepatitis C viral PCR:	Negative
HIV antibody:	Negative

Q.4 What is the diagnosis (A, B, C, D or E)?

A. Previous infection with hepatitis B (HBV)?
B. Chronic HBV?
C. Acute hepatitis C (HCV)?
D. Acute HBV?
E. Chronic HCV?
Liver synthetic function remains normal. She remains nauseated and finds it difficult to eat.

Q.5 How would you further manage this woman (A, B, C, D or E)?

A. Commence antiviral medications?
B. Start an infusion of N-acetylcysteine?
C. Start HBV immunoglobulin?
D. Consider interferon therapy?
E. Ensure good hydration and nutrition?
A few days later her boyfriend visits her with a 4-year-old boy. The boy is the patient's son by another man. They agree to blood tests from the man and the child. The results are as follows:

Investigation 36.4 Boyfriend's test results

Albumin	34 g/L	Bilirubin	20 µmol/L	ALP	150 U/L
GGT	85 U/L	ALT	102 U/L	AST	99 U/L

Virology

Hepatitis B surface antigen:	Positive
Anti-hepatitis B surface IgG:	Negative
Hepatitis B 'e' antigen:	Positive
Anti-hepatitis B 'e' antibody:	Negative
Anti-hepatitis B core IgM	Negative
Anti-hepatitis B core IgG	Positive
Delta antibody:	Negative
Anti-hepatitis C IgG:	Negative

Investigation 36.5 Son's test results

Virology

Hepatitis B surface antigen:	Negative
Anti-hepatitis B surface IgG:	Negative
Anti-hepatitis B core IgG:	Negative
Anti-hepatitis C IgG:	Negative

Q.6 How would you interpret these results?

Answers

A.1 The history is extremely important. It is essential in making the final diagnosis. Her Intravenous drug use (IDU) is a major risk factor in acquiring a blood-borne hepatitis virus (B, C, D). Ascertain if she has shared needles, and when, for clues as to the likelihood and possible length of infection. HBV is more readily transmitted by sex than HCV. Risk of blood transfusion transmission is now rare since blood in developed countries is screened for blood-borne viruses. Tattoos are low risk if done professionally. She could have a faeco-orally transmitted viral hepatitis (hepatitis A or E), but HBV or HCV seem more likely. However, other possibilities should not be dismissed (Table 36.1).

A.2 Initial blood tests should include liver and renal profiles. Jaundice of any cause can lead to dehydration and renal failure. A full blood count must be performed along with a clotting profile. The prothrombin time (or INR) is an essential indicator of liver function.

Here, a diagnosis of viral hepatitis is likely. You should specify the tests that you require. Too often, a blanket request for 'hepatitis virology' is misinterpreted by the laboratory and the wrong investigations are provided.

Blood should be taken for hepatitis A IgM and HBV. A positive hepatitis A IgG is a measure of past, not current, infection. The standard screening test for acute HBV is to

Answers *cont.*

Table 36.1 Risk factors for hepatitis in the acutely jaundiced patient

Diagnosis	Important Points in History
Hepatitis A	Contacts, foreign travel, recent diarrhoeal illness, dietary risk factors, e.g. shellfish ingestion, recreational risk factors, e.g. swimming and surfing, esp. urban beaches
Hepatitis B	Close contacts, sexual history, blood transfusion, IDU, foreign travel, tattoos, body piercing
Hepatitis E	As for hepatitis A
Other viruses, e.g. EBV	Contacts, sore throat, age
Drug-induced hepatitis	Recent medications, although do not get caught out as can be as long as 1–2 months since offending drug was taken – detailed drug history is important; frequently antibiotics, especially flucloxacillin and co-amoxiclav; over-the-counter drugs (especially NSAIDs); complimentary therapies; Chinese medicines; recreational drugs; Ecstasy use
Alcohol-related hepatitis	Alcohol history
Autoimmune hepatitis	Age, female sex, history of other autoimmune disease, e.g. thyroid

measure surface antigen. However, if suspicion is high, a HBV core IgM should also be requested.

HCV rarely causes a severe acute hepatitis; most cases are asymptomatic. In view of her history, evidence of this infection should be sought. Chronic HCV is diagnosed by the presence of HCV IgG antibodies. A PCR (polymerase chain reaction) will confirm the presence of circulating virus. This latter test should only be requested if there is a high suspicion of acute HCV.

Serology for hepatitis E could be sent if the patient is thought to be at risk. This virus, transmitted by the faecal–oral route, is endemic in India, the Middle East, South East Asia and Latin America and Africa. It is also found in Western nations, e.g. the UK. Other viruses can cause an acute hepatitis (e.g. Epstein–Barr virus and cytomegalovirus).

This may not be acute viral hepatitis. The possibility of autoimmune liver disease means that an autoantibody screen and immunoglobulins should be done (positive liver-specific antibodies, such as anti-smooth muscle antibodies, and a raised IgG fraction is in favour of autoimmune disease). Ultrasound is an important test for any patient with jaundice to exclude biliary dilatation and vascular thromboses and allow planning of further investigations. It may help demonstrate features to suggest chronic liver disease (e.g. irregular shrunken liver (cirrhosis) or features of portal hypertension, splenomegaly, etc.).

A.3 These tests suggest a 'hepatitic' cause for her jaundice with predominant elevation of her transaminases (ALT and AST). The only true markers of liver *function* are the bilirubin, prothrombin time (or INR) and albumin.

She has a thrombocytosis which is likely to represent an acute-phase reaction. Lymphocytosis and the presence of atypical lymphocytes raise the possibility of viral infection

A.4 The diagnosis is acute HBV. This is shown by the presence of both hepatitis B surface antigen and core antibody (IgM).

She is at increased risk of other parenterally transmitted viruses. Hepatitis D (delta agent) serology is a 'defective' RNA

Answers *cont.*

virus requiring co-infection with hepatitis B to replicate successfully. Superinfection with the delta agent in a patient with pre-existing chronic hepatitis B may cause an acute hepatitis.

Prevalence of HCV in intravenous drug users is very high (up to 90%). The presence of a positive antibody and negative PCR test mean she has had HCV in the past but has cleared the virus without treatment (spontaneous resolution). This happens infrequently (10% of cases of HCV).

Consent should be sought to test for HIV.

A.5 The correct response is E.

Management is supportive with hydration and nutrition. Most clear the virus completely and develop lifelong immunity (>95% in adults) and will improve enough to be discharged home relatively early. A very small proportion (0.1–0.5%) may develop acute liver failure. Therefore close monitoring is important with regular blood testing. Worrying features include hepatic encephalopathy and coagulopathy. If any of these occurred then she would need transfer to a liver unit. Antiviral drugs in acute HBV do not affect the course or

outcome. The main indication for *N*-acetylcysteine is in paracetamol overdose. It is sometimes used in non-paracetamol related acute liver failure, but should only be used in the liver unit setting. Interferon therapy has no role.

Contact tracing is *extremely* important. Public health or health protection agencies should be informed. There are robust systems to ensure contact tracing. Support for her drug addiction should be offered.

A.6 Her boyfriend is positive for surface antigen and therefore has HBV. The positive IgG antibody and negative core IgM suggest chronic infection. The presence of the e-antigen and absence of anti-e antibodies indicate viral replication. Further tests such as HBV DNA levels and liver biopsy may be required.

Prevent her boyfriend infecting others. HBV can be transmitted to intimate non-sexual contacts, for example by sharing of shaving equipment or toothbrushes. Her son is currently negative for HBV but should be immunized along with close contacts. She needs follow-up in approximately 6 months to check viral clearance with a negative hepatitis B surface antigen.

Revision Points

Hepatitis B Virus
Epidemiology
- In excess of 300 million HBV carriers worldwide.
- Prevalence of chronic HBV between 0.1% and 2% in the developing world to 20% in sub-Saharan Africa.

Clinical Features
Incubation period: 1–6 months.

Acute hepatitis with jaundice presents similarly to our case. Prodromal symptoms are common. Seventy per cent of patients will develop subclinical disease without jaundice.

Revision Points *cont.*

Table 36.2 Understanding hepatitis B serology

Antigen/Antibody	Relevance		When Detectable?
HepBsAg	Hallmark of hepatitis B infection – presence for >6 months implies chronic infection. May be absent in florid acute HBV due to a strong immune response to the virus		First to be detected, usually a few weeks prior to symptoms
HepBsAb (IgG)	Indicates immunity or effective immunization		Appears soon after HepBsAg disappears
HepBeAg	Not necessary for acute diagnosis Marker of active viral replication		Usually after HepBsAg appears
HepBeAb (IgG)	May take years to develop in chronic cases. Usually coincides with disappearance of detectable HBV DNA levels		During resolution phase of acute HBV, before HepBsAg disappearance
HepBcAB	IgM	Presence usually implies acute infection In some cases can be found during flares or reactivation of latent HBV	Appears shortly after HepBsAg
	IgG	Usually seen in resolving infection or chronic infection. Also, present in individuals with previous exposure who have cleared the virus.	
Hep B DNA	Sensitive PCR techniques allow measurement of low levels of virus. Not useful in acute infection. Essential in the monitoring of chronic infection and response to antiviral drugs		

Interpretation of hepatitis B serology is approached with trepidation by undergraduates and postgraduates alike. Its really quite simple (Table 36.2).

Treatment and Course

Some with chronic infection will develop cirrhosis, especially if the virus goes undetected and untreated. There is a significantly increased risk of hepatocellular carcinoma.

Treatment has revolutionized over the last 10 years with the use of interferon and with the advent of powerful oral antiviral medications. Newer drugs (e.g. entecavir, tenofovir) deliver rapid viral suppression with minimal side-effects and are helping to overcome the rising resistance to older antivirals such as lamivudine. In some cases of cirrhosis liver transplantation may be required.

Prevention

HBV is a massive public health problem worldwide. Vaccination of all those at risk, e.g. health workers, high-risk intravenous drug users, children born in highly enedemic areas, results in falls in the prevalence of the disease. Ideally, anyone with HBV should be seen by a qualified doctor and given access to antiviral drugs and surveillance programmes if appropriate. Unfortunately, in areas of the world with the highest prevalence rates, this is too often wishful thinking.

Issues to Consider

- The A to G of viral hepatitis.
- The risk of HBV transmission in healthcare workers.
- What other health problems do you foresee for intravenous drug users? What issues may be problematic for health professionals involved in their care?
- The role of the immune system in the pathogenesis and subsequent clearance of acute HBV.
- How do antiviral drugs work? How can a virus adapt to develop immunity?

Further Information

www.britishlivertrust.org.uk

www.digestive.niddk.nih.gov/ddiseases/pubs/hepb_ez

www.hepb.org.uk

A 47-year-old man with lethargy and hypertension

Mark Gilchrist

A 47-year-old car salesman attends the emergency department with a spontaneous epistaxis. His nose is packed before undergoing cautery by the ENT surgeons. He remarks that he has not been feeling particularly well over the last few weeks. He feels he is somewhat lacking in energy which he had attributed to not eating due to a lack of appetite. This has led to him having to bring his belt in by two notches. On questioning he admits to more frequent headaches than usual. He has not experienced any dysuria or symptoms of prostatism. He has had no vomiting or diarrhoea. He has not had any abdominal pain.

He has never attended the hospital before and thinks the last time he saw his general practitioner was as a child for a sore throat. He takes no regular medication apart from paracetamol for his headaches. His alcohol consumption averages around 30 units per week. He smoked 20 cigarettes per day until 6 years ago.

Examination reveals a rather unwell-looking gentleman. He is apyrexial, and neither cyanosed, jaundiced nor clinically anaemic. His heart rate is 68 beats per minute in sinus rhythm and his heart sounds are normal. Blood pressure is markedly elevated at 214/112 mmHg. His jugular venous pulse is not visible. Auscultation of his chest reveals vesicular breath sounds throughout with no added sounds. Palpation of his abdomen reveals no masses nor are there any ascites. There are, however, some excoriations which the patient believes are due to a new detergent his wife is using. There is no ankle oedema. Fundoscopy shows grade two hypertensive retinopathy. Neurological examination yields no abnormality.

Q.1 What are the possible cause of this man's symptoms?

You decide to admit him for further investigation.

Q.2 Which simple non-invasive bedside test will you perform?

The following blood results become available.

Investigation 37.1 Summary of results

Haemoglobin	91 g/L	White cell count	4.0×10^9/L
MCV	84 fL	Platelets	195×10^9/L
MCH	30 pg		
Sodium	140 mmol/L	Calcium	2.03 mmol/L
Potassium	5.5 mmol/L	Phosphate	1.84 mmol/L
Chloride	98 mmol/L	Total protein	69 g/L
Bicarbonate	18 mmol/L	Albumin	38 g/L
Urea	34 mmol/L	Globulin	31 g/L
Creatinine	570 µmol/L	Bilirubin	24 µmol/L
eGFR	16 mL/min	ALT	44 U/L
Glucose	6.5 mmol/L	AST	45 U/L
Cholesterol	5.0 mmol/L	AlkPhos	164 U/L

Q.3 How would you interpret these results?

Q.4 What would your initial management of this patient include?

Q.5 Which non-invasive investigation would you now like to request?

Q.6 In the longer term what are the main facets of this patient's management?

Q.7 When would you think of starting dialysis?

Answers

A.1 The symptoms described are non-specific and could be attributed to a number of causes. The presence of significant hypertension, visible evidence of vascular damage (retinopathy) and pruritus should raise the possibility of chronic renal failure.

A.2 Dipstick urinalysis is a vital part of the assessment of the hypertensive patient or those with suspected renal disease. The presence of protein would support the presence of renal disease.

Combined with examination of the urinary sediment urinalysis can point to the cause of renal impairment. For example, glomerular disease or vasculitis will produce urine with haematuria and red cell casts whereas a negative urinalysis with few cells or casts suggests renovascular disease.

Answers *cont.*

A.3 There are numerous abnormalities. The patient has renal failure evidenced by the significantly raised urea and creatinine with corresponding low eGFR. There are a few clues to suggest that this patient's renal failure is chronic rather than acute. These are:

- His normochromic, normocytic anaemia reflects reduced erythropoietin production.
- Hypocalcaemia and hyperphosphataemia along with an elevated alkaline phosphatase are a consequence of the failure of hydroxylation of vitamin D and secondary hyperparathyroidism.

Other abnormalities include a mild metabolic acidosis and slightly elevated potassium.

A.4 While the blood tests suggest this is chronic renal failure it may be that there is a reversible component. Therefore it is important to look for potential factors which may have precipitated an acute deterioration.

A detailed drug history is vital, looking for any potentially nephrotoxic drugs. In particular ask about over-the-counter NSAIDs. The second aspect of the drug history is to identify any drugs which may need to be stopped or the dose adjusted given the renal impairment.

An accurate assessment of volume status should be made. Are there any signs of dehydration which may need to be corrected? Is there any evidence of fluid overload?

A.5 The initial investigation of choice is renal ultrasound.

Assessment of renal size will indicate the likely chronicity of the renal impairment. Bilateral small kidneys suggest irreversible renal failure. A biopsy may be of value in normal-sized kidneys. Asymmetric kidneys may be due to unilateral renal artery stenosis or ureteric reflux.

The pelvicaliceal system can be evaluated for the presence of hydronephrosis and renal stone disease

A.6 He needs to be seen early by a nephrologist in order to ensure he is able to access the range of specialist services he will now require. Management will broadly fall in to the following categories:

- Preventing or slowing further decline in renal function. This is achieved by maintaining tight blood pressure control and aggressive management of other co-morbidities like diabetes which may accelerate a fall in GFR. ACE inhibitors and angiotensin receptor blockers are effective in reducing proteinuria and slowing disease progression.
- Preparing for the possibility of needing renal replacement therapy. This begins with patient education, often with specialist nursing staff. Haemodialysis and peritoneal dialysis can be discussed with appropriate patients. Ideally dialysis access, i.e. arterio-venous fistulas, should be in place before the patient becomes dialysis dependent. Transplantation can be discussed. For some individuals the existence of a matched related donor may mean transplantation is a viable first-line option.
- Management of the distal consequences of renal failure. Renal anaemia will require correction with subcutaneous injections of erythropoietin. Some individuals require iron infusions. Renal bone disease will need to be addressed. Calcium and phosphate homeostasis will need to be achieved using a combination of diet, phosphate binders, hydroxylated

Answers *cont.*

derivatives of vitamin D, and attention to parathyroid hormone levels.

- Attending to cardiovascular risk. Patients with renal failure are at a high risk of athero-embolic events. Thus attention to additional cardiovascular risk factors such as hyperlipidaemia is vital. Again meticulous control of blood pressure and diabetes are essential.

- He will need to see a renal dietician. Advice will be required on balancing restricted protein, phosphate and potassium intake with achieving adequate nutrition.

- Education is key. A patient who is engaged in their care will fare much better in achieving a longer time to dialysis dependence and avoiding the complications of chronic renal failure.

A.7 It will often depend on the patient's symptoms. Some patients tolerate a much higher level of uraemia very well where others may be highly symptomatic with a lower blood urea. A patient should begin dialysis before urgent indications develop.

Factors that may precipitate dialysis on an urgent basis include:

- Uraemic complications such as pericarditis, encephalopathy or neuropathy.
- Fluid overload which fails to respond to diuretics.
- Metabolic disturbance such as persistent hyperkalaemia or metabolic acidosis which cannot be corrected medically.

Revision Points

Chronic Renal Failure

Common Causes

- Chronic glomerulonephritis.
- Diabetes.
- Hypertension.
- Reflux nephropathy.
- Ischaemic nephropathy.

Symptoms

- Non-specific.
- Lethargy.
- Pruritus.
- Weight loss.

Investigation

- Urinalysis: dipstick testing and microscopy.
- Blood tests: urea, creatinine, calcium, phosphate, haemoglobin.
- Blood tests 2: autoantibody screens, complement levels, myeloma screen.

- Ultrasound is the imaging modality of choice.

Management

- Patient education is key!
- Address any underlying pathology.
- Remove reversible factors.
- Slow progression with rigorous blood pressure and diabetic control.
- Manage metabolic derangements: calcium/phosphate homeostasis, acidosis, hyperkalaemia.
- Address anaemia with epo and iron if required.
- Prepare for need for renal replacement therapy.

Renal Replacement Therapy

- Institute before life-threatening manifestations occur or symptoms unacceptable.

Revision Points *cont.*

- Most will have hospital haemodialysis.
- Peritoneal dialysis, either continuous ambulatory peritoneal dialysis or automated peritoneal dialysis, can offer greater control of their own management for those who are capable and who want it.
- Transplantation either from living or cadaveric donors potentially offers a much better quality of life. Complications include rejection, infection and malignancy.

Issues to Consider

- What are the advantages and disadvantages to both the patient and to healthcare services of the different modes of renal replacement therapy (renal transplantation, haemodialysis, continuous ambulatory peritoneal dialysis, automated peritoneal dialysis)?
- Why do we monitor parathyroid hormone levels?
- How can we increase the number of renal transplants?

- What are the implications of an increasingly obese population with an increasing prevalence of type II diabetes mellitus for provision of renal replacement therapy services? How will healthcare services meet this challenge?

Further Information

http://www.kidney.org/Professionals/kdoqi/
Links to guidelines on the various facets of the management of chronic kidney disease.

A 35-year-old woman with hypertension

Anne Tonkin

A 35-year-old woman presents to the emergency department complaining of 5 days of progressive generalized headache and nausea. Her blood pressure is measured and is recorded at 250/140 mmHg. The patient states that she has a family history of hypertension and was noted to be hypertensive for the first time 2 years ago. She had no investigations, but was treated with verapamil 80 mg tds. The patient stopped taking this after a few months because it made her constipated.

Q.1 What condition(s) may be responsible for this patient's presentation? What further history is required from her?

The patient does not have any relevant previous illnesses and had a tubal ligation 6 years ago. She complains of sweating, palpitations and anxiety. She takes no drugs, but smokes 10 cigarettes a day and consumes 100 g alcohol a week.

Q.2 What would you look for on examination?

On examination the patient is anxious and sweaty, but otherwise appears fit. Her pulse rate is 120 bpm and regular and her blood pressure 250/140 mmHg. Significant abnormalities include a forceful but undisplaced apical cardiac impulse without evidence of left ventricular failure, and a bruit in the left side of her abdomen. Urinalysis reveals 1+ (0.3 g/L) albumin only. Her retina is shown in Figure 38.1.

Figure 38.1

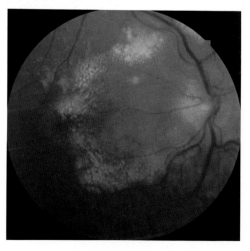

Q.3 What does this retinal photograph show?

The changes seen on fundoscopy are consistent with the clinical picture of severe hypertension.

You insert a radial arterial line for accurate monitoring of blood pressure and admit her to the high dependency ward. Her blood pressure improves with your chosen therapy, and you now have time to think about the possible cause of her hypertensive crisis.

The patient's complete blood picture, ESR, biochemistry, urine microscopy and culture and chest X-ray were normal. The ECG showed a sinus tachycardia and left axis deviation, but was otherwise normal. Urinary catecholamines were within normal limits.

Q.4 What type of treatment should immediately be instituted?

Q.5 What are the possible causes of this woman's hypertension and what investigations would you like to organize?

A renal ultrasound scan is normal. A radionuclide scan of the kidneys is performed, showing delayed perfusion and delayed function of the left kidney and then late hyperconcentration of the isotope in the left kidney. The right kidney contributes 65% of total renal function and the left kidney contributes 35%.

The patient went on to have the investigations shown in Figure 38.2 and Figure 38.3.

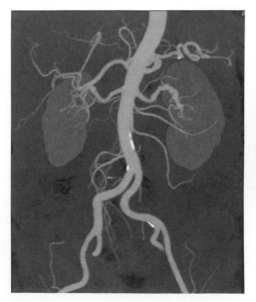

Figure 38.2

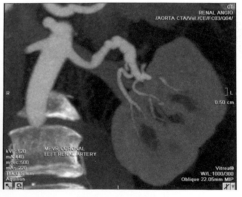

Figure 38.3

> ## Q.6
> What is the investigation and what does it show? How can this condition be treated?

These results strongly suggest left renal artery stenosis, but the diagnosis should be confirmed by either MRAngiography or intra-arterial renal angiography.

The patient had the most marked stenotic segment dilated via percutaneous transluminal balloon angioplasty, with a dramatic improvement in her blood pressure.

An important lesson in this case is that the patient was inadequately assessed on her first presentation with hypertension 2 years earlier. At that time the minimum investigation should have included urinalysis, serum biochemical analysis, ECG and possibly echocardiography (to assess for left ventricular hypertrophy), chest X-ray and lipid profile. In addition, there should have been careful follow-up and counselling to stop smoking.

In view of her young age, a specific underlying cause of her hypertension should have been considered. Further, if the abdominal bruit had been listened for (and been present and found) at her initial presentation, her fibromuscular dysplasia may have been diagnosed and the subsequent emergency avoided.

Patient education is vital to prevent loss to follow-up. If unacceptable side-effects occur, a switch to an alternative medication will promote compliance. Otherwise, their hypertension may go untreated for long periods.

Answers

A.1 She may have poorly controlled essential hypertension or hypertension secondary to underlying kidney disease, and an intercurrent problem such as a viral illness which has produced the headache and nausea. However, she has marked hypertension for a young person and may be in a hypertensive crisis. In this situation encephalopathy can occur which would be suggested by the headache and nausea. Her past medical history will be important as she may give a history of known poorly controlled hypertension or renal disease. You must inquire as to whether she may be pregnant (pre-eclampsia), although such severe hypertension would be very uncommon in early pregnancy.

You should ask her about the severity of her previously diagnosed hypertension, and whether she knows of her recent blood pressure readings – if it has been progressively increasing over several months the immediate risk is lower than if this has been a sudden rise over a few days or weeks.

Ask her about other symptoms associated with hypertensive encephalopathy such as irritability, visual disturbances, confusion, altered consciousness and seizures.

Ask about symptoms that might suggest an underlying disorder to account for her hypertension, such as:

- Renal disease: thirst, polyuria, nocturia, dysuria, haematuria, colic, lethargy and general malaise of uraemia.
- Phaeochromocytoma: sweating, palpitations, anxiety and tremor, particularly occurring in paroxysms.
- Cushing's syndrome: truncal weight gain, thinning of skin, easy bruising, weakness of proximal limb muscles, striae, hirsutism.

You will also need to ask about symptoms suggestive of hypertensive damage to the retina (visual deterioration) or the cardiovascular system, including

Answers *cont.*

acute myocardial ischaemia or cardiac failure (angina, dyspnoea, orthopnoea, ankle swelling), and aortic dissection (back pain).

A drug history is vital, including past use of analgesics (particularly NSAIDs: analgesic nephropathy), current use of drugs associated with hypertension, e.g. oral contraceptive pill, sympathomimetics (e.g. nasal decongestants), steroids, some antidepressants (including venlafaxine) and combinations of antidepressants associated with a risk of serotonergic syndrome (e.g. SSRIs and monoamine oxidase inhibitors). The patient's use of tobacco, alcohol and illicit drugs, particularly cocaine and amphetamine derivatives, should also be explored.

A.2 On examination you will need to look for evidence of hypertensive damage to:
• The CNS (level of consciousness, visual fields, focal neurological deficits).
• The retina (hypertensive retinopathy, especially haemorrhages, new exudates or optic disc swelling).
• The heart (left ventricular hypertrophy, left ventricular failure).
• The aorta (unequal pulses in aortic dissection).
• The kidney (haematuria or proteinuria on urinalysis).
Note: the presence of any acute features, especially neurological symptoms or signs, retinal haemorrhages, exudates or optic disc swelling, and abnormalities on urinalysis, suggests the presence of accelerated/malignant hypertension requiring emergency treatment.

You also need to look for features to suggest the underlying aetiology if the patient has secondary hypertension:
• Cushingoid habitus.
• Delayed femoral pulses in coarctation of the aorta.

• Palpable hydronephrotic or polycystic kidneys.
• Abdominal bruits.
• Appearance of uraemia.
• Sweating, tremor and tachycardia, and rarely, abdominal masses in phaeochromocytoma.
• Generalized oedema and/or abnormal urinalysis in glomerulonephritis.
• Evidence of a connective tissue disorder such as SLE or skin manifestations of vasculitis.

A.3 Figure 38.1 shows:
• Hard exudates.
• Cotton wool spots.
• Flame haemorrhages.
This is grade 3 hypertensive retinopathy. There is considerable hard exudate in the posterior pole with formation of a partial macular star.

In grade 4 retinopathy optic disc swelling would also be present, but there is no evidence that clinical outcomes differ on the basis of the fundoscopic findings and both grade 3 and grade 4 should be regarded as indicators of hypertensive emergency.

A.4 This is a hypertensive crisis because of the very high blood pressure readings together with symptoms and signs of impending or progressive target organ dysfunction. It is a medical emergency, and requires immediate admission to hospital, preferably to intensive care.
• She requires strict bed rest, continuous cardiac monitoring and intra-arterial blood pressure monitoring, together with frequent assessment of neurological status and urine output.
• Her blood pressure should be lowered gradually over several hours, aiming for no more than a 20–25% reduction in mean arterial pressure within the first hour, followed by further reduction to no

Answers *cont.*

lower than 160/100–110 mmHg, over the next 2–6 hours. A careful balance is required between reducing the pressure rapidly enough to prevent or reverse hypertensive encephalopathy and reducing it too rapidly so that perfusion is reduced with the attendant risk of cerebral hypoperfusion and infarction (stroke).

- Blood pressure reduction using a short-acting parenteral agent, titrated according to the blood pressure response, is safer than fixed doses of intravenous, oral or sublingual antihypertensive agents.
- The preferred agents include labetalol (combined alpha and beta blocker), esmolol (short-acting beta blocker), nicardipine (calcium channel blocker) and fenoldopam (a vasodilator that acts by selectively blocking dopamine D_1 receptors). Sodium nitroprusside can also be effective, but has significant toxicity and should generally be avoided. The use of oral nifedipine capsules is no longer recommended because they have a rapid onset of action and reach very high peak plasma concentrations, resulting in the potential for sudden uncontrolled blood pressure reduction and precipitation of stroke.
- Once blood pressure is lowered, a combination of oral antihypertensive agents will probably be needed to maintain good control, the choice depending on the characteristics of the patient. Initially, sodium and volume depletion may be present, and diuretics should not be used until these have been corrected. Combinations of other first-line drugs including angiotensin converting enzyme (ACE) inhibitors, angiotensin receptor blockers, and calcium channel blockers and could be considered. Beta blockers are no longer regarded as

first-line antihypertensive drugs unless indicated for a concomitant condition.
- This patient has a renal bruit; in patients with clinical evidence of possible renal artery stenosis, calcium channel blockers and beta blockade may be safer and more effective than therapy based on an angiotensin converting enzyme (ACE) inhibitor or angiotensin receptor blocker while the diagnosis is pursued, although in the longer term, renin-angiotensin system inhibitors provide renoprotection if acute kidney injury is avoided.
- Note that beta blockers can cause a paradoxical and possibly dangerous rise in hypertension in the presence of phaeochromocytoma, while angiotensin converting enzyme (ACE) inhibitors (e.g. captopril) can precipitate a marked deterioration in renal function in patients with bilateral renal artery stenosis.

A.5 This woman may have essential (primary) hypertension as she does have a positive family history and the hypertension may be exacerbated by smoking and alcohol. However, the severity of her hypertension at her young age suggests a specific underlying cause. The common causes of secondary hypertension include:

- Renal parenchymal disease:
  - unilateral, e.g. pyelonephritis, obstructive or reflux nephropathy, dysplasia, trauma
  - bilateral, e.g. any cause of chronic renal failure, obstructive or reflux nephropathy, diabetes mellitus, analgesic nephropathy, polycystic disease, pyelonephritis, glomerulonephritis, interstitial nephritis.
- Renovascular disease: renal artery stenosis secondary to atheroma, fibromuscular hyperplasia (especially in younger patients), trauma.

Answers *cont.*

- Pregnancy: pre-eclampsia.
- Adrenal disorders: e.g. phaeochromocytoma, Cushing's syndrome, primary aldosteronism (Conn's syndrome).
- Drug associated: e.g. oral contraceptive pill (common), corticosteroids, sympathomimetics, alcoholism.
- Cardiovascular: e.g. coarctation of the aorta.

With her anxiety, sweating and resting tachycardia, it is prudent to exclude a phaeochromocytoma, but her abdominal bruit suggests the possibility of renal artery stenosis. Baseline investigations should include:

- Complete blood picture and ESR.
- Electrolytes, including blood glucose, urea and creatinine.
- Urine microscopy (for casts and cells).
- Chest X-ray and ECG (to detect left ventricular hypertrophy); echocardiography could also be considered.

The next investigation of choice would be a non-invasive screening test for renal artery stenosis. Several different tests can be done, and these include, duplex ultrasound scanning (with or without contrast enhancement), spiral CT angiography and gadolinium-enhanced magnetic resonance angiography (MRA), and radionuclidescans with ACE inhibitor challenge. MRI studies are becoming more technologically advanced and are now able to provide details of morphological damage and function of the kidney itself, allowing better prediction of the potential outcomes of reperfusion. Radionuclide studies are no longer recommended as first line screening because of poor sensitivity and specificity. Catheter angiography of the renal arteries is the 'gold standard' and can identify disease in the branch vessels as well as in the main renal arteries. The site of stenosis varies depending on the nature of the disease, with atherosclerotic renal artery stenosis being more likely to occur at the origin of the renal artery, and fibromuscular dysplasia more likely to be found in the middle or distal part of the artery.

Given the clinical context, this patient should also be screened for a phaeochromocytoma by assessing production of catecholamines. This is usually done by performing a 24-hour urine collection, assayed for excreted catecholamines and their metabolites (creatinine, total catecholamines, vanillylmandelic acid, and metanephrines). Ideally, uring should be collected during a hypertensive crisis where hormone levels are at their highest. Serum plasma metaneprhines is also a useful test, which is more sensitive but less specific.

A.6 Figure 38.2 is a CT angiogram defining the abdominal aorta and its main branches, including the two renal arteries. There are several narrowed segments in the left renal artery, with a pattern referred to as 'beading'. This is typically caused by Fibromuscular Dysplasia. There are no changes to suggest significant atheromatous disease of the renal arteries (although there is mild calcific plaque seen in the aorta below the renal arteries). Figure 38.3 is a close-up image of the left renal CT scan, demonstrating the charictieristic beadin pattern. Figure 38.4 shows a renal MR Angiogram of a different patient with right renal artery fibromuscular dysplasia. MR Angiography is beoming more commonly performed, as gadolinium is less reno-toxic than iodine-based contrast agents (unless the patient has severe renal impairment, in which case all forms of imaging contrast have risks).

Answers *cont.*

The preferred treatment for Fibromuscular Dysplasia is percutaneous balloon angioplasty +/– stenting of the diseased segments.

Figure 38.5 is an invasive renal angiogram of the same patient shown in Figure 38.4, during preparation for balloon angioplasty and stenting procedure.

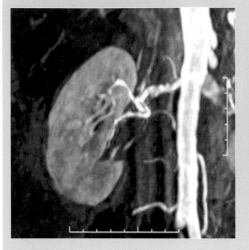

Figure 38.4

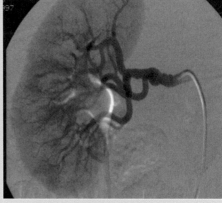

Figure 38.5

Revision Points

Hypertensive Emergencies

Incidence

Less than 1% of all cases of hypertension; secondary hypertension accounts for about 5% of all cases of hypertension but 25–50% of cases of hypertensive emergency.

Risk Factors

• For hypertension: family history, obesity, alcohol abuse.

• For hypertensive crisis: secondary hypertension (esp. renal disease, renovascular disease), oral contraceptive pill, smoking.

Presentation

Headache, visual impairment, dizziness, anxiety, disorientation, tremor, seizures, nausea, vomiting, abdominal pain.

Clinical Features

• Usually severe hypertension (diastolic BP >120) but organ dysfunction may occur at moderate BP levels if BP has risen rapidly from a low baseline.

• Grade 3 or 4 retinopathy (haemorrhages, exudates ± optic disc swelling).

• Proteinuria is common.

• May be focal neurological findings, acute left ventricular failure.

Prognosis

Untreated prognosis is very poor, with 5-year survival about 1%; with antihypertensive treatment 5-year survival is about 75%.

Early Management

• Investigations: plasma electrolytes, urea and creatinine, blood picture, ESR;

Revision Points *cont.*

ECG; chest X-ray; urinalysis and urine microscopy.
- Intra-arterial BP monitoring and intensive care, with infusion of short-acting antihypertensive (labetalol, nicardipine, esmolol or fenoldopam) titrated to response, aiming for no more than 20–25% reduction in BP over first hour.

Later Management

Investigations for secondary hypertension as clinically indicated and specific management if a cause is found.

Combination oral antihypertensive drug therapy according to clinical features (usually require at least two drugs for initial control). ACE inhibitors, long-acting calcium channel blockers, atenolol, and prazosin have all been used successfully. Thiazide diuretics could be used if not volume depleted.

Renovascular Hypertension

Epidemiology

- Accounts for approximately 5–10% of all cases of hypertension and about 15% of cases of hypertensive emergencies.
- Atheromatous renovascular disease is the most common form (seen mainly in elderly patients, men more than women, with vascular risk factors).
- Fibromuscular hyperplasia may account for about 10% of cases and is diagnosed most commonly in women between the ages of 30 and 50 without other vascular disease (bilateral in about 50%).

Diagnosis of Renal Artery Stenosis

- Non-invasive screening initially: duplex ultrasonography, contrast-enhanced magnetic resonance angiography or spiral CT angiography.

- The captopril-challenged isotopic renal scan gives information about individual renal function, but is no longer recommended because of poor sensitivity and specificity.

Ultrasound, CT and MRA have reasonable sensitivity and specificity when performed skilfully, and both renal perfusion scanning and MRI techniques can also indicates functional significance of any stenosis. If isotopic scanning is used and is highly suggestive of renal artery stenosis, then an angiographic method should be used to establish the anatomy of the lesion. Fibromuscular dysplasia has a characteristic 'string of beads' appearance, while atherosclerotic lesions usually present as smooth stenoses close to the origin of the renal artery. Intra-arterial angiography can be followed immediately by angioplasty (plus stenting in the case of significant atherosclerotic disease) following diagnosis.

Treatment

Indications for treatment are uncontrollable hypertension and deteriorating renal function.

Best treated by balloon angioplasty, or surgery if this is unsuccessful; in fibromuscular dysplasia, 60% of patients treated by percutaneous balloon angioplasty will remain cured at the end of 12 months and long-term prognosis is good. Patients with atherosclerotic renal artery stenosis have been shown to do as well with intensive medical management as with angioplasty.

Issues to Consider

- What non-pharmaceutical methods can hypertensives employ to lower their blood pressure?
- How would you control hypertension secondary to a phaeochromocytoma?
- How would the clinical scenario be likely to differ in a case of atheromatous renal artery stenosis? (Consider likely epidemiology and time-course of development.)

Further Information

http://www.clevelandclinicmeded.com/medicalpubs/diseasemanagement/nephrology/hypertensive-crises/

www.ash-us.org *Website of the American Society for Hypertension with lots of links.*

http://emedicine.medscape.com/article/1161248-overview. *Fibromuscular dysplasia – updated 2007.*

Plouin, P.-F., Bax, L., 2010. Diagnosis and treatment of renal artery stenosis. Nat. Rev. Nephrol. 6, 151–159.

A young man with depressed conscious state and seizures

Michelle Kiley

A young man is brought into the emergency department early one morning. He was found 'unconscious' in the street and an ambulance called. There were no witnesses. Immediate assessment shows that his airway is intact and patent, he has normal colour, respiratory rate and pulse oximetry. There is no circulatory compromise. There are no obvious injuries.

He is stuporose and responds with sluggish but purposeful limb movements to painful stimuli. He groans, but does not make any comprehensible sounds. His Glasgow coma score is 6 (E1, V2, M3). He has a temperature of 37°C and cardiorespiratory examination is normal. The pupils are mid-position, equal and reactive and the optic fundi are normal. The plantars are downgoing. He has no neck stiffness and Kernig's sign is negative. No focal neurological abnormality can be elicited. The rest of the physical examination is normal.

Q.1 What test should immediately be performed on arrival in the emergency department and what else should be sought on examination?

The test does not help elucidate the cause of the patient's collapse. The man is reasonably well kempt but there is a faint smell of alcohol on his breath. On closer inspection there is a superficial laceration over the occiput and bruising of the right lateral aspect of the tongue. The patient's underpants are found to be damp with urine.

Before any further assessment is performed the patient suddenly lets out a grunt, all four limbs extend and his spine arches. He stops breathing and rapidly becomes cyanosed. After 30 seconds, violent rhythmic contractions of the limbs begin and persist for at least 5 minutes

Q.2 What is the diagnosis, and what should be done for the patient?

The seizure is aborted after 10 mg intravenous diazepam. At this stage a brother, who had been contacted by the nursing staff, arrives and provides further information. The patient is 24, has had epilepsy since his mid teens, and has been on regular anticonvulsant medication, although the brother is unsure as to the medication's name.

Q.3 What are the causes of this condition? What are the likely causes in this patient?

The brother states that the patient has seizures every few months and his local doctor has told him that due to his poorly controlled epilepsy he is currently ineligible to drive and that it is the patient's responsibility to inform the local licensing authorities. Over the last few days the patient has had several late nights, despite having an upper respiratory tract infection, including the previous night in which he had been out with his brother drinking until the early hours of the morning. He seemed reasonably well when he left the bar, saying that he would walk home.

The patient slowly regains consciousness over the next hour. His last recollection was leaving the bar with his brother the night before. He confirms his brother's account and admits he has not taken his anticonvulsant medication (carbamazepine) for 2 days. In addition to occasional generalized tonic seizures the patient reports isolated myoclonic jerks of the arms and trunk, which usually occur first thing in the morning or later at night, particularly when tired.

Q.4 How will you manage this patient in the short term?

An electroencephalogram (EEG) is performed (Figure 39.1), as one had not been done since diagnosis many years ago. This shows 4–5 Hz paroxysmal generalized polyspike and wave discharges consistent with the diagnosis of primary generalized epilepsy.

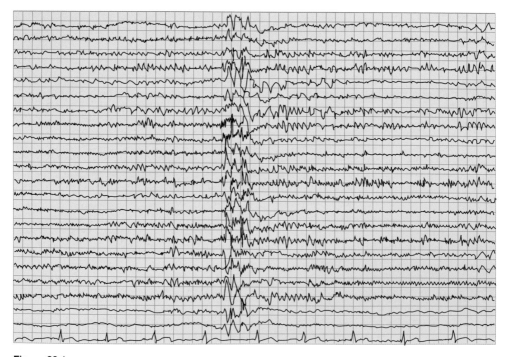

Figure 39.1

Q.5 How are you going to manage his medications?

You counsel the patient about the medications you feel most appropriate for his needs, and spend some time talking to him about his illness.

Q.6 What other advice will you offer him?

Q.7 The patient asks you when he is likely to be able to stop taking anticonvulsant medication. What is your reply?

Answers

A.1 Hypoglycaemia should be promptly excluded by blood glucose estimation.

Further examination should be undertaken for evidence of:

- Drug abuse (needle tracks) and/or drugs or drug paraphernalia on his person.
- Seizure (tongue biting or incontinence).
- Medication usage (medical alert bracelet, personal details in pockets, any information about medications such as sedatives, antidepressants or illicit drugs).
- Signs of chronic liver disease.
- Head injury.
- Assess if the patient is kempt or unkempt and asssess the breath for the smell of alcohol.
- Look for a form of identification or any other personal items that will enable you to contact relatives or friends. Most importantly, these people may be able to give a history.

A.2 The initial clinical picture is consistent with a post-ictal state. The subsequent event was a generalized tonic–clonic seizure. He has not regained consciousness between seizures and the second seizure persisted for at least 5 minutes. He fits the operational definition of convulsive status epilepticus. This is defined as continuous or recurrent generalized seizure activity of greater than 5–10 minutes. There is some evidence that a convulsive seizure of at least 5 minutes duration is unlikely to self-abort. Repeated and or prolonged tonic–clonic seizures are life-threatening

and require prompt treatment to avoid refractory status epilepticus which carries a 30% mortality.

Management consists of:

- Clear and maintain the airway and call for support.
- Monitor cardiac and respiratory status.
- Give high-flow oxygen by face mask and connect a pulse oximeter.
- Establish intravenous access × 2 with large-bore cannulae.
- Give an intravenous benzodiazepine – ideally lorazepam 4 mg (0.7 mg/kg), but if not available then diazepam (5–10 mg at a rate not exceeding 5 mg/min) OR midazolam (1–5 mg at a rate not exceeding 2 mg/min).

  If immediate IV access can not be gained then give midazolam 5 mg intramuscularly and consider insertion of a central line.
- Check for respiratory depression.
- Collect blood for glucose, electrolytes, complete blood picture, toxicology screen and if applicable anti-epileptic drug levels. Also obtain arterial blood gas and pH estimation.
- If lorazapam* is not the benzodiazepine given then load with intravenous

*Lorazepam has a much longer half-life than diazepam or midazolam and thus phenytoin is only required if lorazepam fails to stop the seizure. Due to the higher risk of recurrent seizure activity with shorter-acting benzodiazepines, phenytoin should be given prophylatically. One of the leading causes of refractory status epilepticus is early under-management.

Answers *cont.*

phenytoin via separate IV access
(15–20 mg/kg given at a rate of 50 mg/
min, unless elderly or known history of
cardiac or hepatic impairment in which
case the rate should be reduced to
25 mg/min).
• If seizures persist despite the above,
  prepare to intubate and ventilate the
  patient.

A general anaesthetic agent (thiopental/
propofol/midazolam) can then be used to
control refractory seizures. There is no
evidence that any one of these agents is
superior to any other – they all have both
advantages and disadvantages.

If facilities are not available to intubate/
ventilate, but seizures persist despite
loading with phenytoin, consider IV
phenobarbital (10 mg/kg given at a rate of
no greater than 50 mg/min).

Once a patient with status epilepticus is
intubated and ventilated it is imperative that
EEG/consultant neurologist advice is sought
to assist in guiding ongoing treatment.

Only when control of the seizure is
obtained can the underlying cause be
sought and treated.

A.3 Common causes of status
epilepticus in adults include:
• Epilepsy exacerbated by non-compliance
  with medications, intercurrent illness,
  other lifestyle factors such as alcohol
  abuse, use of other recreational drugs or
  sleep deprivation. The lifetime incidence
  of convulsive status epilepticus in adults
  with epilepsy is 5% and the most
  common cause is low anti-epileptic drug
  levels.
• Head trauma.
• Space-occupying lesion, e.g. brain
  tumour or metastases.
• Stroke including both cerebral infarction
  and haemorrhage.

• Central nervous system infection.
• Metabolic disorders.
• Medication effects including drug
  withdrawal.

Any of these causes are possible in this
patient. Although there are no signs of
meningism or focal neurological signs,
meningitis, encephalitis or a subarachnoid
haemorrhage are still possibilities.
Withdrawal from alcohol or sedative
medications should also be considered.
Further history would be the most helpful in
determining the cause and will determine if
further investigations, such as a CT scan of
the brain, are necessary. If the patient is
not a known epileptic then this investigation
should definitely be undertaken. If recovery
is slow or there are focal neurological signs
in the setting of known epilepsy then
imaging should be strongly considered.

A.4 The additional information from the
patient's brother and the patient's rapid
recovery diminishes the need for further
investigations. As above, in the absence of
a history of epilepsy and/or focal signs/slow
recovery, the next investigation would be a
CT scan. A negative CT would be followed
by a lumbar puncture.

In this instance the underlying cause of
the status epilepticus was longstanding
primary generalized epilepsy exacerbated
by:
• Non-compliance with medication.
• Intercurrent viral illness.
• Alcohol abuse.
• Sleep deprivation.

An EEG may be useful, not to determine
whether a seizure has occurred – this will
be apparent from the history – but to
provide information about the type of
epilepsy, i.e. partial/focal or generalized,
and thus guide further investigation
(particularly if a focal discharge is found)

Answers *cont.*

and the choice of anticonvulsant (as in this case).

A.5 This patient has generalized tonic–clonic and myoclonic seizures and an EEG pattern of idiopathic generalized epilepsy (IGE) with 4–5 Hz polyspike and wave discharges, rather than focal epilepsy with secondary generalization. The history and EEG findings are consistent with juvenile myoclonic epilepsy (JME), the most common form of IGE. This diagnosis influences the optimal choice of anticonvulsant. Single-drug therapy with sodium valproate would be more appropriate than carbamazepine in this instance (carbamazepine is not advised for JME as it may exacerbate myoclonus). The effectiveness of drug therapy, once the patient is compliant, is best assessed by the clinical reduction in seizure frequency. Serum blood levels can be used to monitor compliance if that is in doubt, but serum levels for sodium valproate are very variable and are not advised routinely. Serum levels for carbamazepine are of greater consistency and thus may help guide dosing. If seizures persist, alternative and/or adjunctive therapy should be considered. The more highly effective agents, in addition to sodium valproate, for IGE include lamotrigine, levetiracetam and topiramate. Carbamazepine is the drug of first choice for partial/focal seizure disorders and serum carbamazepine levels are consistent and helpful in determining therapeutic dosage. At this stage referral to a neurologist is advisable.

A.6 The patient has had a life-threatening exacerbation of his epilepsy. This is a good time to discuss the importance of better illness management with him. You should emphasize that the combination of non-compliance with medications, sleep deprivation and alcohol, or in fact any of the above in isolation, will significantly lower seizure threshold. Therefore, he must:

• Be compliant with medication.
• Use alcohol in moderation, e.g. 1–2 drinks daily.
• Avoid alcohol excess, particularly binges.
• Avoid sleep deprivation and fatigue.
• Give up driving until his epilepsy is controlled. The length of time he is not able to drive will be determined by local/ national guidelines and the advice of a consultant neurologist.
• Take precautions at work and with recreation (particular care with fire/ heights/water).
• Wear a medical alert bracelet and carry information concerning his diagnosis and medication on his person at all times.

A.7 Up to 90% of patients with idiopathic generalized epilepsy will achieve freedom from seizures with anticonvulsant therapy. Lifestyle factors (especially avoidance of sleep deprivation) are also extremely important in maintaining seizure control. The chance of seizure freedom with partial seizure disorders is not quite as good, about 65% with monotherapy and up to 75–80% with polytherapy. In considering when to stop anticonvulsant medication, the chance of continued remission after anticonvulsant withdrawal is greatest in those who have been seizure free for more than 2 years on anticonvulsants, have a single seizure type, a normal neurological examination, no underlying structural abnormality of the brain and a normal EEG (of greater relevance in IGE, persisting focal changes in partial seizure disorders are not helpful in guiding the withdrawal of medication). Conversely, those with a structural brain abnormality, an abnormal

Answers *cont.*

EEG, more than one seizure type and poor seizure control requiring more than one anticonvulsant medication, have a high risk of seizure recurrence if medication is stopped. The risk of having further seizures and the impact of seizures on daily activities (for example driving) should be taken into account before recommending withdrawal of anticonvulsants.

Revision Points

Management of the First Seizure

Emergency Care

Check **ABC**: i.e. airway, breathing and circulation. Stop seizure of greater than 5 minutes' duration with intravenous benzodiazepine, e.g. diazepam.

Aetiology

The likely cause depends on the patient's age. Idiopathic generalized epilepsy is unlikely to present for the first time in the elderly but is a common cause in young adults, as is drug and alcohol abuse. Space-occupying lesions, stroke and metabolic disturbance are all more common causes in the elderly, but all causes can occur at any age.

History

From the patient retrospectively, plus an eyewitness account is invaluable:
- How did the seizure start?
- Any aura?
- Any focal or lateralizing features at seizure onset?
- Seizure duration?
- Time taken to recover?
- Past history of head trauma, neurological illness, other diseases (e.g. cardiovascular or cancer), drug and alcohol consumption.
- Family history.
- Associated symptoms, e.g. recent headaches, fever.

Investigations

Always search for an underlying cause:
- Neurological disorder:
  - meningitis/encephalitis
  - space-occupying lesion (tumour)
  - stroke/subarachnoid haemorrhage
- Metabolic disturbance:
  - hypoglycaemia
  - hyponatraemia
  - hypercalcaemia.
- Drug and alcohol abuse.
- Head injury.

Investigations depend on suspected underlying cause but all patients should have complete blood picture, glucose, electrolytes and CT scan. Further investigations may include LP, MRI, EEG, toxicology.

Management

Depends on underlying cause. All patients should be given strict advice about driving according to national regulations.

Issues to Consider

- What advice would you give about driving to a young man presenting with a witnessed first fit?
- What non-pharmacological treatments are available for the treatment of debilitating epilepsy?
- What are the detrimental effects of long-term phenytoin therapy?

Further Information

http://www.epilepsysociety.org.uk/ Forprofessionals *A superb resource for professionals interested in epilepsy from the National Society for Epilepsy. Hundreds of articles, references, literature reviews.*

www.epilepsy.org.uk *A good website from the British Epilepsy Association with lots of information for patients, carers, professionals. Lots of links.*

A middle-aged man with sudden visual loss

Sumu Simon and Robert Fitridge

A 61-year-old man presents to the emergency department with complaints of sudden transient right monocular visual loss. During the interview, he gives a history of two such episodes over the past 24 hours, the last being just about an hour ago. During each episode, his vision became grey and washed out and cleared completely within 5–10 minutes. He denies other symptoms such as headache, nausea, ocular pain, redness, aura or visual haloes. You have been treating this patient for essential hypertension for approximately 5 years, although he has not been completely compliant with medication and follow-up for blood pressure monitoring. He has no other significant medical history, and his only medication is atenolol 50 mg daily. He is obese and is a habitual smoker. He is feeling physically fit, and you are unable to elicit any additional complaints in a review of symptoms. He has a bruit heard in the right neck.

Q.1 What condition is the patient describing? What are the possible aetiologies?

On examination, you measure the blood pressure at 150/95 mmHg. There is no evidence of postural hypotension. Vision, visual fields, pupillary responses, anterior segment examination, gonioscopy and applanation tonometry findings are normal. Visualization of the retina with a direct ophthalmoscope reveals the finding illustrated in Figure 40.1.

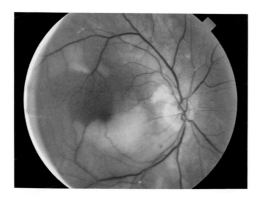

Figure 40.1

Q.2 What sign is present in this fundus photograph? What additional physical examination would you perform as part of your initial assessment?

Q.3 What additional investigations would you order at the same time?

After completing the clinical examination, you arrange carotid Doppler ultrasonography. This indicates a severe (85%) stenosis of the origin of the right internal carotid artery. There is also mild stenosis (no more than 50%) in the region of bifurcation of the left common carotid artery.

Q.4 What treatment would you recommend to this patient?

After evaluating the results of all investigations, you discuss possible medical treatment and surgical intervention with the patient. The patient tells you that on the evening prior to the review appointment, while he was sitting watching television, his left arm became weak and he was unable to pick up his coffee cup. On trying to stand, he found his left leg was dragging, and he was forced to sit down. The episode lasted approximately 10 minutes.

The patient decides in favour of the suggested surgical procedure. In preparation for this, the surgeon orders the radiological study illustrated in Figure 40.2.

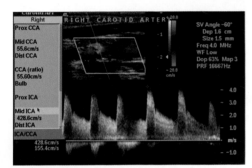

Figure 40.2

Q.5 What is this study? Are the findings consistent with the proposed surgical procedure?

The patient undergoes successful carotid surgery. Postoperatively he is maintained on aspirin and is referred to the cardiac rehabilitation service to improve his lifestyle.

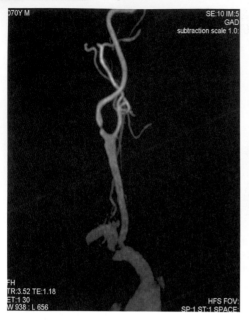

Figure 40.3

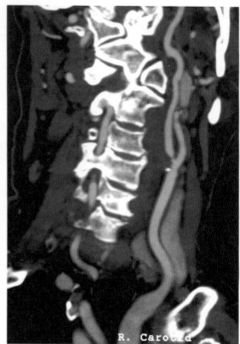

Figure 40.4

Answers

A.1 This patient has presented with transient monocular visual loss (TMVL) or 'amaurosis fugax'. TMVL is characterized by sudden onset of unilateral visual loss lasting no longer than 24 hours. Commonly of ischemic aetiology, the vascular condition can be in the eye or its vicinity, or can be remote.

TMVL can be due to impaired arterial perfusion (retinal, choroidal or optic nerve ciliary arteries) or to venous stasis. Impending central retinal vein occlusion and central retinal vein occlusion can present with TMVL.

Common causes include arteriosclerosis, hypercoagulable and hyperviscosity states. Though rare, vasculitis and retinal migraine (vasospasm of the retinal arteries) can present with transient visual loss. It is important to consider the possibility of

temporal arteritis which may involve the ophthalmic arteries, and has the potential to lead rapidly to arterial occlusion and devastating bilateral blindness. This is most often seen in elderly patients, and other symptoms may include headache, scalp tenderness often apparent when brushing the hair, and jaw claudication, which may occur on chewing food. Polymyalgia rheumatica may co-exist.

TMVL that lasts only for a few seconds is called transient visual obscurations and is typically seen in optic disc oedema (with or without drusen) and in congenital anomalies of the optic disc. The most frequent remote cause for TMVL is *carotid stenosis* (due to atherosclerosis) rather than cardiac source emboli. The site of carotid stenosis is usually at the termination or at the bifurcation of the common carotid artery or

Answers *cont.*

at the origin of the internal carotid artery. Cardiac emboli are associated with atrial fibrillation, mural thrombi (after myocardial infarction) and diseased valves. Other remote causes includes stenosis of the aortic arch and ophthalmic arteries, systemic hypotension and diminished cardiac output. Rarely carotid artery dissection can present with TMVL and may be associated with neck pain and Horner's syndrome.

Ocular disorders such as intermittent angle closure glaucoma, hyphaema, optic nerve demyelination (Uthoff's phenomenon) and keratoconus can also mimic transient visual loss and need to be ruled out by ophthalmologic evaluation.

A.2 Figure 40.1 illustrates an embolus at the branch of a retinal artery.

This is most likely a cholesterol embolus or 'Hollenhorst plaque', originating from the carotid arterial system.

When evaluating a patient with transient monocular visual loss, a careful cardiovascular examination is essential, including measurement of pulse and blood pressure, examination of carotid and temporal arteries, and assessment of the heart. Remember that the absence of a carotid bruit does *not* rule out significant carotid disease. Indeed, the most severely diseased carotids often do not have an associated bruit. This patient has an elevated blood pressure, possibly reflecting poor compliance with antihypertensive medication, which is a risk factor for carotid atherosclerosis.

A.3 Essential investigations should include:
- Urinalysis and fasting serum glucose level.
- Fasting serum lipid profile.
- ECG.

- Carotid duplex ultrasound.
  Other investigations which may be useful:
- Echocardiography (transthoracic/ transoesophageal) is indicated if a significant cardiac abnormality, aortic arch atheroma, atrial appendage thrombus or mural thrombi is suspected.
- Erythrocyte sedimentation rate (ESR) is an important part of evaluation for vasculitis.
- C-reactive protein: CRP is more sensitive (100%) than ESR (92%) in detecting giant cell arteritis. The specificity rate for combined ESR and C-reactive protein in temporal arteritis is 97%.
- In a young person, or if clinical examination suggests an unusual cause, other tests such as autoimmune screening, coagulation studies and tests for hyperviscosity syndromes should be considered to rule out vasculitis and hypercoagulable/hyperviscosity states.
- Doppler of ophthalmic artery – this can reveal stenosis or occlusion of the ophthalmic artery.
- Fundus fluorescein angiography – to evalute choroidal and retinal perfusion abnormalities.

A.4 This patient has suffered a second episode of right monocular blindness and left-hand weakness, while awaiting confirmation of the diagnosis. He is at high risk of having a stroke.
- Aspirin (100–300 mg daily) has a proven role in reducing the risk of stroke. In the absence of contraindications, this medication can be started immediately if the diagnosis of carotid atheroma is suspected.
- Carotid duplex ultrasound scan (Figure 40.2) of the right internal carotid artery shows a peak systolic velocity of 428 cm/s, end diastolic velocity of 155 cm/s. This equates to a severe

Answers *cont.*

internal carotid artery stenosis in the range of 80–99%.

- Contrast-enhanced MR angiogram (Figure 40.3) shows a high-grade stenosis at origin of the right internal carotid. A CT angiogram (Figure 40.4) confirms this lesion as a high-grade stenosis with focal mixed calcified and soft plaque at origin of the right internal carotid, with plaque extending into the common carotid artery (note: not all three imaging modalities are required, but they are presented here in a single patient for educational purposes).
- Carotid endarterectomy is definitive therapy when performed by a skilled vascular surgeon who has an acceptable complication rate. Endarterectomy significantly reduces the risk of subsequent stroke for patients with retinal or cerebral ischaemic symptoms related to severe (70–99%) carotid stenotic lesions. Patients with moderate stenoses (50–69%) may benefit from this surgery, but are generally managed medically. Patients with mild stenoses (less than 50%) have no benefit from intervention. The role for carotid endarterectomy in the treatment of asymptomatic carotid arterial stenosis is still debated. In this patient, with a high-grade symptomatic right internal carotid arterial stenosis, right carotid endarterectomy would be recommended.
- Carotid artery stenting, via a percutaneous approach, is an emerging procedure and has been shown to have similar outcomes to surgery in high-risk patients. Using this approach in lower-risk patients is currently being evaluated in clinical trials. Some controversy exists regarding patient selection for surgery versus stenting.
- Pharmacological stroke prevention should be continued after the surgery.
- Risk factor reduction is essential. This patient has a number of significant cardiovascular risk factors.
- Control of blood pressure is important, and tight control will reduce his absolute risk of stroke and of cardiac disease. Cessation of smoking is another important preventative measure. If the glucose measurement indicates diabetes mellitus or the lipid profile is abnormal, appropriate dietary and pharmacological measures should be instituted.

A.5 As an imaging tool performed prior to carotid endarterectomy, invasive carotid angiography has been replaced by spiral CT angiography and magnetic resonance angiography. These latter two procedures are much less invasive and pose less risk to the patient. Carotid Doppler examination is still widely used and, in expert hands, remains a sensitive tool for the detection of carotid disease.

In this patient, the CT angiogram confirms a severe stenosis at the take-off of the right internal carotid artery, consistent with his symptoms of right amaurosis fugax and left-sided weakness. Yet the artery remains patent. This is an important observation, as endarterectomy cannot be performed on a completely occluded vessel. In other words, the angiographic findings are consistent with the proposed surgical procedure.

Revision Points

Transient Monocular Vision Loss

Definition
Transient ischaemic attack with sudden complete monocular loss of vision with complete recovery within 24 hours.

Differential Diagnoses
- Cardiac disease.
- Aortic arch atheroma.
- Temporal arteritis.
- Hypercoagulability syndromes.
- Vasculitis.
- Optic disc oedema and congenital disc anomalies.

History Focus
- Hypertension.
- Smoking.
- Diabetes mellitus.
- Hyperlipidaemia.
- Cardiac disease.

Examination Focus
- Pulse.
- Blood pressure.
- Rhythm (atrial fibrillation).
- Carotid arteries.
- Temporal arteries.
- Ocular examination.

Investigations
- Carotid Doppler ultrasound.
- CT angiography or MR angiography if intervention contemplated.
- Urinalysis.
- Fasting serum glucose.
- Fasting serum lipid profile.
- Electrocardiogram.
- Consider erythrocyte sedimentation rate, C-reactive protein.

Treatment
- Treat reversible risk factors.
- If no contraindications, commence aspirin (300 mg daily).
- Consider carotid endarterectomy.

Issues to Consider

- Revise the anatomy of the cerebral circulation. For each major vessel, what would be the clinical effect of a transient occlusion (TIA) in that vessel?
- How does warfarin compare with aspirin in the secondary prevention of ischaemic strokes?
- What complications of endarterectomy would you warn the patient about when seeking consent?
- What is the current evidence for stenting versus surgery for carotid disease?

Further Information

Amick, A., Caplan, L.R., 2007. Transient monocular visual loss. Comprehensive Ophthalmology Update 8 (2), 91–98.

Biousse, V., Trobe, J.D., 2005. Transient monocular vision loss. American Journal of Ophthalmology 140, 717–722.

http://neurosurgery.mgh.harvard.edu/ *The website of the neurosurgical vascular service at Harvard with lots of information about carotid endarterectomy.*

www.emedicine.com/emerg/topic604.htm *Transient ischaemic attacks.*

www.pvss.org *Website of the Peripheral Vascular Surgical Society with information for patients and professionals including case studies, an atlas and intraoperative photographs.*

'Jack has leg weakness'

Gabriel Lee

Jack is a 39-year-old electrical engineer. In the past few months, he has noticed that his left leg feels weak. There is intermittent numbness. His wife tells you that Jack has been 'walking funny'.

Q.1 What other questions would you like to ask Jack to clarify the history further?

On specific enquiry, Jack says that he has experienced some headaches recently. These are not associated with nausea and vomiting. He has no spinal pain or sciatica. He has no significant family history. His general health has been excellent.

Q.2 What relevance has his headache in the context of his leg weakness?

You examine him carefully. He is a well-looking man who appears slightly anxious. His temperature is 37.1°C. His blood pressure is 140/80 mmHg and heart rate 85 bpm. Chest and abdominal examination findings were unremarkable.

Neurological examination shows an abnormal gait with an obvious limp. There were no cranial nerve deficits. Upper limb examination shows no focal deficits. Lower limb examination shows a pyramidal pattern of weakness which is most prominent distally (NHMRC power graded 3/5) and increased tone in the left lower limb. Left lower limb reflexes were hyper-reflexic (right lower limb reflexes normal). There was sustained myoclonus present at the left ankle. Sensory testing to light touch and pin-prick were within normal limits. Distal proprioception was normal bilaterally. Plantar response was equivocal on left and flexor on the right.

Q.3 What do the examination findings indicate?

You put your examination findings together, and think about what to do next.

Q.4 What investigations should you consider?

You perform your investigation of choice.

Q.5 What do the following images show?

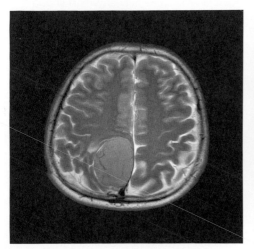

Figure 41.1

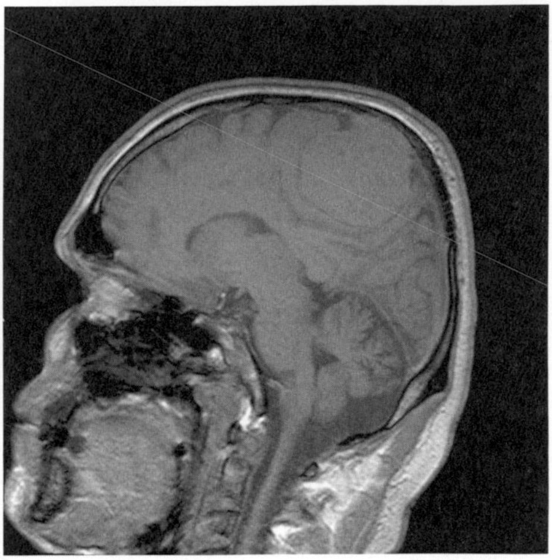

Figure 41.2

Figure 41.3

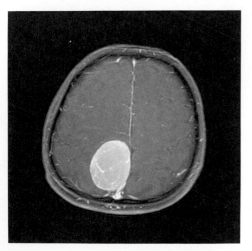

You admit Jack to hospital in the neurosurgery unit, and commence him on oral dexamethasone. This resulted in mild improvement of his lower limb weakness. He undergoes a right craniotomy and excision of the intracranial lesion. The surgery was uncomplicated. Postoperatively, Jack's lower limb weakness was significantly improved over the previous week, and he attends rehabilitation classes with good recovery of function. The histopathology was consistent with meningioma.

Answers

A.1   The clinical history is of utmost importance in the assessment of a neurological illness. In a patient presenting with unilateral limb weakness and sensory disturbance, questions should be directed at gaining clues to aid in neuroanatomical localization. Jack has left leg weakness and numbness, which may potentially be attributed to a lesion(s) in the: 1) right cerebral hemisphere; 2) brainstem; 3) spinal cord; 4) left lumbosacral nerve roots and plexus; 5) peripheral nerves of the left lower limb.

You should clarify whether the neurological complaints are confined to the left lower limb. If Jack has also experienced symptoms in his left upper limb (i.e. hemiparesis) it suggests that the lesion may be localized above the cervical spinal cord, e.g. internal capsule of the right cerebral hemisphere. On the other hand, if Jack has also noted symptoms in his right lower limb (i.e. paraparesis) it is likely that he has a thoracic or lumbar spinal cord lesion. However, it should be noted that bilateral leg weakness may rarely be attributed to a parasagittal intracranial lesion centred on the sensorimotor cortex.

History-taking is also important in establishing a differential diagnosis of possible underlying aetiologies. The onset of the limb weakness is important. A sudden onset raises the possibility of a vascular cause, e.g. stroke. If there was history of preceding trauma, stretch-induced or direct peripheral nerve injuries need to be considered. A gradual and progressive history raises the possibility of a neoplastic lesion. A history of fevers and lethargy should be sought to exclude the possibility of an infective lesion.

The past medical history of the patient needs to be clarified. For example, diabetes mellitus may be associated with myriad neurological presentations which the clinician should be familiar with. A known history of previous malignancy raises the possibility of metastatic cerebral disease. Autoimmune disorders are less common but may also result in neurological deficits. HIV/AIDS is associated with cryptococcal meningitis (fungal infection), as well as lymphoma. A positive family history of neurofibromatosis raises the possibility of nerve sheath tumours, which could account for Jack's neurological complaints.

A.2   In a patient presenting with an intracranial mass lesion there may be associated symptoms of headaches. Classically, headaches secondary to increased intracranial pressure are described as generalized headaches which may be worse in the mornings and can be associated with nausea and vomiting. Furthermore, these headaches may also be exacerbated by straining or Valsalva manoeuvres. Depending on the location of the mass lesion, there may be other associated neurological deficits. Patients presenting with brainstem lesions typically experience other associated debilitating symptoms such as diplopia, facial numbness and weakness, bulbar dysfunction, etc. The commonest clinical pathologies affecting the spinal canal (e.g. disc prolapse, tumours) generally cause local spinal pain and/or radicular pain (sciatica/femoralgia) which aids in the clinical diagnosis. The absence of pain in the history raises the possibility of non-surgical aetiologies, e.g. demyelination, diabetes, etc.

A.3   The neurological findings are highly suggestive of an upper motor neurone lesion. The classical findings include hypertonia, hyper-reflexia, myoclonus and

Answers *cont.*

an extensor plantar response, but may not all be present in a patient. These should be contrasted with the findings found in association with a lower motor neurone (at the level of the anterior horn cell or distal) which are characterized by hypotonia, hyporeflexia and equivocal/flexor plantar response. In Jack's case, the signs support an upper motor neurone lesion.

Given that the abnormal neurological findings of an upper motor neurone pattern were completely confined to the left lower limb, in theory Jack may have 1) an intracranial lesion centred on the motor cortex or 2) a thoracic spinal cord lesion. In clinical practice, most thoracic spinal cord lesions will result in a sensory level and bilateral abnormal neurological findings, e.g. Brown–Séquard syndrome.

A.4 The clinical diagnosis on the basis of history and examination findings points to an upper motor neurone lesion, i.e. intracranial or spinal. Jack has no history of spinal or radicular pain. He has complained of new-onset headaches. This makes an intracranial lesion more likely.

Pre- and post-contrast CT brain imaging is the initial investigation of choice. This modality is widely available and establishes the diagnosis in the majority of cases where a space-occupying lesion is suspected. MRI brain imaging is more sensitive and offers more sophisticated anatomical delineation in three dimensions, but is limited by cost and availability.

A.5 Figure 41.1 is a T2-weighted MRI image demonstrating the right parasagittal lesion. There is local mass effect with bowing of the falx cerebri. CSF appears 'white' (hyperintense). This sequence highlights any cerebral oedema (also hyperintense) which may be associated with a brain tumour. Relatively little oedema is present. Prominent vessels may be seen within the tumour, suggesting hypervascularity.

Figure 41.2 is a T1-weighted sagittal MRI image (without contrast) demonstrating the extrinsic, durally based tumour causing compression of the sensorimotor cortex. There is extension of tumour into the adjacent skull.

Figure 41.3 is a post-contrast T1-weighted MRI image demonstrating intense contrast enhancement of the tumour.

Revision Points

- Patients with brain tumours may present with 1) symptoms of increased intracranial pressure; 2) neurological deficits; 3) seizures.
- Headaches suggestive of intracranial hypertension should prompt early investigation.
- The most common brain tumours are glial series tumours (gliomas), metastatic cancer and meningiomas. The majority of meningiomas are benign lesions.

- Pre- and post-contrast CT imaging is the initial investigation of choice. MR imaging allows detailed delineation of the brain lesion(s).
- The main aims of surgery are 1) to establish definitive histopathological diagnosis, 2) maximal tumour resection while minimizing the chance of neurological deficits.
- Radiation therapy and chemotherapy may be indicated in patients with higher-grade gliomas and other malignant lesions.

Issues to Consider

- Clinical presentations of brain tumours.
- Neurological localization based on history and examination findings.
- Homunculus of the motor cortex.
- Upper versus lower motor neurone lesions.

Further Information

http://www.cancerbackup.org.uk/Cancertype/Brain

http://www.cancercouncil.com.au/editorial.asp?pageid=1226

Fall during a fishing weekend

Andrew Zacest

A 43-year-old man has been brought by ambulance to the emergency department at the weekend. He had been on a fishing trip on a boat with his friends drinking alcohol and he had reportedly taken Ecstasy. He had fallen backwards, hitting the back of his head. Initially he had lost consciousness. He is now alert but irritable and disorientated. There are no other known injuries. The patient has a past history of hypertension but is taking no regular medication.

Q.1 What are the principles in assessing this patient?

In the emergency department he is drowsy, eye opening to voice, localizes to pain and is orientated. His vital signs are HR 94, BP 110 systolic, RR 12, sats 98% on room air. He has oxygen applied, intravenous fluids commenced and a cervical collar already applied. A chest X-ray shows no abnormality. He complains of tenderness in the right occipital area when palpated but there is no observable laceration or bruise.

Q.2 What are the key features of his neurological examination? What is the Glasgow coma score (GCS) and why is this important?

Q.3 What are the appropriate next investigations?

You perform the most important investigation, shown in Figure 42.1A, B.

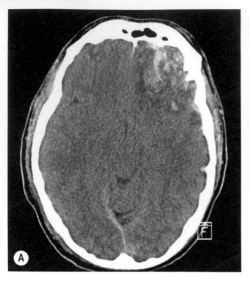

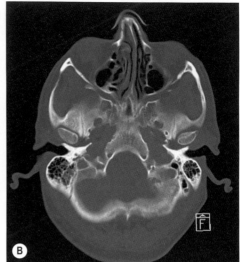

Figure 42.1A   Figure 42.1B

Q.4 What do the tests show and what is the significance of the finding?

The patient's condition improves and he is now eye opening intermittently, obeying commands and orientated, though intermittently drowsy. He is transferred to the high dependency ward for ongoing observation and management.

Q.5 How should he be managed in the first few days?

The patient continues to improve clinically for the first 6 days and is now sitting out of bed, alert and even walking with assistance on the ward. In fact on day 6 the patient absconds from the neurosurgical unit and is discovered hours later at his home! He is brought back to the hospital. The following day, after a morning walk, he is left by his wife to have an afternoon sleep on the ward. Later that afternoon he is found on the floor by nursing staff, unresponsive with a GCS of 4 (E1, M2, V1) extending to pain with fixed and dilated pupils.

Q.6 What is the significance of the clinical signs and what should be done?

Q.7 The patient is intubated emergently and an urgent CT head scan is performed. What does Figure 42.2 show?

Figure 42.2

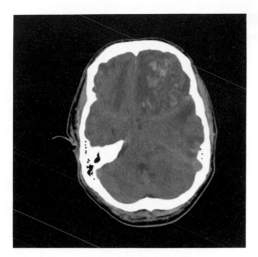

The patient is taken to the operating room and undergoes emergency frontal craniectomy, durotomy and insertion of an external ventricular drain. The intraoperative pathology is shown in Figure 42.3.

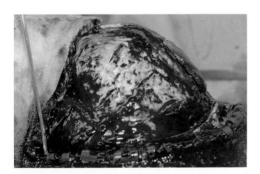

Figure 42.3 The intraoperative photograph shows that a bifrontal craniectomy has been performed and looking from a lateral position the dura over the frontal and temporal lobes is tight from raised pressure. Dural slits have been made to decompress the dura. Through them contused cortex can been seen. An intracranial pressure monitor will be placed prior to scalp closure.

The patient is then transferred to the intensive care unit postoperatively intubated and ventilated. Although initially fixed and unreactive, the pupils eventually become reactive and purposive movement is observed to painful stimulus.

The patient is extubated after 5 days and discharged to the ward. The patient makes a slow recovery while on the ward but eventually is transferred to a rehabilitation facility. He returns in 8 weeks to have the bone flap replaced and is discharged back to the rehabilitation facility, mobilizing freely but with significant impairment in judgement and impulse control.

Q.8 His family ask what his prognosis is. What do you tell them?

Answers

A.1 The patient has sustained a traumatic brain injury and should be assessed using the standardized guidelines for all trauma patients. These include assessment of airway, breathing and circulation (**A**, **B**, **C**), immobilization of the cervical spine and the performance of a brief neurological examination (primary survey). Following this a more detailed secondary survey may be performed to look for further injuries. These principles are detailed in the emergency management of severe trauma (EMST) course manual available through the Royal Australasian College of Surgeons (Committee on Trauma, American College of Surgeons 2008).

A.2 The Glasgow coma score (GCS), originally reported by Drs Teasdale and Jennett in 1974 (Teasdale and Jennet 1974), is an attempt to quantify the level of consciousness of a patient with a head injury in a form which is standardized and hence comparable from place to place, from time to time, and from person to person. The three summed components include the response to eye opening (E), motor response (M) and verbal response (V) (Table 42.1).

This patient is eye opening to voice (E3), localizes to painful stimulus (M5) and is orientated to place (V5) with a GCS of 13. The main utility of the GCS is to allow serial standardized neurological assessment of the head injured patient.

A.3 CT head and neck. Most trauma imaging protocols now have cranial and spinal imaging performed at the same time which allows exclusion of a significant bony spinal injury in the trauma patient.

A.4 The CT head scan shows a right occipital fracture with some intracranial air and a contrecoup left and right frontal haemorrhagic contusion. There is some mass effect with shift of the left frontal lobe toward the right (subfalcine herniation). There is also some blood on the tentorium cerebelli. These findings suggest that the patient has fallen, first striking the right occipital area and then through translation of the force contused the frontal lobes. This scan is concerning because of the size of the original contusion and already present mass effect and the propensity for these lesions to expand with time as a result of further haemorrhage and secondary oedema. Delayed neurological deterioration and even death can occur with such lesions.

A.5 Clinical management of traumatic brain injury is primarily concerned with the prevention of secondary injury including ischaemia, hypoxia, cerebral oedema, raised intracranial pressure, hydrocephalus,

Table 42.1 Glasgow coma scale		
Eye Opening	**Motor Response**	**Verbal Response**
4 Spontaneous	6 Obeys command	5 Orientated
3 To voice	5 Localizes to pain	4 Confused
2 To pain	4 Withdraws from pain	3 Inappropriate words
1 None	3 Flexion to pain	2 Incomprehensible
	2 Extension to pain	1 None
	1 None	

Answers *cont.*

infection and seizure. Serial neurological observation (GCS) by trained nursing and medical staff and investigations including HR and BP, oxygen saturations, serum electrolytes and serial CT head scans provide the data on which to make evidence-based clinical judgement. All patients should have supplemental oxygen, careful fluid balance control to ensure euvolaemia and avoidance of hyponatraemia as well as seizure treatment or prophylaxis if clinically warranted, as in this patient.

A.6 Fixed dilated pupils and extensor posturing are late stages of brainstem herniation, implying disturbance at the level of the midbrain. The most common cause is raised intracranial pressure secondary to a mass lesion causing compression of the upper brainstem. As stated before, emergency care proceeds in a stepwise fashion of airway, breathing and circulation correction before diagnostic investigations. In this patient emergency intubation and ventilation is necessary. The patient may have had a seizure alone or progression of the intracranial mass lesion secondary to oedema, hyponatraemia or further haemorrhage resulting in cerebral herniation. If life-threatening raised intracranial pressure is suspected, as here, temporary hyperventilation to reduce CO_2 and intravenous mannitol 1 g/kg should be given on the way to CT.

A.7 The CT shows increased oedema around the left frontal, right frontal and left temporal contusions and more mass effect (subfalcine herniation) and also compression of the brainstem and hydrocephalus.

A.8 The patient has had a severe traumatic brain injury with resultant marked frontal lobe dysfunction. This is likely to remain a problem for the rest of his life and he will require extensive rehabilitation input. He is unlikely to return to his previous independent functional level because of impaired judgement and lack of insight. This is a tragic outcome, with enormous cost to patient, family and community.

Revision Points

Traumatic brain injury (TBI) is a significant public health problem. It is the number one cause of death in people under 40 and affects mainly young males and the elderly. In addition 2% of the population live with the sequelae of TBI in the community contributing to a major societal burden. Unfortunately, in spite of an enormous amount of research and development of evidence-based guidelines for the treatment of TBI, there are limited proven therapies for stopping the progression of the initial injury and the mortality from severe TBI has remained unchanged for the last two decades.

The cornerstone of clinical TBI management is the prevention of secondary injury. A thorough neurological assessment of the patient's initial injury, including spinal injury, will establish a baseline. Evidence-based guidelines for both the medical and surgical management of traumatic brain injury are published and used in clinical practice. As highlighted in this case, even with close supervision on a neurosurgical unit a patient can deteriorate suddenly (talk and die) and may require life-saving surgery. Anticipation, prevention or timely treatment of secondary injury is therefore essential.

Issues to Consider

- What are the most common causes of traumatic brain injury (TBI) where you live?
- Where do patients undergo rehabilitation after TBI? Can you arrange to spend a day on the unit as an observer?

References

Committee on Trauma, American College of Surgeons, 2008. ATLS: Advanced trauma life support program for doctors, 8th edn. American College of Surgeons, Chicago. Available through Royal Australasian College of Surgeons.

Teasdale, G., Jennett, B., 1974. Assessment of coma and impaired consciousness. A practical scale. Lancet 2 (7872), 81–84.

Further Information

Bullock, M.R., Povlishock, J., 2007. Guidelines for the management of severe traumatic brain injury. Journal of Neurotrauma 24 (Suppl 1).

Bullock, M.R., Chestnut, R., Ghajar, J., et al, 2006. Guidelines for the surgical management of traumatic brain injury. Neurosurgery 58 (3), S2–vi.

An unwell young man in the emergency room

Jonathan Mitchell and Mohammed M. Rashid

A 33-year-old man presents to the emergency department after informing his partner that he had ingested some tablets 24 hours ago. He is initially alert and fully conscious but obviously upset, complaining of headache and asking for sedation.

Q.1 What questions are particularly important?

Q.2 What investigations would you like to organize first?

The following results become available:

Investigation 43.1 Summary of results

Sodium	148 mmol/L	Potassium	3.4 mmol/L
Urea	18.6 mmol/L	Creatinine	220 µmol/L
ALT	1856 U/L	Bilirubin	35 µmol/L
PT	26 seconds	Hb	14 g/dL
WCC	16.1×10^9/L	Plats	367×10^9/L
Salicylates	Negative	Paracetamol	38 mg/L

Q.3 How would you interpret these results? What would you like to do next?

He is commenced on IV acetylcysteine and fluids and admitted to the ward. Six hours later, you are called urgently to the ward. The nursing staff are barely able to rouse him and he is groaning and very sweaty.

Q.4 What are you going to do immediately? Describe and justify what you should look for on examination?

Q.5 What are the common causes of coma? What are the likely causes in this patient?

He is unresponsive and sweaty. Pulse 110/min, respiratory rate of 14 breaths and blood pressure 100/60 mmHg. Axillary temperature is 37°C. He is not responding to painful stimulus but his pupil size is normal. He accepts a Guedel airway. A blood glucose is 2.1. You give him 50 mL 50% glucose and start a 10% dextrose infusion. He becomes responsive and fully conscious.

Eight hours later you are called again. He is agitated, confused, aggressive and wants to self-discharge. He has no neck stiffness. He is generally hyper-reflexic. His pupils are equal in size and reactive to light.

Q.6 What is the likely cause for his confusion?

Q.7 What should you do now?

He is taken to the intensive care and intubated. Blood tests now reveal the following:

Investigation 43.2 Summary of results

Sodium	151 mmol/L	Potassium	3.1 mmol/L
Urea	23.7 mmol/L	Creatinine	0.34 mmol/L
ALT	3469 U/L	Bilirubin	97 µmol/L
PT	76 seconds	Hb	14 g/dL
WCC	24.7×10^9/L	Plats	367×10^9/L

Q.8 What is happening?

Answers

A.1 All patients with an overdose need a through history including the timing of ingestion, the amount of drugs and if the drugs were taken with alcohol. A collateral history is also important, as is an overdose history. It is useful to classify episodes of attempted self-harm by lethality and by intent, depending on the method used and the patient's intentions. A paracetamol overdose may be a low intent but often high lethality overdose, as patients may not realize how dangerous large quantities can be.

A.2

• All patients should have an immediate blood glucose measurement.

Answers cont.

- A 12-lead ECG should be performed. Drugs that cause an abnormal ECG include tricyclic antidepressants and antipsychotics. ECG abnormalities can vary but remember that, a normal ECG on admission should not be overly reassuring especially if suspicion is high. Also, remember that a sinus tachycardia may be the only warning sign of a toxic overdose. If in doubt, monitor!
- Renal and liver function tests are essential. In paracetamol overdose, check the prothrombin time.
- An arterial blood gas may reveal acidosis and hyperlactataemia in many patients, a large proportion of whom are grossly dehydrated at presentation.
- Salicylate and paracetamol levels should be measured in *all* patients with a suspected overdose.

A.3 He is dry and in renal failure. This urgently needs to be corrected with aggressive fluid resuscitation and monitoring of fluid balance. Following a paracetamol overdose, the patient is often grossly dehydrated which contributes to renal failure and lactic acidosis.

His very high ALT signifies significant hepatic necrosis but is not, in itself, a prognostic marker. Most importantly, he has a prolonged PT signifying early hepatic failure.

He has high levels of paracetamol. N-acetylcysteine should be commenced without any delay, as it is the only intervention that can prevent multi-organ failure in these patients.

- The paracetamol nomogram (Figure 43.1) indicates the risk of hepatic injury associated with a paracetamol

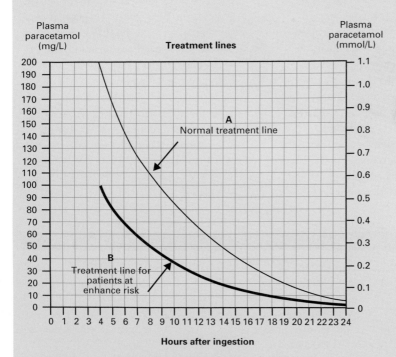

Figure 43.1 Paracetamol treatment chart. (Courtesy of the Clinical Services Unit of the Royal Adelaide Hospital.)

concentration at a known time after ingestion and this should be used as guidance for administering acetylcysteine

- In theory, if the paracetamol concentration lies above the treatment line, N-acetylcysteine should be given. N-acetylcysteine should ideally be started within 8 hours of ingestion.
- In practice, the timing of drug overdose is notoriously unreliable. If the patient has taken a substantial amount of paracetamol (>7.5 g in an adult) or if there is any doubt whatsoever, or if the patient has abnormal liver enzymes despite a paracetamol level below the treatment line then treatment should be started immediately. Always seek expert advice.

All patients with deliberate self-poisoning should be assessed by psychiatric services.

A.4 This is a medical emergency.

A: Check and safeguard his airway

B: Check for spontaneous breathing, apply high-flow oxygen and measure his respiratory rate. Roll the patient on to his side (the 'coma position'). Markedly abnormal breathing patterns are seen in brainstem damage. Compensatory hyperventilation is seen early in metabolic acidosis (e.g. diabetic ketoacidosis, salicylate, methanol, ethylene glycol and other poisonings). Hypoventilation is common in all cases of generalized CNS depression.

C: Measure blood pressure, pulse and assess him for signs of shock. Insert a large bore intravenous cannula, noting his response to painful stimuli. Take blood for laboratory analysis. Commence intravenous isotonic saline. Monitor cardiac rhythm.

Measure blood glucose immediately. He has taken a paracetamol overdose and may have become hypoglycaemic secondary to acute liver failure.

Hypoglycaemia is easily treated, easily missed, and can be fatal. If there is delay or any doubt, administer 50 mL 50% glucose intravenously. This will not do any harm and, if the patient is hypoglycaemic, may save their life.

Consider an opiate overdose or over-prescription (unlikely in this patient). Naloxone is not harmful and will reverse an opiate coma, but it should be given in small increments (e.g. 200 mg doses) as sudden reversal of an opioid overdose may lead to severe and dangerous withdrawal symptoms and an aggressive, uncooperative and delirious patient.

Call the anaesthetic team if his airway is threatened and he may need intubation.

The degree of unconsciousness should be determined by calculating and recording his Glasgow coma score (GCS), as shown in Table 43.1.

Table 43.1 The Glasgow coma score

Eye Opening	Motor Response	Verbal Response
4 Spontaneous	6 Obeys commands	5 Orientated
3 To voice	5 Localizes to pain	4 Confused
2 To pain	4 Withdraws from pain	3 Inappropriate words
1 None	3 Flexion to pain	2 Incomprehensible sounds
	2 Extension to pain	1 None
	1 None	

Answers *cont.*

Spontaneous movements indicate a lesser degree of unconsciousness. Twitching and jerking might indicate seizure activity or serotonergic toxicity. Decorticate or decerebrate posturing or asymmetric responses to pain may indicate neurological injury or dysfunction.

The eyes should be held open and the pupils, spontaneous eye movements and fundi examined. Large pupils are common in overdose of sympathomimetic (e.g. amphetamines) and anticholinergic (e.g. antihistamines, tricyclic antidepressants) drugs. They also occur with drugs that cause retinal toxicity (e.g. quinine, methanol). Small pupils are common with opioid, anticholinesterase and antipsychotic drug overdose. Both large and small pupils can also occur with midbrain or brainstem damage. A unilateral fixed dilated pupil indicates an ipsilateral third nerve palsy, which occurs when raised intracranial pressure leads to tentorial herniation. This may occur in this patient due to cerebral oedema arising from acute liver failure.

The limbs should be tested for tone, response to painful stimuli and reflexes.

A.5 Causes of coma vary, depending on the initial examination findings. The following list is by no means exhaustive. All unconscious patients should receive the same initial emergency management.

1. Localizing cerebral hemisphere signs:
   - Closed head injury.
   - Intracranial haemorrhage (intracerebral, extradural or subdural, subarachnoid).
   - Raised intracranial pressure due to a space-occupying lesion.
2. Signs of brainstem dysfunction alone:
   - Brainstem haemorrhage or infarct.
   - Pressure on the brainstem from above (coning) or from the posterior fossa.
3. Meningism:

- Subarachnoid haemorrhage.
- Meningitis or encephalitis.
4. No specific neurological features:
   - Toxic encephalopathy – poisoning.
   - Metabolic encephalopathy – hypo- or hyperglycaemic coma, hepatic encephalopathy, hyponatraemia.

The main causes of death from poisoning out of hospital include:
- Carbon monoxide.
- Opioids.
- Tricyclic antidepressants (TCAs).
- Alcohol.
- A variety of sleeping tablets.

Many of these respond well to supportive care alone. In hospital the poisons which remain a major concern are those that:
- Are cardiotoxic (e.g. most antiarrhythmic drugs, tricyclic antidepressants, chloroquine).
- Have delayed onset of toxicity (e.g. paracetamol, iron and any overdose on 'slow-release' medications).
- Are designed to kill (e.g. pesticides, herbicides, cytotoxic drugs, bleach).
- Frequently lead to long-term morbidity (e.g. heavy metals, carbon monoxide, theophylline).

Note that most of these substances are not detected by the average 'drug screen'.

Patients with a GCS <8 usually need to be intubated and admitted to an intensive care unit. At the very least, they warrant urgent anaesthetic/ITU review.

Overdoses produce various physiological effects which need to be treated, such as tachycardia, seizures or hypotension. Current teaching is to 'treat the patient, not the poison'. Recent thinking employs the concept of 'toxidromes' which are groups of symptoms and signs producing a clinical picture in different overdose settings. Table 43.2 illustrates the different groups of 'toxidromes'.

Answers *cont.*

Table 43.2 Toxidromes

Stimulant (e.g. Amphetamines)	Sedative/ hypnotic (e.g. Alcohol)	Opiate (e.g. Heroin)	Anticholinergic	Cholinergic (Opposite of Anticholinergic)
Restlessness	Sedation	Pinpoint pupils	Blurred vision	Salivation
Excessive speech	Confusion	Unresponsiveness	Mydriasis	Lacrimation
Excessive motor activity	Paraesthesia	Slow respiratory rate	Dry skin	Urination
Tremor	Diplopia	Shallow respiration	Urinary retention	Defaecation
Insomnia	Blurred vision	Bradycardia	Flushing	Diarrhoea
Tachycardia	Slurred speech	Decreased bowel sounds	Fever	Vomiting
Hallucinations	Ataxia	Hypothermia	Tachycardia	Bradycardia
	Nystagmus		Hallucinations	
	Hallucinations		Psychosis	
	Coma			

Box 43.1 Grades of encephalopathy

Grade I: altered mood, impaired concentration and psychomotor function, rousable
Grade II: drowsy, inappropriate behaviour, able to talk
Grade III: very drowsy, disorientated, agitated, and aggressive
Grade IV: coma, may respond to painful stimuli

This patient has developed hypoglycaemia secondary to liver failure from a paracetamol overdose and he should be given IV glucose promptly.

A.6 He may be hypoglycaemic once more but encephalopathy secondary to acute liver failure is likely and may develop very rapidly indeed

A.7 As before: **A B C** Check his blood glucose once again. Take blood for renal function, liver enzymes, including PT, arterial gases and lactate. Ask for senior help immediately and call for an anaesthetic assessment.

A.8 He has a massive transaminitis secondary to hepatic necrosis, a rapidly rising prothrombin time due to liver failure and renal failure.

The patient has developed hyperacute fulminant hepatic failure. This is encephalopathy occurring in a patient less than 7 days after the onset of jaundice. In paracetamol overdose, this often occurs much more rapidly, sometimes within 48 hours, and the encephalopathy can precede the onset of clinical jaundice.

If the encephalopathy occurs between 7 and 28 days after the onset of jaundice, the condition is termed acute liver failure. If the intervening period is between 28 days and 8 weeks, the term subacute liver failure is used.

Encephalopathy (Box 43.1) due to fulminant hepatic failure is secondary to brain oedema due to cerebrovascular dilatation and rapid swelling of neurones. Early signs may include hyperreflexia, clonus, extensor posturing, teeth grinding as well as irritability. It is not uncommon for

Answers *cont.*

these early signs to be misinterpreted as a lack of cooperation or anxiety in such a patient.

Advanced cerebral oedema may lead to pupillary abnormalities due to midline shift or raised intracranial pressure, sustained arterial hypertension, bradycardia and eventually deep coma and death.

Patients with early signs of brain oedema should be managed in ITU and intubated to reduce agitation and allow the administration of anaesthetic agents such as propofol. This patient is confused and agitated so he is moving from stage II to stage III encephalopathy (see Box 43.1). His hypoglycaemia hours earlier was a warning sign that this was to be the likely outcome. A liver transplant centre should be contacted urgently.

Revision Points

Coma

Definition

Coma is a state of deep unconsciousness where the patient does not wake up with external stimuli.

Emergency Care

ABC (airway, breathing and circulation): i.e. secure the airway and ensure adequate respiration, check pulse and blood pressure, insert an intravenous line and connect to a cardiac monitor so as to identify arrhythmias.

Risk Factors

Examples of coma which lead rapidly to very different pathways of investigation and management include patients who:

- Have severe medical disorders (e.g. chronic obstructive airways disease with respiratory failure, chronic liver disease or uraemia, diabetes).
- Collapsed after suffering a sudden onset severe headache (subarachnoid haemorrhage).
- Have pinpoint pupils and needle tracks (narcotic overdose).
- Are found surrounded by empty pill bottles.

- Have localizing neurological signs, necessitating emergency CT scan of the brain and neurosurgical review.

Self-poisoning is a very common cause of coma and two-thirds of patients ingest more than one substance, and may manifest confusing signs from the combined effects of multiple drugs.

Routine screening for drugs is rarely useful and is expensive.

Management

The management of the comatose patient due to a drug overdose is largely supportive but must begin with **A B C**! Some specific measures to consider include:

- Early consideration of intubation to prevent aspiration and manage airway.
- Gastric lavage only if seen soon after drug ingestion.
- Administration of activated charcoal if possible within a few hours of paracetamol ingestion.
- Exclude and treat hypoglycaemia.
- Naloxone is routinely given, but should be titrated slowly in a known opioid overdose.

Revision Points *cont.*

Paracetamol Overdose (POD)

Epidemiology

- Paracetamol is the most frequently ingested drug in the Western world.
- POD is the most common drug overdose in the UK and if untreated can be lethal. However, since the sale of the drug has been restricted in the UK, deaths from POD have dropped significantly.

Pharmacology

Overdose saturates the normal metabolic pathways of conjugation by the hepatocytes. Paracetamol metabolism is then diverted to the oxidative pathway (CYP450) leading to toxic intermediate metabolites which accumulate to cause lethal hepatotoxicity.

Treatment

The use of the paracetamol nomogram (see Figure 43.1) is important in determining the need for *N*-acetylcysteine therapy. The nomogram indicates the risk of hepatic injury associated with a paracetamol concentration at a known time after ingestion. An adequate history to establish time of ingestion is therefore very useful, but often unreliable. *If in doubt, treat as the 'worst-case scenario'.*

N-acetylcysteine is an effective antidote, which should ideally be given within 8–10 hours of ingestion. It is still helpful in overdoses presenting late and in patients with established hepatotoxicity. It works by liberating cysteine allowing for resynthesis of hepatic glutathione. In patients intolerant of *N*-acetylcysteine, oral methionine is a less effective alternative.

Peak hepatotoxicity may not occur for some days. Following a significant overdose, the INR should be monitored for 24–48 hours. Patients with signs of significant hepatotoxicity should be discussed early with a liver unit. These signs include a worsening coagulopathy, rising creatinine, acidosis and the development of hepatic encephalopathy. A small proportion of patients will develop acute liver failure and some come to liver transplant (Box 43.2).

Follow-up of patients with deliberate self-poisoning and attempted suicide is an important area, and coordination of mental health and support services is essential to prevent the patient undergoing further self-harm, and to treat the underlying causes.

Box 43.2 King's College criteria for listing for liver transplantation

- Acetaminophen patients
  pH <7.3, *or*
  prothrombin time >6.5 (INR) *and*
  serum creatinine >300 µmol/L and grade III or worse encephalopthy.
- Non-acetaminophen patients
  prothrombin time >6.5 (INR), *or*
  any three of the following variables:
    1. age <10 years or >40 years
    2. aetiology: non-A, non-B hepatitis, idiosyncratic drug reaction
    3. duration of jaundice before encephalopathy >7 d
    4. prothrombin time >3.5 (INR)
    5. serum bilirubin >300 µmol/L.
- Lactate >3.5 before fluid resuscitation or >3 after adequate fluid resuscitation.

Issues to Consider

- What step could the drug industry and governments take to almost eliminate deaths from paracetamol overdose?
- In what circumstances might a liver transplant for a patient with paracetamol-induced liver failure be deemed inappropriate?
- What are other possible causes of hyperacute, acute and subacute liver failure?

Why might the amateur forager be susceptible?

Further Information

www.hypertox.com *Downloadable toxicology software*.

www.pharmweb.net

A 68-year-old woman with a left hemiplegia following a conscious collapse

Timothy Kleinig

A previously independent, right-handed 68-year-old woman slid to the floor while eating lunch with her husband. She did not lose consciousness, but immediately noticed severe left-sided weakness. She could not get up unassisted, yet kept repeating 'I'm all right' to her husband. The ambulance was called and she was taken to hospital. It is now 150 minutes since her collapse.

She has a background history of type II diabetes mellitus, hypertension and dyslipidaemia. She has peripheral vascular disease, but no other micro- or macrovascular complications. Her medications include metformin, gliclazide, perindopril and atorvastatin.

Q.1 What is the most likely cause? What other possibilities should you consider?

You continue your history and examination.

Q.2 What are the important features of the examination and ancillary history?

The patient's blood pressure is 164/92 mmHg. She is a febrile, alert and in sinus rhythm. Her eyes are conjugate, but deviated to the right. She has a left homonymous hemianopia. Her speech is dysarthric without dysphasia. She has a dense left hemiparesis with only a flicker of movement at the hip. Sensation is absent on the left. She appears to be unaware of her neurological deficit and is trying to get out of bed.

Cardiovascular and general examination is normal.

Q.3 What investigations would you order?

Apart from a blood sugar of 9.6 mmol/L and evidence of left ventricular hypertrophy on ECG, her blood tests and ECG are unremarkable. Other investigations are shown in Figure 44.1–3.

304

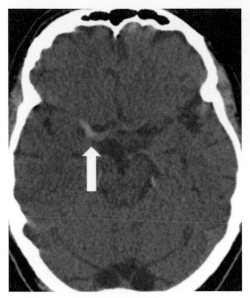

Figure 44.1 Hyperacute CT scan.

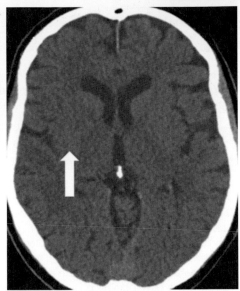

Figure 44.2

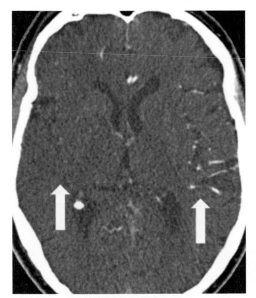

Figure 44.3 A CT angiogram.

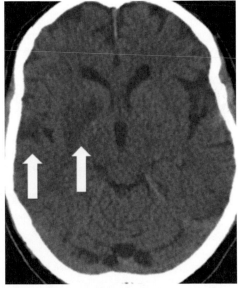

Figure 44.4 Repeat CT 2 days after omission.

Q.4   What do the CT and CTA show? It is now 2 hours and 50 minutes post stroke onset. How would you proceed?

You initiate emergency management, and commence an infusion of thrombolytic as per your stroke unit protocol. After 30 minutes she regains partial power in her left arm and leg, regains sensation to painful stimuli (but not light touch), and she no longer has a conjugate gaze defect.

Q.5   What in-hospital care should this patient receive and what further investigations should be performed?

CTA performed at admission demonstrated only mild atherosclerotic carotid disease. A follow-up CT scan demonstrated a moderate area of infarction within the basal ganglia, and several small cortical areas of infarction (see Figure 44.4), somewhat less than would have been expected from her initial scan. The MCA appeared patent. Transthoracic echocardiography demonstrated an enlarged left atrium, but no thrombus. Fasting blood glucose was 6.2 mmol/L and a HBA1C was 7.8%. Total cholesterol was 5.2, with an LDL of 3.2 mmol/L and HDL of 0.8 mmol/L. While on the ward, 3 days after admission, a rapid and irregular pulse was noted. ECG confirmed atrial fibrillation.

Q.6   What are some possible complications which may arise in the subacute stage?

The patient improved over the ensuing week, and was able to mobilize with assistance. Progress was limited by the left-sided 'neglect' commonly seen with a non-dominant MCA stroke. She was accepted for ongoing inpatient therapy at a specialized rehabilitation facility.

Q.7   What chronic treatment should this patient receive?

You initiate appropriate long-term medical management, counsel the patient and her husband on the risks of recurrence. She does well in rehabilitation, and is able to return to home with assistance from her husband and community supports.

Answers

A.1   It is most likely that this patient has had a stroke. Other causes of a rapidly progressive focal neurological deficit include migraine with aura, epilepsy with a post-ictal Todd's paresis, a conversion disorder and hypoglycaemia, although the lack of observed ictal activity and the sudden onset of symptoms would make acute stroke the most likely cause. This is an emergency – 'Time is brain', and you need to work swiftly in order to provide the best therapy.

A.2   The acute evaluation of a patient with a presumed stroke is guided by the need to determine, as quickly as possible:
• Did she actually have a stroke?
• If so, was it ischaemic or haemorrhagic?

Answers *cont.*

- Does she have any contraindications to thrombolysis?

Other features which are important to establish, but which should not slow a decision regarding the institution of thrombolysis, include:

- What is the severity of the neurological deficit? (This is important to establish a baseline to compare spontaneous or treatment-induced improvement or deterioration.)
- Where is the underlying lesion located?
- What is the underlying cause?

Any observed ictal activity should raise the possibility of a Todd's paresis (although seizures can also occur at acute stroke onset). A history of intracerebral haemorrhage, recent major trauma, surgery or bleeding, recent myocardial infarction or recent ischaemic stroke should be determined, as these may contraindicate thrombolysis.

Vital signs should be noted. Elevated blood pressure is common post stroke and persistently elevated blood pressure (>185/110) may contraindicate thrombolysis. A fever may suggest an underlying cause, such as bacterial endocarditis. Note should be taken of pulse irregularity (atrial fibrillation is an important cause of stroke).

A directed neurological examination should be performed. Depressed conscious state suggests brainstem ischaemia or bihemispheric emboli. A gaze preference to one side suggests an ipsilateral frontal lobe or contralateral pontine stroke. Dysconjugate gaze suggests vertebrobasilar disease, as does vertical or horizontal nystagmus. Visual fields should be assessed. The presence of a dysphasia or dysarthria should be noted. Facial and limb strength should be tested, as should facial and limb sensation. Crossed or bilateral deficits suggest brainstem disease. The presence of ataxia should be noted. In the setting of preserved sensation and vision, evidence of inattention may be found (a failure to perceive bilateral simultaneous stimuli).

Underlying cardiovascular risk factors should be established, and a general examination performed.

A.3 The two most important investigations are a blood sugar level and a CT (preferably CT angiogram). CT perfusion studies are also increasingly used, as they help distinguish stroke core (dead tissue) from penumbra (salvageable tissue). Hypoglycaemia can mimic acute stroke, and hyperglycaemia is a contraindication to thrombolysis. The CT scan determines whether the acute stroke is haemorrhagic or ischaemic. Unless the patient is also on warfarin (an elevated INR contraindicates thrombolysis), these two tests provide sufficient results to proceed with thrombolysis.

Other investigations which should be obtained at this stage include a full blood examination and serum electrolytes (a low haemoglobin may suggest occult bleeding and a platelet count below 100×10^6/L contraindicates tPA). An ECG should be performed to look for previous silent myocardial ischaemia and atrial fibrillation (both potential stroke causes).

A.4 The CT scan is normal, except for a linear hyperdensity in the region of the right middle cerebral artery (see Figure 44.1) (the so-called 'string sign'), and subtle blurring of grey–white differentiation of the medial lentiform nucleus (see Figure 44.2). The CTA demonstrated occlusion of the proximal MCA (not shown) and, more superiorly, significant hypoperfusion of the

307

Answers *cont.*

entire right MCA territory (see Figure 44.3). These findings are consistent with ischaemic stroke. Plain CT is insensitive for cerebral ischaemia in the acute phase, but hypoperfused and infarcted areas can be demonstrated with CT angiography and perfusion imaging. Extensive areas of CT hypodensity represent already infarcted tissue; thrombolysis in this setting is unlikely to be effective, and is more likely to cause haemorrhagic transformation of the infarcted area.

The benefit from thrombolysis with alteplase within $4\frac{1}{2}$ hours of stroke onset has recently been confirmed in multicentre trials. She should receive the accepted dose (0.9 mg/kg over an hour with the first 10% as a bolus).

Her blood pressure should *not* be lowered, as this may decrease perfusion to the threatened, hypoperfused brain (the 'ischaemic penumbra'). Aspirin should not be administered acutely until 24 hours post-tPA. Conversely, ischaemic stroke patients not receiving tPA should receive aspirin at admission; aspirin treatment leads to both short- and long-term reductions in recurrent stroke, death and disability.

A.5

- Patients should be observed closely for the first 24 hours post thrombolysis, as the risk of neurological deterioration and of haemorrhage in this time-frame is considerable.
- Patients should receive antiplatelet therapy plus subcutaneous low molecular weight heparin from 24 hours onwards to minimize the risk of deep venous thrombosis.
- There is overwhelming evidence that admission to a stroke unit improves stroke outcome, minimizing the risk of

death and disability. Although it is unclear which of the components of a stroke unit are most beneficial, likely candidates include better stroke diagnosis and secondary prevention, improved prevention, recognition and treatment of complications and early rehabilitation/mobilization.

- Patients with unilateral anterior circulation ischaemic stroke should undergo imaging of the carotid vessels, if not performed at the admission CT scan. Routine echocardiography has a low yield, but is commonly performed, and may detect intracardiac thrombus. Transoesophageal echocardiogram can detect a probable cause of stroke in many patients, although it is uncertain whether any of these findings (e.g. aortic arch atheroma, patent foramen ovale) should influence management. Holter monitoring can sometimes detect atrial fibrillation as a stroke cause.
- All patients should have fasting lipids and blood glucose measured, although in the setting of acute stroke, the former may be artificially low and the latter artificially high. In young patients with cryptogenic stroke, testing for antiphospholipid disease may be beneficial. Genetic testing should also be considered in young stroke patients.

A.6

Patients' neurological status may deteriorate in the subacute setting due to several reasons, including:

- Propagation of thrombus in a culprit vessel.
- Recurrent emboli.
- Haemorrhagic transformation of the infarction (either spontaneous or treatment-related).
- Progressive oedema.
- Secondary seizures.

Answers *cont.*

Progressive neurological deterioration in the setting of a large anterior circulation stroke has a mortality rate, untreated, of around 80%. This figure can be significantly reduced (in patients less than 60 years of age) by decompressive craniotomy. Some patients who would have died will make an excellent recovery, although some additional patients will survive, but with a severe neurological deficit.

Stroke patients are also prone to develop infections, including aspiration pneumonia, urinary tract infections and pressure sores. The chances of these occurring may be lessened by screening patients for dysphagia, avoiding catheterization and appropriate bedding/turning.

Post-stroke fever is common, and is linked to worse outcome. Although not of proven benefit, administration of antipyretics is recommended in this setting. Patients with stroke, particularly those with decreased mobility, are at increased risk of deep venous thrombosis and pulmonary embolism. This risk can be lessened by antithrombotics, compression stockings, avoidance of dehydration and early mobilization. Malnourishment is a common complication. Post-stroke depression is extremely common, undertreated, and possibly preventable by prophylactic antidepressant therapy.

A.7 The likely aetiology of this patient's stroke is cardioembolism from atrial fibrillation. Her risk of recurrent stroke (untreated) is around 10% per year: this can be reduced to around 3% with warfarin (as opposed to 8% with aspirin). Warfarin is also significantly better in this setting than a combination of aspirin and clopidogrel. It is uncertain in this setting when warfarin should be commenced, as the benefit of early treatment (prevention of further emboli) may be more than offset by the risk of symptomatic haemorrhagic transformation. Most doctors would commence treatment at some point between 10–14 days post stroke (depending on infarct volume).

She may benefit from both more intense lipid-lowering therapy and more intense antihypertensive therapy. Lipid-lowering goals post stroke are uncertain, although a significantly lower risk of stroke was seen in non-hypercholesterolaemic patients following 80 mg/day of atorvastatin versus placebo. However, cardioembolic stroke patients were excluded from this trial. Likewise, in the PROGRESS trial, a combination of perindopril and indapamide was beneficial in stroke prevention, but it is unclear whether this benefit applies to patients already on multiple agents who have already met blood pressure goals. The benefit of lowering her HBA1c levels below 7.8% for stroke prevention is likewise uncertain.

Revision Points

Stroke is the second most common cause of death and disability worldwide. While stroke is more common with increasing age, 20% of strokes occur in patients aged less than 60.

Ischaemic stroke is the commonest form of stroke. Other causes include intracerebral haemorrhage and subarachnoid haemorrhage. Cardioembolism, large artery

Revision Points *cont.*

thromboembolism and small vessel disease are the main aetiological subtypes of ischaemic stroke. Hypertension, advancing age, previous stroke or transient ischaemic attack (TIA), smoking, atrial fibrillation and diabetes mellitus are the most potent risk factors. Hypertension is the most important. The epidemiological relationship between stroke and hypercholesterolaemia is weak, but statin therapy in hypercholesterolaemic patients clearly lowers stroke risk.

Acute stroke is a medical emergency, as is a TIA (10% of TIA patients will have a stroke within a month, most within 2 days). Thrombolysis within 4.5 hours of stroke onset improves outcome when administered to patients without contraindications. Earlier treatment leads to increased chances of benefit. For an outcome of complete or almost complete recovery, the number needed to treat is around eight for treatment within 3 hours and 12 for between 3 and 4.5 hours. Thrombolysis carries a small risk of symptomatic haemorrhagic transformation (2–7%, depending on definition used).

Level 1 evidence supports the following acute interventions in ischaemic stroke:
- Thrombolysis in patients presenting within 4.5 hours without contraindications.
- Admission to a stroke unit.
- Aspirin therapy (administered within 48 hours, although ideally sooner).
- Hemicraniectomy for brain swelling in patients younger than 60 with massive stroke.

Patients with minimal or no neurological deficit and ipsilateral carotid atherosclerosis (>70%, and perhaps greater than 50% in males) should be treated by endarterectomy as soon as possible to prevent further strokes. It is not yet proven whether stenting is equivalent to an open procedure.

Other proven secondary prevention interventions include:
- Antihypertensive therapy, regardless of baseline blood pressure.
- Warfarin for patients with stroke caused by atrial fibrillation.
- Antiplatelet therapy for all other ischaemic stroke patients (ideally clopidogrel, or an aspirin/dipyridamole combination).
- Statin therapy, regardless of baseline levels, for patients with non-haemorrhagic and non-cardioembolic stroke.

Smoking cessation, moderation or cessation of heavy alcohol intake, dietary modification (e.g. a 'Mediterranean' diet) and aerobic exercise are all likely to reduce the risk of recurrent stroke.

Issues to Consider

- How do the causes of stroke differ in younger patients?
- Are the risk factors for intracerebral haemorrhage and ischaemic stroke the same?

Further Information

Donnan, G.A., Fisher, M., Macleod, M., Davis, S.M., 2008. Stroke. Lancet 371, 1612–1623.

http://www.stroke.org

A 31-year-old woman with vertigo

Timothy Kleinig

A 31-year-old teacher presents to your general practice with a 2-day history of a sensation of the room spinning and unsteadiness while walking. The sensation is continuous and partially relieved by lying down. These symptoms have prevented her from going to work. She feels her hearing is normal and she has no tinnitus. Her only medication is the oral contraceptive pill.

Q.1 What are the principles of assessing a patient with vertigo?

Q.2 How do you differentiate central from peripheral causes of vertigo? What are some causes of each?

On examination she appears fit and well. She is afebrile and her cardiovascular examination is normal. The ear canals and tympanic membranes appear normal. There is no evidence of hearing impairment on clinical testing. Visual acuity testing reveals 6/6 vision on the right but 6/9 on the left. The pupils are symmetrical, but you think there is an afferent pupillary defect on the left. On fundoscopy the left optic disc appears pale compared to the right.

On testing the external ocular movements there is nystagmus on looking to the right and on vertical gaze. The nystagmus is independent of head position and is not fatigable. The remainder of the cranial nerve examination is intact. Limb tone, power and reflexes are normal. However, on finger-nose testing there is an intention tremor of the right arm with mildly reduced coordination.

She recalls having problems taking a photograph using her left eye while on holiday 3 months previously. This had resolved spontaneously over 1 week and she did not pursue the matter.

There is nothing else in the history and from the examination that helped elucidate the cause of the patient's current problem.

Q.3 How do you interpret this woman's neurological signs?

Given the probable site of the problem, the patient is referred to a neurologist. Her vertigo had improved but has not resolved completely. Various tests were performed. Figure 45.1A, B was taken from one of the tests.

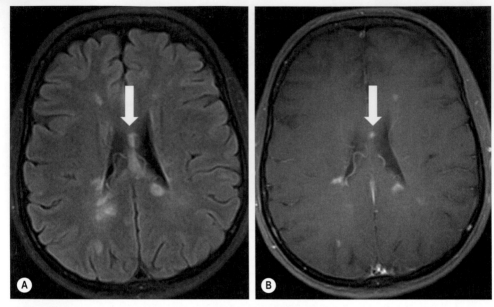

Figure 45.1A   **Figure 45.1B**

Q.4 Name the investigation and describe the abnormalities.

Q.5 What is the likely diagnosis and what other tests could be done to further support the diagnosis?

The cerebrospinal fluid demonstrated a mild elevation of mononuclear cells, normal protein and glucose and an elevated IgG:albumin ratio. Oligoclonal bands, unmatched in a serum specimen, were detected.

After the diagnosis is made, the patient returns to see you. Her symptoms have largely resolved. She asks what her prognosis is and if any treatment is available.

Q.6 What is your reply?

Answers

A.1 Vertigo is a sensation of movement, typically spinning or rotating, either of the environment or the patient in relation to the environment. This spinning sensation distinguishes vertigo from pre-syncopal 'dizziness' which occurs in cardiac arrhythmias, postural hypotension, anaemia or hypoglycaemia. A history of loss of consciousness suggests syncope or epilepsy.

Patients with vertigo present in three main ways: spontaneous onset of persistent vertigo, recurrent vertigo associated with changes in posture, and recurrent episodes of spontaneous vertigo. The major task in the assessment of vertigo is to decide whether the cause is peripheral (related to the vestibular apparatus) or central (vestibular nuclei and connections). Central causes of vertigo are generally more sinister, and a thorough neurological examination is required in patients presenting with new-onset vertigo.

On examination attention should be paid to a full neurological examination looking for focal signs suggesting a central cause. In particular:

- Examine the eyes looking for nystagmus.
- Examine the external ear, including the tympanic membrane and hearing.

You will also need to perform a careful general physical examination.

A.2 Signs suggesting central nervous system involvement include:
- Vertical nystagmus.
- Dysarthria.
- Facial sensory loss.
- Upper motor neurone signs and limb or gait ataxia.
- Internuclear ophthalmoplegia (lateral gaze induces horizontal nystagmus in the abducting eye and incomplete or slowed adduction of the contralateral eye) – due

to a lesion of the medial longitudinal fasciculus, which connects the abducens nucleus (CN VI) to the contralateral oculomotor nucleus (CN III).

Examples of central lesions causing vertigo include:
- Vertebrobasilar ischaemia.
- Demyelination (e.g. multiple sclerosis).
- Cerebellar disease.
- Migraine.
- Temporal lobe epilepsy (rare).
- Cerebellopontine angle tumour (more commonly associated with deafness, ataxia and other neurological signs such as facial sensory loss).

Examples of peripheral causes of vertigo include:
- Benign paroxysmal positional vertigo.
- Vestibular neuronitis.
- Ménière's disease.
- Middle ear disease.

A.3 This woman has *multiple* signs of CNS pathology supporting a central cause of vertigo. The vertical nystagmus suggests brainstem dysfunction, the pale left optic disc suggests optic nerve disease, and intention tremor of the right arm suggests a disorder of the right cerebellar hemisphere or its connections.

She has no tinnitus, deafness or nausea and does not find that head turning precipitates vertigo. She is otherwise well. This would be unusual for any of the common peripheral causes of vertigo.

A.4 Magnetic resonance imaging (MRI) of the brain. Both FLAIR (fluid attenuation inversion recovery) and post-gadolinium T1-weighted sequences are shown. T1 MRI scans are good at showing anatomy (i.e. grey matter is greyer than white matter). FLAIR imaging is very sensitive at demonstrating pathology. Gadolinium

Answers *cont.*

enhancement demonstrates areas of acute blood–brain barrier disruption.

There are multiple hyperintense periventricular FLAIR signal foci, as well as callosal hyperintensities and several juxtacortical lesions. Several lesions were also seen in the posterior fossa and spinal cord (not shown). Some, but not all lesions demonstrated gadolinium enhancement (see Figure 45.1B), suggesting that lesions are of differing stages. This picture is almost pathognomonic for multiple sclerosis (MS), particularly with this clinical presentation.

A.5 This woman has a number of features in her illness that point to central nervous system disease:

- Left optic atrophy (previous optic neuritis).
- Vertigo and nystagmus (brainstem dysfunction).
- Poor control of right arm movement (cerebellar disturbance).
- Multiple white plaques on MRI.
- A pleocytosis and oligoclonal bands in cerebrospinal fluid.

The presence of multiple symptoms, occurring over time, related to different sites within the central nervous system, and the finding of multiple demyelinating lesions within the central nervous system make multiple sclerosis (MS) the most likely diagnosis.

Vertigo is an unusual presenting symptom in MS, although one-third of patients will experience this symptom during the course of the illness.

Cerebrospinal fluid (CSF) obtained at lumbar puncture can be helpful. The most characteristic finding in MS is an increase in the CSF IgG:albumin ratio (suggestive of intrathecal immunoglobulin synthesis), which fractionates into oligoclonal bands on electrophoresis, seen in around 90% of patients. Evoked visual response testing would not be relevant in this case because the patient has optic atrophy. Therefore we know already that this is a site of disease.

A.6 Multiple sclerosis commonly presents in a relapsing and remitting pattern, with complete or near complete recovery after each relapse. Approximately half will eventually develop progressive disease. A smaller proportion are left with permanent deficits after each relapse. In a further group, predominantly aged over 40, the disease is slowly progressive from the outset with spinal cord dysfunction being the major feature. Currently, the average survival is at least 30 years from the diagnosis, which represents an average shortening of life expectancy of around 5–10 years.

There is no curative treatment for the disease. Acute episodes can be treated with high-dose intravenous methylprednisolone. This hastens recovery of function but does not alter the degree of recovery from acute relapses or the longer-term prognosis.

In established relapsing-remitting MS, immunomodulation with interferon beta has been shown to reduce the rate of clinical relapse by 30%. Glatiramer acetate produces an equivalent effect. Natalizumab, which specifically interferes with leucocyte transmigration into the central nervous system, is a new and potent therapy for multiple sclerosis; however, there is an associated increased risk of progressive multifocal leucoencephalopathy, caused by the JC virus. The long-term effect of these agents on secondary disease progression remains uncertain. Mitoxantrone and cyclophosphamide are both effective in the setting of aggressive relapsing disease uncontrolled by first-line therapies.

Answers *cont.*

Numerous other injectible and oral agents are in development.

All current preventative therapies are administered by self-injection or intravenous infusion. There are no proven therapies for primary progressive multiple sclerosis. Supportive treatments for pain, spasticity (e.g. baclofen and physiotherapy), fatigue, depression constipation and urinary dysfunction are important.

Low vitamin D levels have a strong epidemiological association with both the risk of MS development and relapse. Although still controversial, many doctors recommend maintaining vitamin D serum levels above 100 nmol/L. Psychological support is vital. Patients should be offered counselling, and involvement with national MS societies and support groups.

Revision Points

Multiple Sclerosis

Definition
A demyelinating disease of the central nervous system 'disseminated in time and space'.

Aetiology
The aetiology is uncertain. Genetic and environmental factors (e.g. sun exposure, infectious mononucleosis) both contribute. As the disease progress ('secondary' or 'primary' progression) it assumes a neurodegenerative pattern; immunotherapy at this stage is less effective or ineffective.

Presentation
MS often begins in early adult life and is more common in women. Symptoms and signs correspond to involvement of cerebral hemispheres, brainstem, cerebellum or spinal cord. Associated fatigue and depression are common.

Diagnosis
Dissemination in time and space needs to be demonstrated. If the symptoms and signs can be accounted for by a single lesion then the diagnosis cannot be made. The presence of oligoclonal bands in CSF can help establish the diagnosis in primary progressive disease. MRI scanning can reveal additional lesions that enable the diagnosis to be made.

The differential diagnosis includes:
- Neuromyelitis optica, a severe demyelinating illness characterised by predominant spinal cord and optic nerve involvement, and association with antibodies to aquaporin-4, a brain water channel. Acute disseminated encephalomyelitis (ADEM), a monophasic demyelinating illness, commonly post-infective.
- Vasculitis affecting the central nervous system.
- Multiple ischaemic events (usually easily distinguishable on neuroimaging).
- Inherited or acquired neurodegenerative disorders (if primary progressive presentation).

Optic Neuritis
- Presents as unilateral partial or complete central visual loss associated with pain on eye movement.
- In the acute phase the optic disc will appear normal. Subsequently optic

Revision Points *cont.*

atrophy will occur as evidenced by disc pallor, as in this case.
- It is reversible in two-thirds.
- However, in women, 75% of those with optic neuritis will go on to develop MS.

Vertigo

Clinical symptoms to assist in deciding whether vertigo is of central or peripheral origin are shown in Table 45.1.

Table 45.1 Clinical symptoms of vertigo

	Peripheral	Central
Characteristics	Severe, episodic	Mild to severe, semicontinuous
Precipitants	Head movement, typically turning, lying down in bed	May be exacerbated by movement
Exacerbating factors	Head movement	Head movement
Interval after movement	Few seconds	Immediate
Duration	Seconds to continuous	Continuous
Nystagmus	Mixed horizontal/torsional, suppressed by fixation	Horizontal, vertical, gaze provoked, not suppressed by fixation
Associated features	Deafness, tinnitus	Brainstem signs, e.g. facial numbness, diplopia, ataxia, weakness
Causes	Ménière's disease, vestibular neuronitis, benign paroxysmal positional vertigo, middle ear disease	Ischaemia, demyelination

Issues to Consider

- What other conditions may cause disc pallor and optic atrophy?
- Sudden unilateral loss or diminution of vision has a number of causes – what are they?

Further Information

Compston, A., Coles, A., 2008. Multiple sclerosis. Lancet 372 (9648), 1502–1517.

www.msfacts.org *Multiple sclerosis website with information for patients and health professionals. Many links.*

A 31-year-old man with sudden onset headache and vomiting

Andrew Zacest

You are working in the emergency department and a 31-year-old man is brought in after collapsing and vomiting while watching television at home the previous evening. It was reported that he had a generalized seizure. When he awoke he was complaining of a severe headache. He is known to drink alcohol excessively and has a 20 pack-year smoking history. He had been binge drinking over the weekend. There is no known history of hypertension.

Q.1 What is the differential diagnosis?

Q.2 What are the key features of the neurological examination in this patient?

On arrival he is alert but agitated, disorientated to time and obeying commands. He is afebrile, but has marked neck stiffness. His heart rate is 52/min and blood pressure 130/80 mmHg. Neurological examination shows no cranial nerve or focal neurological deficit. On investigation his haemoglobin is 127 g/L, white cell count 8.4 and platelets 111 000. His serum biochemistry (including calcium and glucose) is within normal limits and a serum troponin is negative. His chest X-ray is normal and an ECG shows sinus bradycardia with T-wave inversion.

Q.3 What is the next appropriate investigation and what difficulties might be encountered in obtaining this?

The patient required intravenous morphine and midazolam for the radiological investigation.

Q.4 What does the CT head scan (Figure 46.1) show?

On the advice of the consulting neurosurgeon, the patient was retrieved to the nearest neurosurgery centre and had further investigations to determine the cause of the subarachnoid haemorrhage.

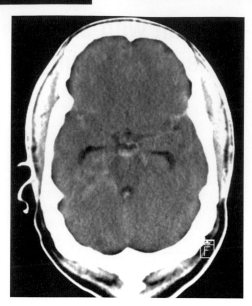

Figure 46.1

Q.5 What are the two investigations shown in Figures 46.2 and 46.3 and what do they show?

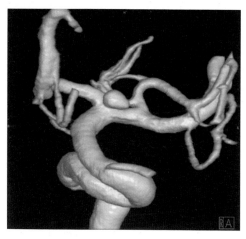

Figure 46.2

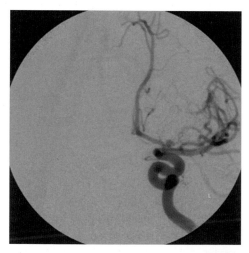

Figure 46.3

Q.6 What treatment options are available for a patient with a ruptured cerebral aneurysm?

Endovascular coiling was attempted in the patient but was technically unsuccessful.

The patient underwent craniotomy and clipping of the aneurysm which was successful. The patient was making good progress until the third postoperative day when he became progressively confused, verbally abusive and drowsy.

Q.7 What are the diagnostic possibilities and what investigations would be helpful?

The patient's blood pressure was 140/80 mmHg, temperature 38.6°C and oxygen saturation 100% on room air. A CT head showed no new intracerebral haemorrhage, no hypodensity consistent with infarction or hydrocephalus. The angiogram did not show any evidence of vasospasm. The serum sodium was 121 mmol/L, potassium 4.6 mmol/L, osmolality 266 mmol/kg (270–300), urine osmolality 116, urine sodium 177 mmol/L (40–100).

Q.8 Discuss the diagnosis, pathophysiology and treatment.

The patient was transferred to the high dependency unit for administration of hypertonic saline, monitoring of arterial blood pressure and fluid balance monitoring and oral sodium replacement. The patient progressively improved and was transferred back to his local hospital 3 weeks following his haemorrhage. He was reviewed 3 months following surgery and was doing well. He was smoking again.

Q.9 What are risk factors for aneurysm formation and subarachnoid haemorrhage and what advice should be given to this patient?

Answers

A.1 This is a young man who has suddenly collapsed with vomiting and headache and therefore subarachnoid haemorrhage (SAH) should be considered the diagnosis of exclusion in this patient. Primary intracerebral haemorrhage, secondary to an arteriovenous malformation or hypertensive haemorrhage should also be considered, given the young age. The possibility of a traumatic intracerebral haemorrhage, e.g. subdural haematoma, particularly in a patient with unclear history and a history of alcohol abuse, needs to be considered. Intracranial infection, e.g. meningitis, would be less likely to present with such an acute ictus.

A.2 The neurological examination of any patient has two key aims – to establish the diagnosis and to determine the site of the lesion.

Focus on:
- The level of consciousness (alert or drowsy).
- Glasgow coma score (GCS) (see Table 42.1).
- Cranial nerve examination, particularly the pupillary size and reactivity and external ocular movements, suggests brainstem compression.
- Signs of meningeal irritation suggesting meningeal blood or infection.

319

Answers *cont.*

- Signs of head trauma – e.g. scalp bruising, laceration or tenderness, CSF leak.
- Limb weakness, e.g. hemiparesis, indicates a contralateral supratentorial lesion usually.
- Vital signs especially HR, BP and temperature.

A.3 A CT head scan with and without contrast needs to be performed urgently in any patient in whom subarachnoid haemorrhage is in the differential diagnosis. If the CT cannot be performed at the receiving facility then the patient should be retrieved to an appropriate facility as soon as possible. Patients who are agitated may require intravenous sedation and even intubation to facilitate or even safely perform this test. It is preferable to avoid intubation to allow careful neurological assessment to be made.

A.4 The CT head shows diffuse subarachnoid haemorrhage around the brainstem.

A.5 The first is a CT angiogram and shows a left terminal internal carotid artery aneurysm. The second test is a cerebral angiogram (digital subtraction angiogram) which shows the aneurysm at the termination of the left internal carotid artery – at the point where it bifurcates into the middle and anterior cerebral arteries.

A.6 Endovascular coiling and craniotomy and surgical clipping of the aneurysm are the two choices. Both techniques can be effective in securing the aneurysm and preventing rebleeding and death. Important variables that may favour one technique over the other include the relative neck to dome ratio (coiling more favourable with a narrow neck), ease of access to the aneurysm location (posterior circulation aneurysms are more difficult surgically), and the presence of active vasospasm and brain swelling (surgical retraction may be more hazardous).

A.7 For 3 weeks following aneurysmal SAH the patient is at potential risk for a rebleed (if the aneurysm is not secured), cerebral vasospasm, fluid and electrolyte disturbance and postoperative surgical and medical complications, including seizures, wound or systemic infection. The history should determine when the deterioration occurred (vasospasm unlikely before 3 days, peaking at 7–10 days and less likely after 2 weeks), whether the deterioration occurred gradually (electrolyte disturbance or progressive ischaemia from vasospasm) or suddenly (acute vascular events or seizures). Vital signs, wound review and a detailed neurological exam will establish important changes from prior baseline. Electrolytes, cardiac enzymes, full blood count, ECG, CXR would be appropriate. An urgent CT with angiography is essential.

A.8 The patient has hyponatraemia. Following SAH hyponatraemia is most commonly due to either cerebral salt wasting (CSW) or the syndrome of inappropriate antidiuretic syndrome (SIADH). The former is currently believed to be due to release of atrial natriuretic (ANF) following SAH which results in the loss of urinary sodium and also water through the kidneys. The distinction can be made by examining the urinary sodium excretion which is well above normal in CSW as well as there being clinical and biochemical evidence of hypovolaemia (reduced CVP, elevated haematocrit). The treatment of

Answers *cont.*

CSW is sodium and volume replacement together and for SIADH, volume restriction. A potential hazardous situation may arise if an erroneous diagnosis of SIADH is made, the patient is fluid restricted and hypovolaemia is exacerbated resulting in inadequate cerebral perfusion and ischaemia. If in doubt treatment for CSW with volume and sodium replacement is safer.

A.9 Risk factors for the formation of aneurysms include a prior aneurysm, smoking, cocaine use, hypertension, a family history of aneurysms and some inherited connective tissue disorders, e.g. Marfan's syndrome. Up to 20% of patients who have one aneurysm may have another at some point in the future. The most modifiable of all the patient's risk factors will be to cease smoking.

Revision Points

Subarachnoid Haemorrhage

Although spontaneous SAH has a number of potential causes, rupture of a cerebral aneurysm is the most common (75–80%) and the most important cause clinically because untreated the 30-day mortality is 46%. The most important management step for the non-specialist is early recognition (by taking an appropriate history and thinking of the diagnosis) and immediate referral to a neurosurgical centre for specialist treatment. As in this case, a differential diagnosis may exist; however, if SAH is in the differential diagnosis there should be no delay. Delay may be life-threatening and/or may compromise the possibility of good-quality survival.

The newest developments in the diagnosis and treatment of cerebral vascular lesions are radiological. CT and MRI angiography, which can be performed non-invasively and reformatted in multiple planes, is now readily available and has improved the resolution of vascular imaging. However, conventional angiography (DSA) still remains the gold standard investigation after a suggestive history, particularly if intervention is planned. Endovascular therapies, including coiling with or without stenting, are rapidly evolving, are available in most neurosurgical centres and can be an effective treatment for aneurysms (ruptured and unruptured); however, each case should be judged on its own merits by the treating neurovascular team.

Issues to Consider

- What measures might be undertaken to reduce the risk of cerebral vasospasm in a patient with subarachnoid haemorrhage?
- What is the role of lumbar puncture in cases of suspected subarachoid haemorrhage?

Further Information

Bederson, J.B., Awad, I.A., Wiebers, D.O., 2000. Recommendations for the management of patients with unruptured intracranial aneurysms. Circulation 102, 2300–2308.

Inagawa, T., Kamiya, K., Ogasawara, H., Yano, T., 1987. Rebleeding of aneurysms in the acute stage. Surgical Neurology 28 (2), 93–99.

Rinkel, G.J., Djibuti, M., Algra, A., van Gijn, J., 1998. Prevalence and risk of rupture of intracranial aneurysms: a systemic review. Stroke 29, 251–256.

Fatigue and bruising in a teenager

Charles G. Mullighan

A usually fit and active 13-year-old boy complains of gradually worsening tiredness for a month. In the last few days, he has noticed bruises, both after minor trauma and without any obvious trauma, to his arms and legs. His past medical history includes a tonsillectomy, adenoidectomy and appendicectomy. He does not take any regular medication, and denies using alcohol, over-the-counter or non-prescription drugs. He has a low-grade fever, is pale and has moderate cervical lymphadenopathy. There are multiple small to moderate bruises in dependent areas, and small haemorrhages at the bite line of the buccal mucosa. The spleen is palpable 5 cm below the left costal margin.

Q.1 What are the possible causes of this boy's signs and symptoms? What investigations should be performed?

The following investigations become available.

Investigation 47.1 Summary of results			
Haemoglobin	61 g/L	White cell count	23×10^9/L
		Neutrophils	0.1×10^9/L
MCV	102 fL	ESR	54 mm/hour
Platelets	23×10^9/L		
Sodium	134 mmol/L	Calcium	2.8 mmol/L
Potassium	5.1 mmol/L	Phosphate	0.35 mmol/L
Chloride	106 mmol/L	Albumin	38 g/L
Bicarbonate	15 mmol/L	Bilirubin	15 µmol/L
Urea	5 mmol/L	ALT	18 U/L
Creatinine	0.09 mmol/L	AST	20 U/L
Uric acid	0.24 mmol/L	GGT	30 U/L
Glucose	4.6 mmol/L	ALP	90 U/L
LDH	354 U/L		

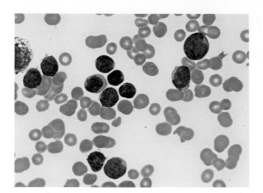

Figure 47.1

Blood film (Figure 47.1) comment:

Macrocytic anaemia. Anisocytosis and poikilocytosis. Abnormal lymphoctes present; possibly atypical, possibly blasts.

Infectious mononucleosis screen (IM): Negative. EBV IgM: Negative.

Q.2 Interpret the blood test results. What further investigations and management should be arranged?

While awaiting transfer to the haematology ward, he develops rigors and is noted to have a temperature of 39°C.

Q.3 What investigations should be performed immediately, and what treatment would you like to start?

An urgent bone marrow aspirate is performed (Figure 47.2). Microscopic examination of the aspirate smears shows over 90% blasts, immature chromatin, few nucleoli, scant cytoplasm and few granules. Immunophenotyping of the bone marrow aspirate shows the presence of a lymphoblast populations staining for CD45, CD5, CD7, and cytoplasmic CD3, but negative for cell surface CD3, negative for the B lymphoid markers CD19 and CD79a, and negative for the granulocytic markers CD13 and CD33.

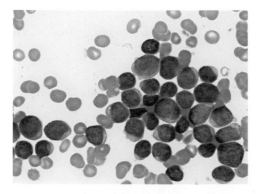

Figure 47.2

Immunophenotyping of peripheral blood yields similar results. Subsequent examination of bone marrow trephine sections shows complete replacement with a homogeneous infiltrate of lymphoblasts.

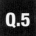 **What is the diagnosis?**

While the patient awaits further investigations, including a lumbar puncture, and prepares for initial treatment, the ward nursing staff are concerned that the he has become short of breath, with a dry cough and difficulty swallowing. You are asked to review him urgently.

Q.5 What are the possible diagnoses? What do you look for on examination and what investigations should be performed?

He is sitting on the edge of his bed with respiratory rate of 25, a peripheral oxygen saturation of 94% on air and mild facial swelling. Chest examination reveals dullness to percussion at the right lung field base, with reduced breath sounds on the right side. You repeat the chest X-ray (Figure 47.3).

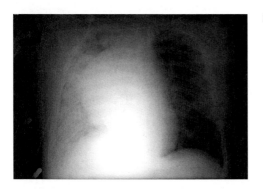

Figure 47.3

Q.6 What does the chest X-ray show, and what is the diagnosis? What additional management is appropriate?

Soon after commencing chemotherapy the patient becomes confused and is noted to have reduced urine output.

Q.7 What complication is likely to have developed? What investigations should be ordered, and what are they likely to show?

Q.8 How should this complication be prevented and managed?

Following stabilization and a good initial response to treatment, the patient and his family enquire as to the prognosis of his disease.

Q.9 What do you tell them?

Answers

A.1 Fatigue, pallor, spontaneous/easy bruising and enlargement of the spleen and lymphoid organs strongly suggests a serious haematological disorder or malignancy. However, primary viral infections such as Epstein–Barr virus (EBV), causing infectious mononucleosis or glandular fever, can also present in this way and must be considered in the differential.

An acute leukaemia or lymphoma should be considered. Aplastic anaemia is less likely given the presence of lymphadenopathy. Appropriate investigations include a full blood count with examination of the peripheral blood film, serum biochemistry and serology for EBV infection (Paul Bunnell/monospot tests and/ or EBV antibodies/PCR).

A.2 He has pancytopenia, i.e. all three cell lineages, red cells, platelets and white cells, are abnormally low. There are abnormal lymphocytes seen on examination on the blood film. The blood film raises the possibility of an acute leukaemia, and a bone marrow biopsy is required.

Poikilocytosis simply means abnormally shaped red blood cells and is seen in a wide range of conditions. It is therefore fairly non-specific.

Anisocytosis, as its name suggests, means there are red cells of different sizes. Again, this can occur in many conditions including those in which folate and ferritin deficiency occur, producing macrocytes

and microcytes. Coeliac disease would be one example of a condition in which this phenomenon occurs.

The EBV serology results are against a diagnosis of acute infectious mononucleosis. Review by a haematologist should be arranged urgently and admission arranged. The creatinine is high for his age and, taken with the elevated LDH and biochemistry results, suggests a degree of spontaneous tumour lysis.

A.3 Fever in a patient with pancytopenia is a potentially life-threatening medical emergency. Clinical re-examination and investigations should be performed quickly and antibiotics commenced without delay. The patient should be examined for any site of infection, including the skin, mouth, teeth, chest, urinary tract and perianal region. *At least* one set of blood cultures should be taken, urine collected and sputum, if available, sent for culture. Broad-spectrum antibiotics should be commenced according to local haematology unit protocols – this usually consists of a third-generation cephalosporin and aminoglycoside (e.g. gentamicin) but the choice of antibiotics varies widely according to local sensitivities. The combination chosen should cover both Gram-positive and Gram-negative bacteria as well as *Pseudomonas* spp. A chest X-ray should be performed for occult infection.

A.4 Acute lymphoblastic leukaemia, T-lineage.

We know you may consider this an unfair question as the interpretation of immunophenotyping is an area of expertise only to be expected from haematology specialists. The key features of the bone marrow exam are, however, the presence of a large population of lymphoblasts. Abnormalities within the nuclear material of these cells suggests that they may be neoplastic in nature. While the total blood count is elevated, there are very few normally functioning white cells, meaning that this young man is very susceptible to infection.

A.5 He may have pneumonia or a mediastinal mass due to lymph node enlargement from leukaemic involvement. A detailed respiratory examination should be performed, and the initial chest X-ray reviewed. A further X-ray may be needed if the initial film was normal.

A.6 The chest X-ray shows gross mediastinal widening with compression of the right lung field. This is consistent with a mediastinal mass from involvement by leukaemia. The facial swelling raises the possibility of superior vena cava obstruction. This is a medical emergency.

The haematologist should be notified and intensive care should be called to assess the patient immediately. A CT is required to evaluate the degree of tracheal compression. The lumbar puncture will require anaesthetic support. The patient should receive a platelet transfusion prior to the lumbar puncture to minimize the risk of a traumatic lumbar puncture (bleeding into the CSF).

A.7 In view of the diagnosis and mediastinal involvement, the patient is at high risk of tumour lysis syndrome after commencement of chemotherapy. Urgent measurement of electrolyte levels and ECG are required. These may show hyperkalaemia, hypocalcaemia, hyperphosphataemia, hyperuricaemia and renal impairment.

A.8 All patients at risk of tumour lysis should receive vigorous intravenous hydration with potassium-free fluids, supplemental sodium bicarbonate and close monitoring of fluid balance. Allopurinol should be given. Treatment of established tumour lysis will depend on the severity of electrolyte disturbance and renal dysfunction, but may require intensive care management, continuous cardiac monitoring for arrhythmias, and more aggressive therapy to correct electrolyte imbalances, hyperuricaemia, and preserve renal function. All nephrotoxic agents (aminoglycosides, non-steroidal anti-inflammatory drugs and intravenous contrast, etc.) should be avoided if at all possible.

A.9 ALL is the commonest childhood cancer and over 80% of children are cured. The prognosis declines in adolescence, and is less favourable in older males with T-lineage ALL. Accurate prediction of outcome will depend on close monitoring of the early response to therapy (for example, by flow cytometry of bone marrow or blood samples to measure levels of minimal residual disease). Treatment usually consists of combination multi-agent chemotherapy and CNS prophylaxis (with intrathecal chemotherapy), and is commonly prolonged, lasting up to 2 years. Strict compliance with therapy is essential to maximize the chance of cure.

Revision Points

- Acute leukaemia is a malignancy of leucocyte precursors. Acute lymphoblastic leukaemia (ALL) is the commonest childhood cancer. Acute myeloid leukaemia is less common in children, but more common in adults. There is a bimodal peak in the incidence of leukaemia – young children and older adults. Acute leukaemia is characterized by recurring chromosomal alterations including aneuploidy (abnormal number of chromosomes) and translocations, but the aetiology in most cases is unknown.
- Acute leukaemia results in proliferation of leukaemic cells (blasts) that fill the bone marrow and suppress growth of non-leukaemic blood cells, resulting in anaemia, thrombocytopenia and neutropenia.
- Appropriate investigations to distinguish acute leukaemia from other disorders resulting in pancytopenia, such as viral infections, severe vitamin deficiencies and drug/toxin effects, are required. A bone marrow biopsy is usually required.

- Acute leukaemia is fatal if untreated, but over 80% of children with ALL are cured. Prognosis is worse for adolescents and adults.
- ALL may arise from B or T lymphocytes. T-lineage ALL more commonly occurs in older males, and is associated with higher-presentation leucocyte counts and solid tumour (most commonly mediastinal) masses.
- The mainstay of ALL treatment is intensive multi-agent chemotherapy, intrathecal chemotherapy to prevent CNS relapse, and careful supportive care. Clinical and genetic features are used to stratify risk and guide the intensity of treatment (including the use of bone marrow transplantation).
- Patients presenting with and undergoing therapy for acute leukaemia are extremely vulnerable to infection, bleeding, and tumour lysis. These require specialized care but awareness of these potential problems is important.

Issues to Consider

- What are the implications of successful treatment of childhood leukaemia when the patient enters adulthood?
- What are the different types of 'bone-marrow transplant'?
- What is red cell distribution width (RDW) and how is it interpreted?

Further Information

Hoffbrand, A.V., Moss, P.A.H., Pettit, J.E. (Eds.), 2006. Acute leukemia. In: Essential haematology, 5th edn. Blackwell, Oxford, ch 12. *This is an excellent book covering normal and malignant disorders aimed at medical students.*

Pui, C.H. (Ed.), 2006. Acute lymphoblastic leukemia. In: Childhood leukemias, 2nd edn. Cambridge University Press, Cambridge, ch 16. *A detailed textbook covering all aspects of the biology and management of ALL.*

www.leukaemia.org *A UK-based web resource for parents and sufferers.*

An 18-year-old girl is brought into the emergency department by ambulance from a youth hostel. She is a backpacker and has been travelling around the country. She is drowsy and unable to give any history. Her airway is clear and her breathing is unhindered. She reacts purposefully to painful stimuli, moving all limbs, and grunts but does not speak. She opens her eyes briefly in response to you shouting her name.

Q.1 What is her Glasgow coma score?

She is of normal build and is well kept. Her temperature is 37.5°C, her pulse rate is 135 bpm and her supine blood pressure is 95/60 mmHg. She has deep sighing respirations with a respiratory rate of 25 breaths/minute. Her mouth is extremely dry and her tissue turgor is reduced. She has no other abnormalities on cardiac and respiratory examination, and she has no focal neurological signs. Her abdomen is not distended but appears guarded and she reacts as if in pain when palpated. Bowel sounds cannot be heard.

Another girl appears who says she is a companion from the hostel. The two have only known each other for 2 weeks and agreed to travel together. The girl claims her friend became unwell over the last week, particularly over the last 2 days. She complained of being very tired. The patient had become lethargic and listless. She had not wanted to eat, but had complained of being very thirsty and had been drinking large amounts of water. Today she stayed on her bunk and was unable to get up. She complained of abdominal pain and vomited three times. The friend had gone out for a few hours and on her return found the patient looking very unwell and an ambulance had been called. The patient is not known to have any major medical problems or to take medications or drugs of any kind.

Q.2 Provide a differential diagnosis.

There are a number of possible causes for this woman's comatose state.

Q.3 What should be done immediately?

A finger-prick blood glucose measurement has been obtained using a bedside glucose meter and reads 'high'. A urinary catheter drains 50 mL urine which, when tested with a strip, registers ketones as ++++. After initial resuscitation, results of the preliminary blood tests come back as follows:

Investigation 48.1 Summary of results			
Haemoglobin	151 g/L	White cell count	18.6×10^9/L
Platelets	289×10^9/L	Neutrophils 57%	10.6×10^9/L
PCV	0.38	Lymphocytes 27%	5.0×10^9/L
MCV	86.9 fL	Monocytes 11%	2.0×10^9/L
MCH	29.5 pg	Eosinophils 3%	0.6×10^9/L
MCHC	340 g/L	Basophils 2%	0.4×10^9/L
Sodium	140 mmol/L	Calcium	2.16 mmol/L
Potassium	6.0 mmol/L	Phosphate	1.15 mmol/L
Chloride	109 mmol/L	Total protein	67 g/L
Bicarbonate	7.0 mmol/L	Albumin	38 g/L
Urea	6.1 mmol/L	Globulins	29 g/L
Creatinine	0.13 mmol/L	Bilirubin	16 µmol/L
Anion gap	28.5	ALT	24 U/L
Glucose	30 mmol/L	AST	28 U/L
Cholesterol	3.8 mmol/L	GGT	19 U/L
LDH	202 U/L	ALP	52 U/L
Arterial blood gas analysis on room air			
pO_2	99 mmHg	pCO_2	15 mmHg
pH	7.0	Calculated bicarbonate	7.0 mmol/L

Q.4 What are the abnormalities? How do they help in clarifying your differential diagnosis?

You have a working diagnosis for this patient who is critically ill.

Q.5 What is your acute management plan?

You institute emergency management. An intravenous line is inserted, and she is managed in the high dependency ward with close nursing care to monitor all vital signs and to keep the airway clear. The patient's urine output is regularly charted to establish that renal function is normal and urine production is taking place. An insulin infusion is commenced.

In addition to your fluid replacements, the electrolytes are checked after 2 hours to measure the potassium concentration. It is now 3.6 mmol/L and you begin to add potassium supplementation to the intravenous infusion at 13.6 mmol and later to 27.2 mmol (1–2 g KCl) per hour. You check her potassium level again at 4 hours and 8 hours. A chest X-ray is performed and urine microscopy sent off to look for any intercurrent infection. After 12 hours the patient's blood glucose is down to 15 mmol/L. The intravenous fluid is changed to 5% dextrose 1 L over 6 hours with 2 g KCl added to each litre of fluid.

Twenty-four hours later your patient's condition has significantly improved. She is fully conscious, no longer vomiting or nauseated and is allowed to start eating. The urine shows only a trace of ketones.

Q.6 How will you change her insulin therapy now?

329

She responds well to your insulin regimen, and is stable for discharge. Further history establishes that she has previously been healthy: now she has a diagnosis of diabetes. She is frightened by what has happened, and anxious about her diabetes management.

Q.7 Describe your ongoing management plan for this patient while she is in hospital and prior to discharge.

The patient decides to curtail her backpacking holiday and return home.

Answers

A.1 Her Glasgow coma score is 11 (E4, V2, M5).

A.2 Given her young age, history of polydipsia and clinical evidence of dehydration and hyperventilation, the most likely diagnosis is diabetic ketoacidosis. Abdominal pain is quite common in this condition and does not indicate any acute abdominal problem (although intra-abdominal problems must be considered in the differential diagnosis). Other diagnoses to consider include poisoning (alcohol, food or drug-related, particularly street drugs) and infection (e.g. meningitis).

A.3 As part of the immediate management, the following must be undertaken:
- Protect the airway.
- Insert an intravenous cannula and take blood for electrolytes, urea and creatinine, blood glucose, complete blood picture, lipase.
- Collect a finger-prick blood sample for glucose estimation and, if available, ketone measurement.
- Perform an arterial blood gas assay to obtain the pH and ascertain if patient is acidotic.
- Insert a urinary catheter and check for urinary ketones and measure the urine output.

- Commence emergency resuscitation with intravenous infusion of isotonic saline. At least 1–1.5 litres should be given over the first hour.

A.4 The patient has a severe metabolic acidosis as characterized by the low serum pH and low bicarbonate level. The low pCO_2 is due to respiratory compensation for the metabolic acidosis. This explains the hyperventilation.

The increased anion gap is due to the presence of anions not measured in the calculated anion gap. This 'hidden' anion here is ketone bodies.

Metabolic acidosis can be divided into:
- High anion gap acidosis (addition of anions to the blood, e.g. ketoacidosis, lactic acidosis and salicylate or alcohol poisoning).
- Normal anion gap acidosis with a high chloride level, usually as a result of loss of alkali (bicarbonate), for example from the gut with severe diarrhoea or in renal tubular acidosis.

The apparent hyperkalaemia is due to the shift of potassium from the intracellular space to the extracellular space caused by the acidosis (potassium in exchange for hydrogen ions). In spite of the elevated serum potassium, these patients are usually depleted of total body potassium. This is an important point to grasp. Large amounts of

Answers *cont.*

potassium are lost via the kidneys as a result of the glucose diuresis and also through vomiting. The serum potassium level will need careful monitoring as it will drop rapidly when treatment with insulin is commenced and the acidosis starts to correct, placing the patient at risk of hypokalaemia and arrhythmias.

Hyperglycaemia is consistent with the diagnosis of diabetes and is a marker of insulin deficiency. The glucose level, though usually elevated in patients with ketoacidosis, may not be particularly high nor at the levels generally seen in patients with hyperosmolar non-ketotic coma.

Leucocytosis is seen quite commonly in association with ketoacidosis and does not necessarily indicate infection. Infections are common triggers for ketoacidosis, and patients should be checked for septic foci once their resuscitation has started.

The combination of the clinical picture, hyperglycaemia, metabolic acidosis with high anion gap and ketones in the urine confirms the diagnosis of diabetic ketoacidosis.

A.5 Diabetic ketoacidosis is an acute medical emergency, requiring rapid diagnosis and treatment. These patients are critically ill and need specialized care and close monitoring. The patient's vital signs must be observed regularly, and recorded along with fluid input and output and bedside blood glucose monitoring. If the patient's potassium concentrations are significantly abnormal cardiac monitoring may be needed. Ketoacidosis may induce gastroparesis and the patient should be kept fasted to minimize the risk from gastric aspiration.

Principal Steps in Management

Urgent:
- Fluid and sodium replacement.
- Correction of the acidosis and hyperglycaemia with insulin.
- Monitoring and replacement of potassium.
  Then:
- Diagnosis and management of precipitating events.
- Prevention of complications of ketoacidosis.
  Once patient is better:
- (Re)establishment of ongoing diabetes management plan.
- Prevention of recurrence of ketoacidosis.

Fluid and Sodium Replacement

- Severe dehydration is common. This is secondary to the osmotic diuresis (hyperglycaemia and ketonuria) compounded by vomiting and hyperventilation. The degree of dehydration needs to be assessed both clinically and biochemically.
- Sodium depletion is common. This is consequent on the diuresis (although the serum sodium level may appear normal).
- Rehydration is started with isotonic saline. For example, give 1 L/hour for 2 hours then a third litre over the following 4 hours. The severely dehydrated patient may need up to 6 litres of fluid in the first 24 hours.

  After 12 hours (or once the blood glucose has dropped to 13 mmol/L), fluid replacement can be changed to 5% dextrose.

  Urine output should be monitored (an indwelling bladder catheter can be placed as part of the initial resuscitation). Hypovolaemia and the risk of acute renal tubular necrosis must be minimized. During

Answers *cont.*

the osmotic diuresis, the urine output must be matched on a regular basis with intravenous fluid replacement. Once the dehydration has been corrected, an output of at least 30 mL/hour must be maintained.

Correction of Acidosis and Hyperglycaemia with Insulin

Insulin therapy will correct both the acidosis and hyperglycaemia.

Continuous intravenous infusion of insulin using an insulin pump at 4–8 units per hour is the best method of delivering insulin. Rapid changes in pH, glucose and potassium are thus avoided, thereby preventing complications such as cardiac arrhythmias and cerebral oedema.

If infusion is not possible hourly intramuscular doses may be used; subcutaneous insulin therapy should not be used in the acute treatment of diabetic ketoacidosis particularly in significantly dehydrated patients because of the unreliable rate of insulin absorption.

Blood glucose must be monitored hourly using a bedside glucose meter while patient is receiving intravenous insulin infusion.

The use of bicarbonate is generally not required in the treatment of diabetic ketoacidosis. The metabolic acidosis is corrected by rehydration and by cessation of ketogenesis with the use of insulin.

Potassium Replacement

Rapid shifts in potassium will occur once treatment for ketoacidosis is started. Use of insulin and correction of the acidosis will cause shift of potassium back from the extracellular to the intracellular space. As the patient is depleted of total body potassium, the drop in serum potassium can be potentially life threatening.

- Replacement potassium can commence with the second litre of saline – provided

the initial serum potassium was in the normal range.
- If the initial potassium level is high, recheck the potassium after 2 hours of intravenous saline infusion and commence potassium replacement as soon as the serum potassium is in the normal range (do not wait till hypokalaemia has occurred to start potassium replacement).
- Potassium replacement in range of 10–20 mmol/L/hour (1 g KCl = 13.6 mmol). This rate is likely to be required for the first 12 hours. Be prepared to increase this rate if serum potassium is not being maintained in the desirable range.
- Check serum electrolytes every 2–4 hours for the first 24 hours. Insertion of a central line allows repeated drawing of blood without venepuncture as well as monitoring of central venous filling.
- Ensure adequate urine output has been established. If the patient is not producing urine they may be in acute renal failure, and potassium replacement may need to be modified.

Diagnosis and Treatment of Precipitating Events

Once resuscitation of the acute metabolic state is underway it is important to look for any precipitating event that may have triggered the onset of ketoacidosis. In this patient's age group the commonest causes are either infection or omission of insulin. Investigations should be performed for chest, urinary tract, skin and gastrointestinal infections.

Prevention of the Complications of Ketoacidosis

- Cerebral oedema is a rare but dangerous complication; it can be prevented by

Answers *cont.*

careful fluid balance and avoiding dramatic drops in blood glucose levels.

- Aspiration of gastric contents can be prevented by careful nursing and keeping the patient fasting until she is fully conscious and has bowel sounds.
- Thrombosis is a relatively common complication; anticoagulation until the patient is mobile may need to be considered.

A.6 You are now able to change the patient to subcutaneous insulin using a bolus of short-acting insulin with each main meal and a long-acting insulin to provide basal cover. (Some patients may wish to consider a subcutaneous insulin infusion pump.)

Insulin infusion is ceased 1 hour after the first dose of subcutaneous insulin is given.

A.7 Once the acute event of the ketoacidosis is over a long-term management plan for the ongoing treatment of the patient will need to be developed. In this patient ketoacidosis was the mode of first presentation of her diabetes. During hospitalization she might not be able to fully comprehend the diagnosis and its implications. She would not be reasonably expected to assimilate all the information that she needs to manage her diabetes. Therefore she should be given the necessary information to enable her to manage her diabetes in the immediate future with further education to occur as an outpatient. Diabetes nurse educators should be contacted to assist with her education.

In Hospital:

- She needs to be commenced on a basal/ bolus insulin regimen using short-acting insulin before each main meal and basal

insulin at bedtime. She should be taught the action of the different insulins that she will be using. (A starting dose of insulin may be estimated using the calculation of 0.3–0.5 unit insulin per kg of body weight per 24 hours split half into basal and half to be divided into the three bolus doses.)

- She needs to be taught to recognize the symptoms of hypoglycaemia and instructed on how to prevent and treat hypoglycaemia.
- She needs to understand that she should not omit her insulin therapy.
- She should be taught how to self-administer insulin using syringes or an insulin pen device. Diabetes nurse educators will be important in helping her cope with these and other issues.
- She should be taught how to use a personal blood glucose monitor and how to interpret the readings that she obtains. She needs to understand what factors affect blood glucose levels, e.g. food, exercise, insulin dose. She should learn to keep a record of her blood glucose.

As an Outpatient

- A diet plan is important with basic knowledge on the appropriate food types. A balanced diet with complex carbohydrates should be encouraged and simple sugars avoided. The diet should have less than 30% as fat. Most importantly she should understand the necessity to eat regularly with an even spread of carbohydrates over the day and not to miss meals. Between-meal snacks and supper will need to be taken.
- She should be advised to be very moderate with alcohol consumption and to ensure that she eats adequate carbohydrate-type food when she drinks alcohol.

Answers *cont.*

- She should be taught how to recognize the symptoms of hypoglycaemia and what the appropriate treatment is.
- She should be given information on how travelling can affect diabetes and what steps she needs to take.
- The patient needs to understand that diabetes is a lifelong disease that needs to be managed well to prevent long-term complications. However, details of long-term treatment and prevention and

monitoring of long-term complications can be given at a later date when she is getting used to her condition.
- She should be strongly advised to seek referral to a specialist diabetes centre on her return to her home country to continue her diabetes management and education.
- If she drives a car, her licence may be affected and she will need to contact the appropriate authority.

Revision Points

Diabetic Ketoacidosis

Diabetic ketoacidosis is an acute medical emergency that is potentially life threatening but completely reversible if diagnosed and treated rapidly.

With aggressive and early management of ketoacidosis in recent years the mortality rate from ketoacidosis has been markedly reduced to less than 5%.

Ketoacidosis can occur as the first presentation of a patient with type 1 diabetes or as a complication in a patient known to have the condition. It occurs in type 1 diabetics when there is absence or insufficiency of insulin due to:

- Failure to administer insulin; *or*
- An increased need for insulin at times of physical stress (e.g. an intercurrent infection, trauma, surgery, etc.).

Aetiology

Insufficient insulin leads to uncontrolled gluconeogenesis and impaired peripheral glucose utilization, both of which result in hyperglycaemia and glucosuria. A severe osmotic diuresis results leading to loss of fluid and electrolytes. Insulin deficiency also leads to the formation of ketone bodies which are strong acids leading to a metabolic acidosis.

Clinical Features

- Polyuria.
- Polydipsia.
- Anorexia, nausea and vomiting.
- Long sighing respiration (Kussmaul breathing).
- Sweet-smelling ketotic breath.
- Clinical signs of dehydration.
- Coma (in severe cases).

Treatment

Intravenous insulin infusion allows a gradual and steady correction of the metabolic abnormalities.

Complications

- Electrolyte disturbances as indicated above (particularly hypokalaemia).
- Hypoglycaemia.
- Infections such as aspiration or stasis pneumonia and urinary tract infection from indwelling catheters.
- Thrombosis risk may require short-term anticoagulation.
- Gastric dilatation and haemorrhage.
- Ominous but fortunately rare complications include adult respiratory distress syndrome and the cerebral dysequilibrium syndrome from cerebral oedema.

Revision Points *cont.*

Follow-up

Patients must be encouraged to learn and perform regular home blood glucose monitoring for day-to-day adjustment of their insulin regimen, while their longer-term glycaemic control can be monitored by measuring the glycosylated haemoglobin (HBA1c).

Macrovascular complications leading to ischaemic heart disease, cerebrovascular disease and peripheral vascular disease can also be significantly reduced by concomitantly treating hypertension and hyperlipidaemia and urging patients to stop smoking.

Patients with type 1 diabetes should be followed in specialized diabetes centres if possible, where multidisciplinary care is available from endocrinologists, diabetes nurse educators, dieticians and podiatrists.

The achievement of optimal control of diabetes is especially important in young patients with type 1 diabetes such as this patient as there are now impressive data to show that the long-term microvascular complications (retinopathy, nephropathy and neuropathy) are significantly reduced with good blood glucose levels.

Young women such this patient should be counselled in avoiding unplanned pregnancy as it is important for the diabetes to be optimally controlled prior to conception to achieve the best outcome for both mother and baby. Contraception should be encouraged if the patient is sexually active and not planning pregnancy. Patients with diabetes may face restrictions with their driving licences and need to apply annually for licence renewal.

Future developments in the management of diabetes range from glucose-monitoring devices which do not require finger punctures, new insulin analogues, new insulin delivery methods such as inhaled insulin, pancreas transplantation, in islet cell transplantation and possible gene therapy to replace insulin-producing cells in patients with type 1 diabetes. However, the current imperatives remain to assist patients in achieving the best control of diabetes to prevent both short-term problems such as ketoacidosis and long-term complications such as blindness, renal failure, etc.

Issues to Consider

- How do you manage a type 2 diabetic patient in hyperosmolar non-ketotic state?
- What new drugs are becoming available for the treatment of type 1 and type 2 diabetes?

Further Information

http://emedicine.medscape.com/article/766275-overview *A tutorial on the emergency management of diabetic ketoacidosis.*

www.diabetesnet.com *A patient-focused website dealing with many of the practical aspects of living with diabetes, including information on the newer insulins.*

A woman with palpitations

David Torpy

A 63-year-old female retired administrative assistant attends your preoperative assessment clinic prior to a diagnostic left knee arthroscopy after several months of unexplained left knee pain. In passing, she mentions palpitations and you note her to have an irregular pulse with a rate of 130/minute with a pulse deficit of 20/minute.

You also note a small asymmetric and slightly irregular goitre. She has no personal history of thyroid disease or other medical conditions although she admits to recent stress and anxiety. Her sister had surgery for an 'enlarged thyroid' many years ago.

Q.1 What is the likely diagnosis? What other symptoms should be enquired about?

She describes a 10 kg weight loss over 2 months, heat intolerance, excess sweating, anxiety, sleep disturbance (although she has attributed this to her knee pain), infrequent but mild palpitations and tremulousness. She denied any change in appetite, has had no diarrhoea and no ocular symptoms.

Q.2 What signs should be looked for on examination and how useful are they?

Physical examination reveals a slim lady of 59 kg, height 164 cm. She has warm sweaty palms. There is no palmar erythema. She has a goitre with the thyroid approximately 5× its normal size. It is irregular and nodular. She has thyroid stare due to lid retraction and lid lag but no exophthalmos. She has atrial fibrillation.

Q.3 What investigations would you like to arrange and how would they assist in your management?

An ECG (Figure 49.1) shows atrial fibrillation.
Laboratory investigations include the following:
A thyroid technetium scan (Figure 49.2) shows an enlarged thyroid with generally increased tracer uptake in a patchy distribution consistent with a multinodular goitre.

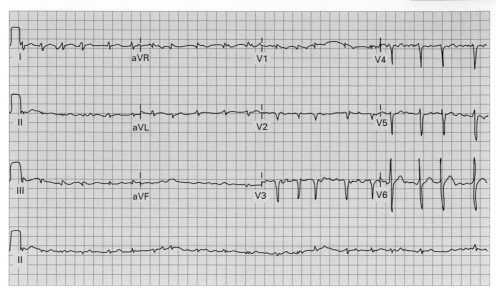

Figure 49.1

Investigation 49.1	Summary of results	
Free T4	64.8 pmol/L	(10–25 pmol/L)
Free T3	12.8 pmol/L	(3.1–5.4 pmol/L)
TSH	<0.01 mIU/L	(0.5–3.7 mIU/L)

Figure 49.2

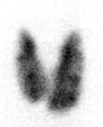

Q.4 What treatment should be started? How might the treatments for the thyroid and heart problems interact? What are the risks of the thyroid treatments and how should the patient be counselled?

The patient is treated with carbimazole 20 mg bd and propranolol 20 mg bd. Warfarin is started and titrated to an INR of 2–2.5. She is seen with thyroid function tests initially at 3-weekly intervals to check that the thyroid hormone levels are falling and to allow reduction of the carbimazole dose.

After 3 weeks, she reports the resolution of most of her symptoms, particularly reduced anxiety. Her heart rate is 60 and irregularly irregular consistent with atrial fibrillation. Blood tests are as follows:

Investigation 49.2 Summary of results		
Free T4	20 pmol/L	(10–25 pmol/L)
Free T3	7.3 pmol/L	(3.1–5.4 pmol/L)
TSH	<0.01 mIU/L	(0.5–3.7 mIU/L)
WCC	3.6×10^9/L	Neutrophils 1.6×10^9/L ($1.8–7.5 \times 10^9$/L)

Q.5 What do these blood tests indicate?

The dose of carbimazole was reduced to 15 mg bd and 3 weeks later to 15 mg daily.

Six weeks later her free T4, free T3 and TSH are all normal although she remains in atrial fibrillation.

Q.6 What are the options now? What are their relative risks and benefits.

Her subsequent clinical course is described in her notes as follows (Figure 49.3):

Radioactive iodine given at 14 weeks, dose 466 MBq Na-I131 by capsule.
Carbimazole interrupted for 4 days before therapy and 6 days after
I131 to maximize radioiodine uptake.

Review 4 weeks post-I131 therapy
TSH 9 IU/mL, free T4 15 pmol/, free T3 3.8 pmol/L
Carbimazole reduced to 5 mg daily

Review 7 weeks post-I131 therapy
TSH 9.6 mIU/L, free T4 14, free T3 3.4 pmol/L.
Carbimazole stopped.

Review 10 weeks post-I131 therapy
TSH 10.1 nIU/L, free T4 12 pmol/L, free T3 3.5 pmol/L.
Thyroxine 50 mcg daily started.

Review 14 weeks post-I131 therapy
TSH 7.1, Free T4 12.5 pmol/L, free T3 3.4 pmol/L.
Thyroxine increased to 100 mcg daily.

Review 18 weeks post-I131 therapy
TSH 3.0 mIU/L, free T4 15 pmol/L, free T3 3.9 pmol/L.
Now in sinus rhythm.
Continued on thyroxine.
Warfarin to stop in 2 months.

Figure 49.3

Answers

A.1 This is consistent with atrial fibrillation (AF). Although AF can occur in otherwise healthy individuals, there is often an underlying cause including ischaemic heart disease, myocardial disease such as a cardiomyopathy, or mitral valve disease. Non-cardiac causes include thyrotoxicosis. Thyrotoxicosis is suggested here by the physical finding of a goitre.

Important historical features to suggest thyrotoxicosis include heat intolerance or excessive symptoms of feeling hot even when others are feeling cool, weight loss often with maintained or increased appetite, tremor, proximal muscle weakness, sweating, sleep disturbance, palpitations, diarrhoea, anxiety and sleep disturbance. It is important to recognize that older people may have fewer symptoms than the young but are more likely to present with cardiac features such as arrythmias, angina pectoris and, when very severe, cardiac failure. All patients with new AF should have thyroid hormone levels checked. Thyroid disease tends to run in families, particularly when there is a history of autoimmune disease. Autoimmune thyroid disease is more common in women.

It is important to ask about the recent use of iodine either as a dietary supplement such as kelp tablets or given as a component of some radiocontrast media. Some medications such as amiodarone and some cough mixtures contain large amounts of iodine which may precipitate thyrotoxicosis – the 'Jodbasedow effect'.

A.2 Thyrotoxicosis is associated with a fine finger tremor, tachycardia, sometimes with arrhythmia which is most often atrial fibrillation, proximal muscle weakness, evident by an inability to stand from a squatting position or abduct the arms above the horizontal, and a thyroid stare accompanied by lid retraction (where the sclera is apparent above the iris on normal forward gaze) and lid lag (where the upper lid does not follow the eye down on rapid downward gaze exposing the sclera above the iris).

In addition, there may be signs of Graves' disease including exophthalmos, proptosis or forward protrusion of the eye due to inflammatory infiltration of the muscles and other tissues behind the eye. The sclera is often apparent below the limbus on norma forward vision in this situation. The degree of eye proptosis can be measured with a portable bedside device known as an exophthalmometer.

An infiltrative skin lesion known as Graves' dermopathy may be present, but this is far less common than thyroid or eye involvement. Graves' dermopathy is also known as pretibial myxoedema with plaques and nodules developing over the shins. Finger clubbing, also known as thyroid acropathy, may also occur in Graves' disease.

Many patients with thyrotoxicosis have a goitre (enlarged thyroid) which may be diffusely enlarged in Graves' disease or have a single nodule in thyrotoxicosis due to a toxic nodule. Alternatively, a multinodular gland may be palpable.

A.3 An electrocardiogram should be obtained to confirm the clinical finding of atrial fibrillation. Measurement of serum free thyroxine (fT4), free triodothyronine (fT3) and thyroid-stimulating hormone (TSH) is necessary to confirm thyrotoxicosis. Primary thyrotoxicosis would be expected to be associated with elevated free T4 and/or free T3 and suppression of pituitary sourced TSH by negative feedback.

A thyroid radioisotope (technetium or I-123) scan will assist in differential

Answers *cont.*

diagnosis. In this case thyroid uptake of tracer, which is treated like normal iodine by the thyroid iodine uptake mechanism, would be expected to be increased in a pattern consistent with multiple nodular hyperactivity although there may also be nodules with reduced uptake.

Check for TSH receptor antibodies. These are antibodies that stimulate the TSH receptor and lead to excessive TSH-independent thyroid hormone hypersecretion and the thyroid gland growth pathognomic of Graves' disease.

A.4 Treatments for primary hyperthyroidism include antithyroid drugs which inhibit thyroid hormone synthesis, thyroid destructive therapy such as radioactive iodine or surgery. Often, antithyroid drugs, from the thionamide class (e.g. carbimazole or propylthiouracil) are used to achieve a euthyroid state. Permanent destructive thyroid therapy can be used once the patient has stabilized.

AF and other tachyarrythmias can be treated with beta blockade. Beta blockade also controls many other thyrotoxic features such as tremor and anxiety which represent excessive activity of the sympathetic nervous system. For this reason, non-selective beta blockers, usually propranolol, are the drugs of choice.

AF entails a significant risk of embolization with a substantial risk of stroke which can be reduced by anticoagulation with warfarin. Doses required to produce therapeutic anticoagulation are generally smaller in thyrotoxicosis as thyroid hormone increases the clearance of vitamin-K dependent clotting factors.

It is necessary to counsel her about the risks of thioamide drugs. Agranulocytosis is a rare but serious complication. She should present promptly if she develops sore throat and fever! More common side-effects include skin rash or nausea. Hepatitis occurs rarely.

A.5 These tests reveal a mild persistent elevation of T3 consistent with persistent thyrotoxicosis but substantial resolution of the hyperthyroxinaemia. The TSH is suppressed by negative feedback from high T4 and T3 levels. This suppressive effect may persist for several months, even after T4 and T3 levels are normalized.

Mild neutropenia is often seen in thyrotoxicosis and does not necessarily signify an idiosyncratic effect of thionamides.

A.6 Options include ongoing antithyroid drugs, radioactive iodine or surgery. Patient preference plays a role in therapy selection and there is marked variation in approaches and acceptance of therapies internationally.

If a permanent thyroid destructive treatment is used, radioiodine is preferred, as treatment has minimal immediate risk. Radioiodine given as I-131 is a beta particle emitter that destroys functioning thyroid tissue after uptake by the sodium-iodine symporter. The mean time to euthyroidism is approximately 8 weeks. Therapy can be given as an outpatient. The half-life of I-131 is approximately 6 days and some precautions are advised to minimize unnecessary radiation exposure to others. No long-term side-effects such as tumours have been observed in treated patients. However, some cases of progression of thyroid eye disease have been described.

Answers *cont.*

Surgery involves subtotal thyroidectomy and risks damaging neighbouring structures such as the recurrent laryngeal nerve leading to hoarseness and the parathyroids leading to hypoparathyroidism, as well as the usual risks of surgery and general anaesthesia. It's useful for those with very large goitres although a reduction in thyroid size is usual after radioiodine.

Revision Points

Causes of Thyrotoxicosis

- Graves' disease.
- Toxic multinodular goitre.
- Subacute (or acute) thyroiditis.
- Toxic nodule.
- Thyroid carcinoma.
- Struma ovarii (ectopic thyroid tissue within an ovarian teratoma).
- Exogenous thyroxine excess.
- TSH-secreting pituitary adenoma.

Treatments for Thyrotoxicosis

- Thionamide drugs (carbimazole or propylthiouracil).
- Radioactive iodine.
- Subtotal thyroidectomy.

Issues to Consider

- Which causes of thyrotoxicosis do not lead to reduced uptake of radiotracer?
- What are the different types of thyroid cancer?
- What is a symporter?
- What is a thyroid storm? How is it managed?

Further Information

http://www.thyroidmanager.org/ *Website covering management of thyroid disease in many sections. Available also via the Endotext website (http://www.endotext.org/).*

http://www.endocrineweb.com *A US based patient centred site but with a lot of well written articles on a whole range of endocrine disorders.*

A collapsed, breathless woman

Andrew W. Perry

You are working in an emergency department overnight and you receive an urgent call from the ambulance service. A paramedic crew is en route to your hospital with a 50-year-old woman who collapsed at home shortly after taking her first dose of antibiotic. Vital signs are: HR 110 bpm, BP 80 mmHg palpable at the radial pulse, oxygen saturation of 92% on room air improving to 98% on high-glow oxygen, Glasgow Coma Scale score (GCS) 14 with some confusion. Facial swelling and wheeze is noted. Nebulized salbutamol and intravenous fluid are being given. Estimated time to arrival is approximately 10 minutes.

Q.1 What will you do in the 10 minutes you have to prepare for the arrival of this patient?

The patient arrives on an ambulance stretcher and is wheeled straight into the resuscitation bay.

The history records that she is a previously healthy mother of two, who was prescribed a course of amoxicillin by a locum family practitioner this evening for sinusitis. She took her first tablet 40 minutes ago and began to feel unwell approximately 30 minutes ago. She complained of tingling and swelling of her mouth, tongue and lips, tightness in her chest and abdominal pain followed by one episode of vomiting. She has taken penicillins before with no reaction, and has no known allergies.

Q.2 What system would you follow to examine this patient?

You note the following on a rapid focused examination of the patient:

Airway: mild stridor and hoarse, soft voice. There is swelling of the face and tongue. There are no airway adjuncts being used.

Breathing: respiratory rate 32 with use of accessory muscles. She can speak in short phrases. There is no tracheal tug. Air entry is moderate, with widespread expiratory wheeze. She continues to saturate between 96 and 98% on 15 L oxygen via a Hudson mask.

Circulation: pulse is thready, tachycardic and regular. She has poor capillary refill of >5 seconds and is cold, sweaty and pale. Her HR is 130 bpm (post salbutamol) and BP is 80/40 mmHg. She has one 18G IV cannula in situ and has received approximately 750 mL of normal saline thus far.

You note an urticarial rash starting to develop over her trunk. Abdominal examination reveals a generally tender but relatively soft abdomen.

Her GCS is still 14 with one point lost for some confusion. Blood glucose is 6.2 and Hb 140 g/L. An arterial blood gas shows a metabolic acidosis with borderline oxygenation.

Q.3 What is the likely diagnosis?

Q.4 What is your immediate management?

You institute rapid treatment of this woman as described and she responds well. Most significant symptoms settle within an hour without requiring either intubation or invasive monitoring. While her rash has largely settled she complains of ongoing itch.

Q.5 What other medications could be used in the management of this acute allergic reaction?

Q.6 How long will you keep her in hospital, and why?

You admit your patient to the emergency short-stay ward for observation overnight. Your patient recovers well and is grateful for your treatment. You see her on the ward the next morning, and make arrangements for her discharge.

Q.7 What will you tell her prior to discharge, and what important arrangements must be in place before she leaves hospital?

You discharge your patient, armed with an adrenaline (epinephrine) pen (EpiPen® or Anapen®) and the knowledge of how to use it, letters to her local doctor and her immunologist, and with the paperwork to apply for a medical alert bracelet having been sent off in the post.

Answers

A.1 The purpose of advance notification by ambulance services is to allow emergency departments to optimally prepare for their arrival by notifying all relevant personnel both in the emergency department and also other staff, e.g. anaesthetists, radiographers. They should also ensure that an adequate location in the emergency department is available (a resuscitation bay), and that equipment and all medications are present and ready for immediate use. A team leader (usually the

Answers *cont.*

most senior emergency doctor) is chosen, and both medical and nursing staff allocated with defined roles (airway, breathing and circulation, documentation). Staff should be waiting in the resuscitation bay before the patient arrives.

A.2 This is a life-threatening situation so your examination (and treatment) needs to follow the resuscitation algorithm of **ABC** – Airway, Breathing and Circulation (you can add DEFG – 'Dont Ever Forget Glucose!').

Airway. Is it patent, or fully or partly occluded? Is there stridor, or snoring if the patient is unconscious? Do they have obvious swelling or rash of their perioral region, mouth, lips, tongue or neck?

Breathing. Respiratory rate? Effort of breathing including use of accessory muscles? What is the volume of speech they are able to produce? Is it full sentences, phrases or words? What does their chest sound like – is there equal air entry and are there added sounds, e.g. wheeze, or is it silent? (Silent is a bad sign.) Oxygen saturations, noting the oxygen flow rate and delivery method? Arterial blood gas?

Circulation. Palpable pulse? Rhythm (on monitor)? Blood pressure? Are they peripherally shut down, as often assessed by capillary refill time, and colour and temperature of peripheries? What is the blood pressure? What does cardiac monitoring and a 12-lead ECG show? What intravenous access do they have? How much of what fluid has been given so far?

A Glasgow Coma Scale score estimation is also performed as a guide of cerebral function.

Documentation and timing of events is important, and in retrospect may prove

vital. In the resuscitation scenario, management, e.g. airway-opening manoeuvre (e.g. chin thrust), is often occurs at the same time as examination is taking place, especially as issues are identified.

A.3 This is most likely an anaphylactic reaction to her antibiotics. Anaphylactic reactions are life threatening – you should call for immediate assistance (an arrest code may be appropriate depending on the level of expertise in your emergency department). Re-assess your **ABC**!

Airway. Intubation may be required before the obstruction worsens and intubation becomes impossible. Facial and tongue oedema may make endotracheal intubation extremely difficult. Alert the staff (and yourself) that the patient may require a cricothyroidotomy or emergency tracheostomy.

Breathing. Continue high-flow oxygen via a non-rebreather mask (i.e. aiming for as close as possible to 100% FiO_2). Continuous nebulized beta agonists in the form of salbutamol or adrenaline (epinephrine) to treat the bronchoconstriction. Adrenaline is particularly useful in this setting because it treats both bronchoconstriction and hypotension via beta-1 and -2 adrenergic effects (see Table 50.1). Note that pulse oximeters are prone to falsely low readings from inadequate application to the patient's finger and peripheral shutdown. In this case application of a special earlobe probe may be beneficial.

Circulation. Ensure the patient has sufficient IV access – this usually consists of two large-bore (18G or larger) IV cannulae. Your patient only has one cannula so a second should be inserted. Crystalloid (e.g. normal saline) solutions are generally preferred over colloid (e.g. albumin or

345

Answers *cont.*

Table 50.1 Adrenaline's main effects on adrenoreceptors

Adrenoreceptor	Location of Receptor	Action When Stimulated	Effect
α-1	Vascular smooth muscle	Vasoconstriction	Increased blood pressure via increased peripheral vascular resistance
β-1	Heart	+ve inotrope and chronotrope	Increased blood pressure through increased cardiac output (via increased stroke volume and heart rate)
β-2	Bronchial and vascular smooth muscle	Relaxation of affected smooth muscle	Relief of bronchoconstriction (in high doses α-1 effects on peripheral vascular resistance predominate)
	Mast cells and basophils	Decreased histamine and other mediator release	Decreased vascular permeability leading to decreased mucosal oedema and increased circulating blood volume

hetastarch) because of similar efficacy and low cost. Normal saline is preferred over dextrose (because of rapid tissue uptake) or compound sodium lactate (a.k.a. Hartmann's solution) or lactated Ringer's solution; the lactate contained in both may contribute to the metabolic acidosis which occurs in anaphylaxis.

Removal of allergen (e.g. removal of the venom sac from bee or wasp stings or cessation of the medication infusion or blood product). Do not induce emesis even if the causative agent (e.g. medication or food) is in the gut. Provoking emesis increases the risk of aspiration.

A.4

Adrenaline – the Silver Bullet in Anaphylaxis

Adrenaline (epinephrine) is the first-line treatment of severe anaphylaxis. It exerts its effects as a non-selective agonist of both alpha and beta adrenoreceptors. There are no absolute contraindications to use of adrenaline because the risk of death or significant disability outweighs its adverse effects. Several case series have implicated

the failure to administer early adrenaline as a consistent cause in anaphylaxis-related deaths.

- 500 μg of adrenaline (0.5 mL of 1:1000 adrenaline) intramuscularly is recommended, although smaller doses intravenously and titrated to effect can be used, as can endotracheal and subcutaneous routes.
- Repeat doses at 3–5 minute intervals, due to the very short half-life.

A.5 *Adrenaline* is the first-line agent in severe anaphylaxis and no other agent can replace it. However, a number of other medications may be used as adjuncts to treat certain symptoms. The majority of these agents have poor evidence to support their efficacy in anaphylaxis but are included because of their long history of empirical use.

Bronchodilators: beta-2 agonists such as salbutamol may be used to assist or as an alternative to adrenaline to relieve bronchoconstriction.

Antihistamines: systematic reviews of the literature do not show any randomized controlled trials supporting the use of H1 receptor subtype antihistamines in anaphylaxis other than to reduce pruritus and urticaria. This patient is reporting significant itch so use of these agents is probably warranted.

H2 receptor blockers (e.g. ranitidine) have been given in the past on the theoretical basis of completing the histamine blockade; however, there is minimal evidence to support their use.

Steroids: glucocorticoids have no role in the immediate treatment of anaphylaxis, due to the time lag between their administration and effect. However, these agents are routinely given on an empirical basis with the rationale that they may help to prevent the biphasic reactions that occur in up to 20% of individuals. Hydrocortisone IV 6-hourly is often commenced, followed by a discharge supply of oral prednisolone for no more than 4 days. The rationale for 4 days is on the basis that all biphasic reactions reported to date have occurred within 72 hours.

A.6 This patient has had a life-threatening anaphylactic reaction, and must be closely observed until completely symptom free. If treated properly most anaphylactic episodes are short-lived with symptoms resolving within hours. There is, however, a phenomenon of *biphasic anaphylaxis* which is defined as a recurrence of symptoms that develops following the apparent resolution of the initial anaphylactic event. The pathophysiological basis of this phenomenon is thought to be related to the delayed release of mediators that are manufactured by mast cells and basophils in response to the initial allergen exposure. Biphasic reactions have been reported to develop in 1 to 20% of anaphylactic reactions and typically occur within 8 hours after resolution of the initial symptoms,

although recurrences up to 72 hours later have been reported.

A.7 Anaphylaxis may be recurrent – hence all patients with suspected anaphylaxis should be referred to an allergy/immunology specialist for investigation and provision of a comprehensive anaphylaxis management plan.

- Patients at risk of anaphylaxis should wear an identifying MedicAlert® (or similar) bracelet, which will increase the likelihood that adrenaline will be administered in an emergency.
- Patients in whom episodes are unpredictable, who are allergic to foods that are extremely difficult to avoid, or when the cause cannot be identified should carry injectable adrenaline and be trained in its use, and should always carry a mobile telephone.
- Patients should consider notifying family, friends and work colleagues or school teachers about their allergy and if they carry an adrenaline pen inform them of its location and provide instructions on adrenaline use. Carrying a pocket/wallet card describing an anaphylaxis action plan (Figure 50.1), such as that supplied by the Australasian Society of Clinical Immunology and Allergy (ASCIA – see further information at the end of the chapter) which contains all this information is recommended.
- In some circumstances it may be possible to reduce the severity of allergy by specific immunotherapy.
- Where there is doubt or confusion about whether an anaphylactic reaction has occurred or the inciting agent is uncertain, immunologists can perform a number of blood and skin tests and follow up tryptase levels.

ACTION PLAN FOR
Anaphylaxis

ascia
australasian society of clinical immunology and allergy inc.
www.allergy.org.au

Name: _____

Date of birth: _____

Photo

Allergens to be avoided: _____
_____
_____

Family/carer name(s): _____
_____

Work Ph: _____

Home Ph: _____

Mobile Ph: _____

Plan prepared by:
Dr _____
_____

Signed _____

Date _____

for use with EpiPen® or EpiPen® Jr adrenaline autoinjectors

MILD TO MODERATE ALLERGIC REACTION

- swelling of lips, face, eyes
- hives or welts
- tingling mouth, abdominal pain, vomiting

ACTION

- stay with person and call for help
- give medications (if prescribed) ....
- locate EpiPen® or EpiPen® Jr
- contact family/carer

▼ **Watch for any one of the following signs of Anaphylaxis**

ANAPHYLAXIS (SEVERE ALLERGIC REACTION)

- difficult/noisy breathing
- swelling of tongue
- swelling/tightness in throat
- difficulty talking and/or hoarse voice
- wheeze or persistent cough
- loss of consciousness and/or collapse
- pale and floppy (young children)

ACTION

1 Give EpiPen® or EpiPen® Jr
2 Call ambulance*- telephone 000 (Aus) or 111 (NZ)
3 Lay person flat and elevate legs. If breathing is difficult, allow to sit but do not stand
4 Contact family/carer
5 Further adrenaline doses may be given if no response after 5 minutes (if another adrenaline autoinjector is available)

If in doubt, give EpiPen® or EpiPen® Jr

EpiPen® Jr is generally prescribed for children aged 1-5 years.
*Medical observation in hospital for at least 4 hours is recommended after anaphylaxis.

How to give EpiPen® or EpiPen® Jr

1
Form fist around EpiPen® and PULL OFF GREY SAFETY CAP.

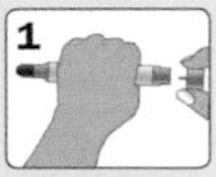

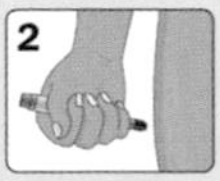

2
PLACE BLACK END against outer mid-thigh (with or without clothing).

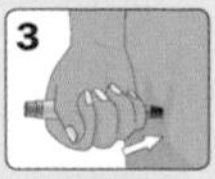

3
PUSH DOWN HARD until a click is heard or felt and hold in place for 10 seconds.

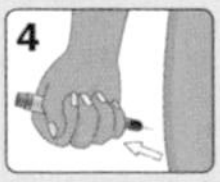

4
REMOVE EpiPen® and DO NOT touch needle. Massage injection site for 10 seconds.

© ASCIA 2009. This plan was developed by ASCIA

Additional information _____
_____

Figure 50.1 This information has been reproduced with permission from the Australasian Society of Clinical Immunology and Allergy (ASCIA), from the ASCIA website (www.allergy.org.au). ASCIA is the peak professional body of clinical immunology and allergy specialists in Australia and New Zealand.

Revision Points

Classic anaphylaxis involves *previous* sensitization to the allergen. Patients may have had no reaction after past exposures, or mild rash and itch right through to previous anaphylactic episodes. The most common agents to cause anaphylaxis include foods and food additives (notably peanuts, seafood and egg), insect stings or bites and medications (especially antibiotics). Anaphylactic reactions vary in their presentation with the most noticeable symptoms involving the skin and mucosa, respiratory tract and GI tract, and the cardiovascular system, 90% of patients having some combination of urticaria, erythema, pruritus, and/or angioedema.

Issues to Consider

- How do you use an adrenaline pen?
- What are the adverse effects of adrenaline?
- What are the skin and blood tests that can be done to investigate anaphylaxis and allergies?

Further Information

Dunn, R., Dilley, S., Brookes. J., et al. (Eds.), 2003. The emergency medicine manual.

Venom Publishing, Tennyson, Australia. *Textbook with comprehensive notes on the pathophysiology of anaphylaxis.*

www.allergy.org.au *Australasian Society of Clinical Immunology and Allergy (ASCIA): an excellent resource for both doctors and patients on the many issues involved in anaphylaxis including a number of action plans that can be printed off and used by patients.*

Management of a young man who is HIV positive

Karen E. Rowland

A 32-year-old unemployed man presents for a check-up. He and his partner have recently moved from another city 'for personal reasons'. He claims he has no major health problems and takes no medications. He smokes about 30 cigarettes a day and drinks 30–70 grams of alcohol daily. Sensing that there is more to the story, you spend some time talking. During the course of the conversation he reveals that just before moving, he had a positive blood test for human immunodeficiency virus (HIV).

Q.1 **What further information should be gained from the history?**

The patient reveals that previously he and his male partner used intravenous drugs and shared needles for about 5 months. He has not changed sexual partners, and has never had a blood transfusion or travelled overseas. On direct enquiry he recalls a severe flu-like illness about 4 months ago which involved headache, fever, weakness and muscle aches and pains and lasted about 10 days. The patient explains that he and his partner have definitely ceased intravenous drug use and limit their drug use to marijuana. His partner has not had an HIV antibody test as he is 'too scared'.

Q.2 **What may the flu-like illness 4 months ago have represented?**

Q.3 **What should be sought on examination?**

Currently, the patient's health is good. His weight is stable, he has no fevers or sweats and his systems review is unremarkable. The patient is examined. He does not have a fever or skin rash, he has good dentition and his mouth is unremarkable. There is no lymphadenopathy or any abnormalities that might be attributable to his recent diagnosis.

Q.4 **What investigations should be performed?**

Blood screens show a complete blood picture within the normal range, CD4⁺ lymphocyte count of 800 cells/μL (RR 405–2205 cells/μL) and HIV viral load of 4000 copies/μL. He is hepatitis B surface antigen negative and hepatitis C antibody positive. The patient has asymptomatic HIV infection.

The partner is also found to be HIV antibody positive and has similar hepatitis serology. The partner describes a painless lesion on the tip of his penis which has been present for 10 days (Figure 51.1).

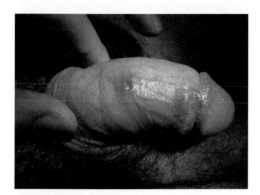

Figure 51.1

> **Q.5** What are the possible causes of the lesion in Figure 51.1? What treatment is required?

> **Q.6** How would you counsel the couple?

They are offered vaccination against hepatitis A and B viruses given their sexual orientation and recent history of injecting drug use. They both receive treatment for the penile lesion. The patient and his partner decline to identify any of their contacts. They are followed every 3 months with a full review of symptoms, examination findings and blood screens. After 12 months they stop attending appointments and are lost to follow-up.

Four and half years later the man presents with a 3–4-week history of feeling unwell. He is tired and lethargic and has lost 6 kg in weight. He has also had a sore mouth. He denies any other gastrointestinal symptoms including diarrhoea and there are no other significant symptoms on systems review.

On examination he appears thinner than previously and looks depressed. He is afebrile. His oral mucosa is coated with numerous thick white plaques (Figure 51.2). He has generalized lymphadenopathy, the nodes being 1–2 cm in size. You refer him to a hospital infectious diseases clinic. His blood screens reveal his haemoglobin has dropped to 112 g/L but his complete blood count is otherwise normal, his CD4⁺ lymphocyte count has dropped to 210 cells/μL and the HIV viral load is >200000 copies/μL.

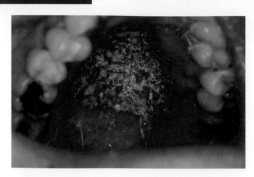

Figure 51.2

Q.7
What does Figure 51.2 show? What has happened? What are the principles of management?

The patient is counselled and commences antiretroviral therapy with tenofovir/emtricitabine 300 mg/200 mg as a fixed-dose combination tablet and boosted atazanavir 300 mg/ritonavir 100 mg all taken once daily. His oral candidiasis is treated with fluconazole 100 mg daily. If his CD4⁺ count drops further (below 200 cells/μL) he will require *Pneumocystis* prophylaxis with co-trimoxazole 160 mg/800 mg daily. He is reviewed monthly.

Q.8
The patient asks if this treatment will cure his HIV infection and whether he has AIDS. Give an appropriate reply.

Answers

A.1
- The patient's understanding of the meaning of a positive HIV antibody test. The implications of the positive test must be explained to the patient in a sensitive manner.
- History of risk factors for the acquisition of HIV infection: intravenous drug use, sexual history (including other sexual partners while in a relationship and condom use), travel and sexual intercourse overseas, blood transfusion prior to 1990, and tattoos and body piercing.
- Whether the partner knows the HIV diagnosis and whether he has been tested.

- History of other sexually transmitted diseases and other blood-borne virus infections.
- A full review of symptoms to elicit symptoms attributable to HIV infection, immune deficiency or opportunistic infections.

A.2 HIV seroconversion illness which is also known as acute retroviral syndrome. This is a mononucleosis-like illness with fevers, malaise, sore throat, lymphadenopathy and rash. It occurs 10 days to 6 weeks after HIV infection and coincides with the appearance of HIV antibodies in the blood. It is estimated that 50–90% of people with acute HIV infection

Answers *cont.*

experience acute retroviral syndrome but, because it is non-specific, it is often not recognized at the time.

A.3

- Evidence of ill health: weight loss, fever, anaemia, marks of recent intravenous drug use.
- Assessment of global neurological function: e.g. mental state examination.
- Skin eruptions: seborrhoeic dermatitis, boils/furuncles, Kaposi's sarcoma, onychomycosis.
- Oral lesions: oral candidiasis, oral hairy leucoplakia, ulceration, periodontal disease.
- Generalized lymphadenopathy.
- Abnormalities in specific systems: respiratory, focal neurological defects.
- Perianal disease: warts/malignancy, herpes simplex ulcers.
- In women: vaginal examination for cervical warts/malignancy.

A.4

1. Investigations to assess HIV infection and readiness for treatment:
   - Repeat HIV serology (including Western blot) to confirm positive.
   - CD4$^+$ cell count, CD4$^+$ percentage, CD4$^+$:CD8$^+$ ratio and HIV viral load.
   - HIV resistance testing.
   - HLA*B5701 genotype: this reliably predicts hypersensitivity to abacavir – a nucleoside analogue.
   - Electrolytes, renal and liver function and complete blood examination.
2. Sexual health screen:
   - Serology for hepatitis A, B and C viruses.
   - Gonorrhoea: throat and rectal swabs for culture and PCR.
   - Chlamydia: urine for PCR.
   - Syphilis serology.

3. Investigations to identify opportunistic infections:
   - Serology for cryptococcal antigen, CMV, EBV, toxoplasmosis.
   - If history/risk of tuberculosis exposure: chest X-ray, CT chest and sputum for TB culture.
   - CT or MRI brain if neurologic deficits found on examination.

A.5 The classic cause of a *painless* genital ulcer is the chancre of primary syphilis. Figure 51.1 shows an erythematous painless ulcer on the edge of the glans (the foreskin is retracted in the photograph). Where the foreskin rests on the primary ulcer, a secondary ulcer has occurred, termed a 'kiss-lesion'. This is a classic appearance of primary syphilis. This ulcer is highly infectious, containing millions of spirochaetes. Even without treatment, this ulcer will heal in 10–14 days, followed later by lesions of secondary syphilis. For many years syphilis has been extremely rare; however, since 2005 there have been increasing numbers of cases of primary syphilis among men who have sex with men. Other possible diagnoses include herpes simplex ulcers (usually painful) or cancer (the history is too short). Diagnosis of primary syphilis requires demonstrating the spirochaetes in the lesion with dark field microscopy or polymerase chain reaction for treponemal DNA. Treatment is one single dose of 1.8 g IM benzathine penicillin. The partner must also receive treatment, even if his serology is negative.

A.6 The patient should be counselled together with his partner. The partner needs to be tested for HIV infection. If the partner is negative, further tests need to be done 3 months after the last risk exposure to ensure he is not in the window period

353

(HIV infected but seroconversion has not yet occurred).

The couple need to be informed of the methods by which HIV is transmitted. They should be informed about post-exposure prophylaxis with antiretroviral therapy in case of accidental exposure.

In many countries, diagnosis of HIV infection requires notification of public health authorities.

A new diagnosis of HIV infection is psychologically challenging for the patient. Issues that may need to be addressed include: his own mortality, fear of illness/disability/death, infidelity in a relationship, occupational issues, parenting in a heterosexual relationship, isolation/loneliness if his social situation is such that he cannot discuss the diagnosis freely for fear of ostracism. It is important the patient is offered access to appropriate support services.

A.7 Figure 51.2 illustrates white plaques of oral candida infection on the hard palate. The patient's CD4$^+$ count is 210 cells/μL indicating advanced immunodeficiency; he has developed accompanying constitutional symptoms, lymphadenopathy and an opportunistic infection (oral candidiasis). He has symptomatic HIV infection with uncontrolled HIV replication as demonstrated by his high viral load. He should be managed in conjunction with a clinic specializing in HIV medicine.

Principles of HIV Management

1. Control HIV replication, aiming for complete suppression so HIV is no longer detectable in plasma. This requires combination antiretroviral therapy for the rest of his life. Antiretroviral drug classes are nucleoside/nucleotide analogues

(tenofovir/emtricitabine), non-nucleoside reverse transcriptase inhibitors (efavirenz), protease inhibitors (atazanavir, ritonavir) and the new classes of integrase inhibitors and CCR5 inhibitors. Combination treatment is necessary as HIV replicates rapidly and mutates to become resistant to therapy with a single agent.

2. Treat and administer prophylaxis against opportunistic infections: necessary when the CD4$^+$ count is below 200 cells/μL. Co-trimoxazole is used to prevent *Pneumocystis jirovecii* pneumonia (previously known as *P. carinii* or PCP) and toxoplasmosis, azithromycin to prevent disseminated *Mycobacterium avium* complex infection, fluconazole to prevent candida infections, and ganciclovir to prevent CMV disease.

3. Monitor for the emergence of malignancies, such as cerebral lymphoma, squamous cell carcinoma of the anal canal or cervix, Kaposi's sarcoma and other malignancies.

4. Manage associated co-morbidities: the HIV-infected person is at increased risk of developing metabolic diseases such dyslipidaemias, diabetes mellitus, coronary artery disease and osteoporosis. Long-term management of HIV patients includes prevention and treatment of these conditions.

5. Support in the terminal phases of HIV infection.

A.8 The treatment will not cure the patient's HIV infection. Pro-viral HIV DNA persists for the lifetime of the person. Antiretroviral therapy prevents active HIV replication. This allows restoration of CD4$^+$ cell counts and recovery of immune function. There is no known mechanism for removal of pro-viral DNA once integration

Answers *cont.*

into the host has occurred. If antiretroviral therapy stops, HIV reappears in the plasma (within days to weeks) and immune damage resumes.

The World Health Organization divides HIV infection into four stages for clinical and surveillance purposes (Table 51.1). This patient has CD4$^+$ count of 210 cells/μL, weight loss and persistent oral candidiasis.

He has stage 3 disease with advanced HIV-associated immunodeficiency. Acquired immune deficiency syndrome (AIDS) is said to be present when a patient has stage 4 immunodeficiency and an 'AIDS defining condition' has been diagnosed. This patient does not have AIDS, but he does have advanced immunodeficiency (stage 3) due to his HIV infection.

Table 51.1 2007 WHO clinical staging and immunological classification for adults with confirmed HIV infection

WHO Stage	Clinical Presentation	CD4 Count cells/μL	HIV Associated Immunodeficiency
Stage 1	Asymptomatic	>500	None
	Persistent generalized lymphadenopathy		
Stage 2	Moderate weight loss <10% body weight	350–499	Mild
	Skin eruptions		
Stage 3	Severe weight loss >10% body weight	200–349	Advanced
	Chronic diarrhoea >1 month		
	Persistent oral candidiasis		
	Severe bacterial infections		
	Pulmonary tuberculosis		
	Anaemia		
Stage 4 AIDS	Presence of an *AIDS defining condition* such as:	<200	Severe
	HIV wasting		
	Pneumocystis pneumonia		
	Oesophageal candidiasis		
	CMV retinitis		
	Disseminated *Mycobacterium avium* complex		
	HIV encephalopathy		
	Cerebral lymphoma or other HIV associated tumour*		

For full list of AIDS defining conditions see WHO case definitions of HIV for surveillance 2007.

Revision Points

HIV Epidemiology

HIV is spread via infected blood, semen, vaginal fluid and breast milk. HIV infects about 33 million people worldwide, the greatest number in sub-Saharan Africa where 22 million people live with HIV and where 72% of AIDS deaths occur. In sub-Saharan Africa, 50% of infected people are female and transmission is through heterosexual intercourse or from mother to child in utero or at birth. Elsewhere HIV prevalence is greatest among men who have sex with men, intravenous drug users and sex workers. Since the introduction of highly active antiretroviral therapy, mortality from HIV infection has greatly improved.

Issues to Consider

• What is the risk to healthcare workers of accidental transmission of HIV? How can this risk be reduced? What policies are there in your hospital to address this risk?
• What measures do you know of to deal with the global AIDS epidemic? What interventions are available for low-income countries? Does circumcision affect HIV transmission?
• What is the risk of an infected mother passing HIV to her child? How does mother to child transmission occur? What can be done to reduce this risk?

Further Information

Deeks, S., Phillips, A., 2009. HIV infection, antiretroviral treatment, ageing, and non-AIDS related mortality. British Medical Journal 338, 288–292.

Hammer, S.M., Eron, J.J., Reiss, P., et al., 2008. Antiretroviral treatment of adult HIV infection. Journal of the American Medical Association 300, 555–570.

Back and leg pain in a middle-aged man

Gabriel Lee

A 50-year-old man experiences a sudden onset of back and leg pain while walking. The pain radiates from the left buttock to his knee and as far as his ankle. There is no recent history of trauma. He has no significant past medical or surgical history. He has been bed-bound for 3 days.

Q.1 What key features need to be sought from the history?

On specific questioning, there is a similar pain which radiates down his right leg although this is of a lesser intensity. The patient has noticed that the pain is aggravated when he coughs or strains. He has noticed some numbness over his buttocks. This is associated with some difficulty in voiding. Prior to the onset of this pain, the patient had not experienced any urinary symptoms. There has been no alteration in bowel function. His general health is good and he has not lost any weight recently. He is not on any medications.

Q.2 What specific features should be sought on physical examination?

A general physical examination is unremarkable. His blood pressure is 130/90 mmHg and his heart rate is 90 bpm. The rest of the cardiovascular system is normal, and in particular all his peripheral pulses are present and of good volume. Abdominal examination is unremarkable except for some dullness to percussion in the suprapubic region. Digital examination of the rectum suggests a rather lax anal sphincter. Examination of his back reveals no significant spinal tenderness. Straight leg raising is restricted to 30° in both legs, with reproduction of leg pain. The power and tone of both legs are normal to testing in the bed but he is unable to stand on his toes, indicating plantar flexion weakness. The ankle jerks are bilaterally absent and his plantar responses are flexor. Hypoaesthesia is present in the lateral and plantar aspects of both feet. In addition, sensory testing to pin-prick reveals some numbness over the buttocks and reduced sensation in the perineum.

Q.3 What is the diagnosis?

The clinical picture fits for an acute neurological problem.

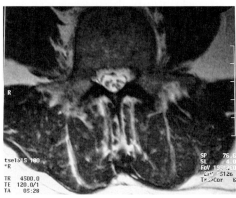

Q.4 How should the patient be investigated?

An investigation is performed as shown in Figures 52.1–52.3.

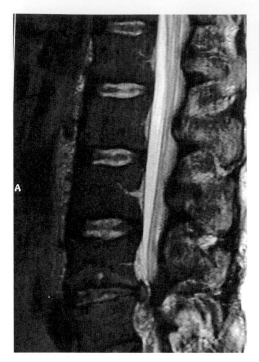

Figure 52.1

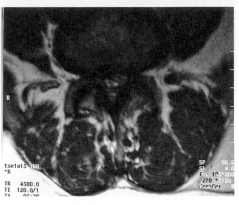

Figure 52.2

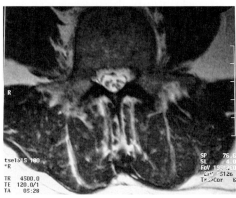

Figure 52.3

Q.5 What is the investigation and what do the three images show?

The patient underwent a microdiscectomy as an emergency procedure. This gave him relief of his pain and his symptoms of cauda equina compression resolved over the next week.

Answers

A.1 The first aim of the history is to try to distinguish between the major causes of limb pain. These include:

- Vascular:
  - intermittent claudication
  - chronic venous insufficiency.
- Musculoskeletal:
  - joint disease
  - muscle/ligament injury
  - stress fracture.
- Neurogenic:
  - sciatica
  - spinal canal stenosis
  - cauda equina syndrome.

This patient gives a typical account of 'sciatica' (which often arises from lumbar disc herniation). It is important to distinguish between radiculopathic pain ('sciatica') and non-specific lumbar pain. Radiculopathic pain refers to pain which radiates into the limb in a myotomal distribution. It arises from compression or compromise of particular nerve root(s). This is typically exacerbated by coughing, sneezing or straining. Surgery to relieve nerve root compression (e.g. lumbar discectomy in the presence of a significant disc prolapse) is generally performed with the key aim of improving radiculopathic pain. Non-specific lumbar or back pain may radiate to the buttock and thigh but not usually beyond the knee. It is usually not helped by surgery.

The clinician may also use the patient's description of radiculopathic pain to deduce the possible nerve roots affected in the majority of patients. For example, an L3 radiculopathy typically results in pain which radiates to the knee. In contrast, an S1 radiculopathy usually causes pain which is felt as far as the ankle/foot. Asking specific questions about the pattern of any sensory changes may further point to specific dermatome(s).

Further history should be directed towards excluding:
- Serious ('red flag') underlying conditions, e.g.:
  - tumour
  - infection
  - coagulopathy.
- Severe neurological compromise, e.g. evidence of:
  - lower limb weakness
  - sensory changes
  - bladder or bowel symptoms.

A.2 On physical examination evidence should be sought of overall state of health, e.g.:
- Fever.
- Recent weight loss.
- Disseminated malignancy (e.g. cachexia, pallor, lymphadenopathy, pleural effusions, breast lumps, hepatomegaly, prostatic enlargement, bone tenderness, unexplained bruises).

Specific features referable to the symptoms and the need to be excluded:
- Peripheral vascular disease (check pulses).
- Musculoskeletal disorders (examine joints).
- Neurological disorders (the examination must focus on the trunk and lower limbs, including the perineum, ensuring that no sensory level is missed).

A.3 This patient has evidence of cauda equina compression. This is judged by symptoms of acute bladder paralysis and buttock numbness. The clinical examination has revealed a distended bladder, reduced anal tone and numbness in the perineal and buttock regions (S2, 3, 4). There are also signs consistent with S1 nerve root compression (absent ankle reflexes and plantar flexion weakness).

Answers *cont.*

A.4 This is a neurological emergency and any delay in treatment may compromise neurological recovery and result in permanent paralysis. An urgent MRI scan of the lumbosacral spine is the investigation of choice, but may not always be available. A CT scan is the more often performed procedure. In the absence of MRI or CT, a lumbar myelogram can also point to the diagnosis. Plain X-rays are generally unhelpful. Lack of appropriate radiological facilities and neurosurgical expertise should prompt an urgent transfer of the patient to a centre where these are available. Cauda equina compression requires prompt surgery to optimize the chances of neurological recovery. In patients with sphincteric dysfunction (bladder/bowel), the recovery process may take many months and is often incomplete.

Blood tests should be done but must not delay emergency treatment. They are of lesser importance in those patients who otherwise appear in normal health, making a benign aetiology more likely. They can be very important in those with presentations suspicious of a sinister underlying problem, e.g. malignancy. An elevated white cell count or inflammatory markers (ESR, CRP) may suggest infection. Other abnormalities in blood counts, liver function tests, total protein or calcium levels could suggest underlying malignancy. Tumour markers

(e.g. PSA) may be helpful. Coagulation studies (INR, APTT) should be performed when there is clinical suspicion of a bleeding diathesis.

A.5 These are MRI scans, with focus on the spinal canal. T2-weighted images show cerebrospinal fluid (CSF) contained within the thecal sac which has a hyperintense (bright) appearance. A compressive lesion (e.g. disc prolapse) is easier to recognize on this sequence.

The sagittal MRI of this patient (Figure 52.1) reveals two problems. First, the patient has a congenitally narrow spinal canal. Any disc prolapse is more likely to cause a cauda equina compressive syndrome. Second, the patient has an L4/5 disc prolapse (Figure 52.2) which explains his clinical presentation. This compresses the thecal sac to the extent that little CSF is visible at this level. This compression leads to compromise of the nerve roots which form the cauda equina. Figure 52.3 is at the level of L3/4 disc and shows the normal appearance of the thecal sac and spinal canal.

Abnormalities involving the vertebral body (e.g. osteomyelitis, metastatic disease) or disc (e.g. infective discitis) will involve careful study of both T1- and T2-weighted MRI sequences. The diagnosis is further aided by post-contrast imaging studies.

Revision Points

Lumbar Disc Disease

Incidence
Benign lumbar disc disease is common in clinical practice.

Management
• Patients who present with uncomplicated 'sciatica' or radiculopathic leg pain may

generally be managed conservatively for 4–6 weeks. Strong oral analgesics may be required.
• In the absence of 'red flag' conditions or severe neurological deficits, back and leg pain arising from lumbar disc disease generally follows a benign course.

Revision Points *cont.*

- Investigations (CT or MRI) are then considered if symptoms are severe and persistent.
- More than 80% of patients improve with conservative management and do not require surgery.
- The main aim of surgery (lumbar microdiscectomy) is to relieve radiculopathic leg pain. Non-specific back pain is not generally an indication for surgery. Spinal fusion for back pain in the absence of sciatica or nerve root symptoms is controversial. Surgical outcomes are inconsistent. More recently, lumbar artificial disc arthroplasty has also become an option. However, its role and indications remain to be clarified. Long-term studies are awaited.
- These patients must be differentiated from those with:
  - severe neurological compromise
  - pathologies other than benign disc disease.
- These latter patients require urgent neurosurgical assessment.

Cauda Equina Syndrome

This is a surgical emergency. It is characterized by:
- Sphincter disturbances.
- Sexual dysfunction.
- 'Saddle anaesthesia': perianal, buttocks, perineum, genitals, thighs.
- Significant motor weakness usually involving more than one nerve root.
- Bilateral sciatica.
- Bilateral absence of ankle jerks.

  Delay in diagnosis and treatment may jeopardize any neurological recovery.

Issues to Consider

- How are the pelvis and the lower limb innervated?
- What other conditions might predispose to the development of a cauda equina syndrome?

Further Information

www.caudaequina.org *A patient-based website with links and patient perspectives.*

Acute respiratory failure in a 68-year-old man

Stephen W. Lam

Having just finished congratulating yourself for managing your last case so well, you are called to see a 68-year-old man brought into the emergency department by ambulance with severe dyspnoea. He is accompanied by his wife, who states that he has had increasing shortness of breath overnight with some symptoms of an upper respiratory tract infection for the last day or so. Over this time he has also had increasing wheeze and a dry cough with 'tightness' of his chest. He has become somewhat agitated this morning.

He is in obvious respiratory distress, unable to utter more than one or two words at a time.

This man obviously needs urgent assessment and treatment. You only have time to elicit the essential parts of the history while you rapidly examine the patient and start the appropriate management.

Q.1 What are the major differential diagnoses to consider immediately?

The patient's breathing is so laboured that he is unable to answer any of your questions.

Q.2 What are the main points of further information that you would like to elicit from his wife and ambulance officers?

The man's wife tells you that he has 'pretty bad' emphysema. He has no known history of cardio-vascular disease.

His medications are:

- Salbutamol inhaler: 2 puffs prn (1–3 times on a typical day).
- Salmeterol: 2 puffs metered dose inhaler bd.
- Fluticasone: 500 μg metered dose inhaler bd.
- Ipratropium bromide: 2 puffs metered dose inhaler bd.

He has smoked heavily for most of his life, but has reduced his current cigarette consumption to about five a day. He does not drink and has no known allergies.

The ambulance officer states that haemoglobin oxygen saturation (measured by pulse oximetry, SpO_2) has been around 80% throughout the journey, and that he has been wheezing loudly. He has been given 5 mg nebulized salbutamol in the ambulance.

As you examine the patient, you observe that on 6 L/min of oxygen by face mask, his SpO_2 is 78%. He seems irritable, obviously dyspnoeic, and grasping the sleeve of your designer shirt, he utters 'help …'.

You persist with the examination. His respiratory rate is 30 breaths per minute with a prolonged expiratory phase. The pulse rate is 110 bpm and regular. His temperature is 36.5°C and the blood pressure 110/75 mmHg. He is well hydrated and peripheral perfusion is adequate. His peripheral pulses are all present and of good volume. In the semi-recumbent position his jugular venous pulsation (JVP) is 3–4 cm above the base of the neck. Both heart sounds appear normal and there are no murmurs. His trachea is in the midline. He is barrel-chested and there are reduced breath sounds throughout. There is a diffuse expiratory wheeze and the percussion note is normal, there are no crepitations. His abdomen is soft and non-tender. His calves are normal and there is no pedal or sacral oedema.

Q.3 What investigations should be performed straight away?

An electrocardiogram is performed which shows a sinus tachycardia. His arterial blood gas (ABG) results are as follows:

Investigation 53.1 Arterial blood gas analysis	
PaO$_2$	48 mmHg
PaCO$_2$	70 mmHg
pH	7.24
Bicarbonate	29 mmol/L

Q.4 What does his arterial blood gas show?

You adjust his oxygen therapy carefully. He is too dyspnoeic for a peak expiratory flow rate (PEFR) measure. You order an urgent mobile chest X-ray and go on to administer emergency medications to treat this man's condition.

Q.5 What should you do immediately with his supplemental oxygen therapy?

Q.6 Outline your options for administering supplemental oxygen to his man.

A chest X-ray is performed and is shown in Figure 53.1.

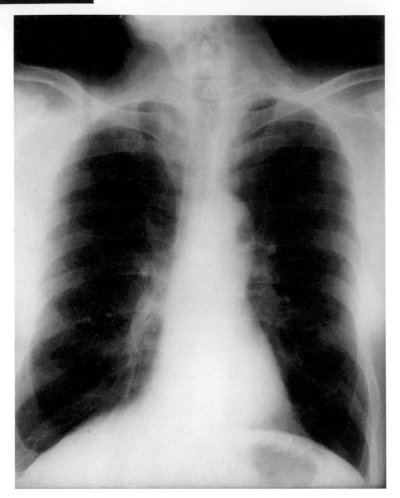

Figure 53.1

Q.7 What does the X-ray show? What is your diagnosis?

Q.8 Describe in detail what you would use to treat this man.

The patient starts to improve, but he is still struggling. You call the intensive care team, who admit him to the intensive care unit (ICU). He receives close monitoring of his gas exchange. He is placed on BPAP (bi-level positive airway pressure ventilation by non-invasive face mask) to support his ventilation. A radial arterial line is inserted to monitor blood gases.

The patient responds almost instantaneously with BPAP, reporting a marked reduction in dyspnoea. Oxygen therapy is carefully monitored and adjusted in the ICU. Bronchodilators are continued and he is commenced on a course of oral prednisolone beginning with 50 mg daily. His blood gases stabilize with improvement in his respiratory condition, achieving almost his baseline level of function over several days with PaO_2 65 mmHg on 1 L/minute via nasal cannulae, $PaCO_2$ 53 mmHg, pH 7.38, bicarbonate 28 mmol/L.

He is discharged after 7 days in hospital to complete a 10-day course of prednisolone (dose to be tapered according to clinical progress), a programme for respiratory rehabilitation and to discontinue smoking, and follow-up appointments in the respiratory medicine clinic with pulmonary function testing.

Answers

A.1 In the absence of an obvious external cause (e.g. chest trauma, upper airways obstruction), the vast majority of cases of acute shortness of breath in adults will be due to one of four conditions:

- Exacerbation of chronic obstructive pulmonary disease (COPD) or asthma.
- Pneumonia/lower respiratory tract infection or irritation (such as aspiration).
- Pulmonary embolism.
- Pulmonary oedema (it is important to look for the underlying causes, e.g. myocardial ischaemia or cardiac arrhythmia, and non-cardiogenic causes).

Spontaneous pneumothorax, while much less common than the conditions above, is also an important diagnosis to consider.

Anaemia and metabolic acidosis may also cause tachypnoea and, along with pulmonary embolism, should be sought particularly in patients with normal-appearing plain chest radiograph.

A.2 You will need to have:

- A brief account of what has happened since the onset of his illness, including his condition on arrival of the ambulance officers and any treatment given so far. It is important to know the current trend of his condition (e.g. rapidly deteriorating, stable, improving, etc.) and response to treatment, as this can give you important clues to the diagnosis and vital information on the urgency and aggressiveness of intervention required.

- A 'problem list' of his active and inactive medical conditions.
- A list of his current medications.
- Information about any allergies.

A.3 The most important immediate investigations are:

- Arterial blood gas (ABG) analysis.
- Mobile chest X-ray.
- ECG.

All are quick to perform, and can be done while the patient is being examined and treated.

ABGs provide results within minutes, can be done in many emergency departments and intensive care units, and provide information on blood gases, acid–base status, most vital electrolytes (including sodium, potassium, chloride, bicarbonate, ionized calcium), blood glucose, and haemoglobin. All of these parameters are important in the assessment of any acutely unwell patient and can immediately influence the course of treatment.

ABGs performed on room air are not necessary, and should not be performed in patients requiring supplemental oxygen to maintain adequate SpO_2.

Complete blood picture, full electrolyte panel and cardiac enzymes should also be requested, but results may take some time to become available.

A.4 The ABGs show severe hypoxaemia. His acid–base status cannot be fully

365

Answers *cont.*

determined with the information available; however, the ABG result is consistent with acute on chronic respiratory acidosis.

The presence of a low arterial blood pH indicates the $PaCO_2$ is acutely raised. As a rough guide, for every acute increase in $PaCO_2$ of 10 mmHg, pH falls by approximately 0.07, and bicarbonate increases by about 1 mmol/L. In 'chronic' hypoventilation, compensatory mechanisms can bring the pH almost back to normal (takes about 2–3 days), with bicarbonate increasing by approximately 3 mmol/L for every 10 mmHg increase in $PaCO_2$.

Working backwards accordingly, it can be estimated that this man's baseline 'chronic' $PaCO_2$ would be around 50 mmHg, and bicarbonate around 27 mmol/L. In addition to acute respiratory acidosis, he also has chronic respiratory acidosis with metabolic compensation.

Insufficient results have been provided for calculation of his anion gap; however, this is always important to calculate in order to detect a concurrent wide anion-gap metabolic acidosis (e.g. from ingested toxins, lactataemia from ischaemic bowel, alcoholic/ starvation/diabetic ketoacidosis, etc.).

A.5 A major error in this patient would be to reduce the supplemental oxygen therapy. Patients do not lose their 'hypoxic drive' (if this phenomenon actually exists) unless they have lost their hypoxia! His PaO_2 is 48, i.e. he is definitely still hypoxaemic, and this is contributing to his agitation and confusion.

- Titrate the O_2 up, aiming for a SpO_2 of around 90–94%, *regardless* of what is happening with his $PaCO_2$.
- Haemoglobin oxygen saturation (SaO_2) is more important as a clinical end point for titration of supplemental oxygen therapy than PaO_2. This is so for three main reasons. First of all, SaO_2 is a much

greater determinant of the actual amount of oxygen in arterial blood being delivered to tissues than PaO_2, where blood oxygen content = $(1.36 \times Hb \times SaO_2) + (0.0031 \times PaO_2)$. Secondly, SaO_2 can be monitored almost continuously and non-invasively using SpO_2 (pulse oximetry). Thirdly, the haemoglobin–oxygen dissociation curve is 'shifted to the right' by both acidosis and high $PaCO_2$, meaning that for any given PaO_2, the SaO_2 is lower. Therefore while the PaO_2 may appear satisfactory at around 60 mmHg, SaO_2 will be <90%, and therefore arterial oxygen content insufficient. For example, with pH 7.24 and $PaCO_2$ 70 mmHg, a PaO_2 of 60 mmHg will produce SaO_2 of around 85%, and PaO_2 of 55 mmHg will produce SaO_2 of around 81%. Clearly, a PaO_2 of 55–60 mmHg is inadequate for such a patient.

- Hypercapnia needs to be followed clinically (rate and depth of respiration, signs of hypercapnia such as drowsiness, vasodilatation, bounding pulses, asterixis) and with periodic ABGs. Remember that good SpO_2 readings do not mean that the patient's ventilation is adequate – alveolar ventilation is monitored by the $PaCO_2$. An arterial line should be inserted to allow frequent ABG analysis. If $PaCO_2$ is either increasing or elevated with associated respiratory acidosis, ventilatory support in the form of non-invasive mechanical ventilation (NIV, including bi-level positive airway pressure – BPAP) or invasive ventilation (involving induction of anaesthesia and endotracheal intubation) may be needed to control this, *not* a reduction in supplemental oxygen (unless SaO_2 is greater than 94%).

A.6

- Nasal cannulae can be used with oxygen flow rates of up to 6 L/min, although

Answers *cont.*

many patients experience discomfort and drying of nasal mucosa with flow rates greater than 4 L/min. Pure oxygen from the nasal cannulae is mixed with room air during inspiration and hence the actual inspired concentration of oxygen (fraction of inspired oxygen, FiO_2) can vary depending on nose versus mouth breathing, as well as several other factors such as the patient's rate and depth of respiration. As a rough guide, nasal cannulae increase the inspired oxygen percentage by approximately 3 for every L/min of oxygen flow (e.g. inspired oxygen of around 28% at 2 L/min).

- If nasal cannulae are insufficient, a face mask (called medium capacity O_2 mask (MCOM)) can be used, with a minumum oxygen flow of 6 L/minute. MCOMs can deliver up to around 50% inspired oxygen, with the same caveats as discussed above with nasal cannulae.
- Non-rebreather masks with 15 L/min oxygen flow can deliver close to 100% inspired oxygen (provided the patient is inspiring at a rate slower than 15 L/min); however, the oxygen is not humidified, and inadequate humidification of inspired gases leads to abnormal mucociliary function.
- Venturi masks can be useful in controlling the FiO_2 in these patients more reliably than nasal cannulae and ordinary MCOMs. Venturi masks deliver gas at a predetermined percentage of oxygen directly to the patient by utilizing the entrainment of a high (and fixed) volume per minute of room air with a fixed flow rate of oxygen. This removes the variability in room air entrainment inherent in gas delivery methods where rate of inspiration is greater than rate of gas delivery.

- 'High flow humidified oxygen circuits' (HFOs) also provide accurate control of FiO_2 by delivering a high volume of gas per minute, thereby minimizing entrainment of room air during inspiration. Because the gas they deliver is humidified, they are the preferred method of providing a high FiO_2 to patients beyond the acute setting.

A.7 The chest X-ray shows flattening of the diaphragms consistent with 'gas trapping', which reflects the inability of gas to escape from the lungs due to airways obstruction. The lung fields are clear, with no evidence of alveolar consolidation or oedema.

This man is having an exacerbation of his COPD.

He is starting to succumb to respiratory fatigue, and hence hypoventilate. The work of breathing is becoming too much for him. This is reflected by his climbing $PaCO_2$, as the carbon dioxide in his alveoli is not being 'washed out' due to inadequate ventilation.

- Remember that cough and wheeze can also be due to pulmonary oedema ('cardiac asthma').

Those with low tidal volumes may not have prominent crepitations or wheeze, due to the low volumes of gas reaching the alveoli and low air flows. Thus, the absence of crepitations does not exclude cardiogenic pulmonary oedema, and a lack of wheeze does not exclude airways disease.

Chest tightness is a symptom commonly described by patients with bronchoconstriction as well as patients with cardiac angina.

For these reasons, acute pulmonary oedema (which may have been precipitated by cardiac ischaemia or infarction) was an important differential diagnosis in this man's presentation, and thus the emergent importance of a CXR and ECG.

Answers *cont.*

A.8

- Beta-2 adrenergic agonists are indicated. The conventional way to use them is to nebulize 2.5–5 mg of salbutamol, diluted to a total of 3 mL with normal saline (to make up an appropriate volume for nebulization), repeated continuously up to three doses in a row (takes about 15 minutes each). The maximal response is usually reached after three continuous doses.

- Ipratropium bromide is also useful, suggested to be particularly so for COPD, at a nebulized dose of 250–500 µg every 4–6 hours.

- If the patient's ventilatory status is poor, the dose of nebulized medication actually reaching the airways (rather than being nebulized into the environment for the medical and nursing staff to breathe) may be markedly reduced. Undiluted nebulized salbutamol and continuous nebulized salbutamol can be used; however, there is doubt over the effectiveness of these techniques.

- All parenterally administered sympathomimetics and methylxanthines (such as aminophylline) are less effective and more hazardous than the inhaled bronchodilators discussed above, and are nowadays rarely used.

- A common mistake is to continue aggressive nebulized or parenteral beta-2 adrenergic agonists in an attempt to completely eliminate wheeze and dyspnoea. In exacerbations of chronic airways disease and asthma, acute mucosal inflammation with oedema and increased mucus production are often significant contributors to airflow limitation. Maximal bronchodilatation is still the goal; however, airflow limitation with wheeze can still be present when this has been achieved. Time for the precipitating event (such as airway irritation or infection) to resolve and airway inflammation to settle (assisted by corticosteroids) is needed before baseline airway patency can be achieved. In the meantime oxygen, bronchodilator therapy and ventilatory assistance are continued as required to support the patient through the exacerbation. Continuing administration of beta-2 adrenergic agonists can lead to significant toxicity with hypokalaemia, tachyarrhythmias, lactic acidosis, tremor and hypoxaemia (beta-2 mediated pulmonary vascular dilatation and consequent ventilation–perfusion mismatch) among their prominent adverse effects.

- Continuous or bi-level positive airway pressure (CPAP and BPAP) are both modalities of 'non-invasive' ventilatory (NIV) support (non-invasive means not requiring endotracheal intubation). NIV utilizes a ventilator machine with a face (or nose) mask to apply pressure during inspiration and expiration. NIV is a vital component of the management of acute exacerbation of COPD, where important contraindications (most notably the need for immediate endotracheal intubation) are not present. When used correctly, NIV can reduce the need for intubation, which is associated with a higher incidence of ventilator-related complications and poorer patient outcome. 'Gas trapping' (gas not exhaled before the next inspiratory breath due to airflow limitation) creates an elevated intrathoracic pressure which must be overcome by the patient's respiratory muscles before air will actually enter the lungs (via a pressure gradient). This 'threshold work of breathing' is countered by NIV at the onset of inspiration. Patients often report an immediate improvement in their

Answers *cont.*

symptoms on correct application of NIV. NIV can also assist inspiration, thereby helping them to achieve better alveolar ventilation and hence a lower $PaCO_2$.

- A short course of systemic corticosteroids starting with 40–60 mg of oral prednisolone or equivalent daily, preferably given in the mornings, and tapered over 7–10 days should be given. Longer courses have been shown to be of no further benefit. Parenteral corticosteroids have not been found to be more effective than orally administered therapy provided that patient is capable of taking oral medication.

- Inhaled corticosteroids (in addition to systemic corticosteroids) may also be helpful, and doses required are around 500–1000 μg of budesonide nebulized every 15–30 minutes. Dose-dependent, rapid-onset non-genomic effects take place within minutes and include vasoconstriction which can reduce hyperaemia in inflamed mucosa and may potentiate the effect of adrenergic bronchoconstrictors. Clinical evidence, however, is not yet sufficient for their use to be included in management guidelines.

- A course of immunosuppressive glucocorticoids can result in the emergence of infectious agents such as fungi, *Pneumocystis* and *Mycobacterium*

tuberculosis (TB). Those with a suspicion of latent (or even active) TB should be referred to the appropriate clinic for further assessment and advice.

- Antibiotics are not always indicated in acute exacerbations of COPD as non-infectious and viral LRTI may be responsible. When antibiotics are commenced empirically, patients with COPD require broader-spectrum coverage (including *Pseudomonas*). Typical antibiotics used for empirical cover include one of either ticarcillin (± clavulanic acid), piperacillin (± tazobactam), cefepime, or a carbapemen (e.g. meropenem) along with a macolide (e.g. azithromycin) to cover bacterial organisms of 'atypical' pneumonia (e.g. *Legionella*, *Mycoplasma*). Outcomes in severe Streptococcus pneumoniae pneumonia may also be improved by the addition of a macrolide antibiotic to 'standard' antibiotic cover for pneumococcus. Newer-generation quinolones such as moxifloxacin provide an important alternative for patients with contraindication to beta-lactam antibiotics, as well as some coverage for 'atypical' bacterial organisms.

- Mucolytics and chest physiotherapy have been shown to be ineffective in acute exacerbation of COPD.

Revision Points

In acute respiratory failure:
- Hypoxia is the enemy.
- It is never correct to reduce oxygen supplementation when severe hypoxaemia and tissue hypoxia are present.

- The minimum amount of oxygen should be used to achieve adequate tissue oxygenation in patients with chronic hypercapnoeic respiratory failure. The usual target in these patients is SaO_2 (measured on ABG and monitored

Revision Points *cont.*

clinically using pulse oximetry, SpO$_2$) of 90–94%, while also ensuring adequate cardiac function. It is *not* correct to conclude that arterial oxygen content is adequate by looking at the PaO$_2$. Many factors alter the haemoglobin-oxygen dissociation relationship (including acid–base status and PaCO$_2$), and haemoglobin-oxygen saturation (SaO$_2$) is a much greater determinant of blood oxygen content than PaO$_2$.

- Not all people with a diagnosis of COPD are 'CO$_2$ retainers' with 'hypoxic drive'.

  Fatigue from sustained and severely elevated work of breathing is a common cause for rising PaCO$_2$ in patients with acute severe exacerbation of COPD; however, a loss of 'hypoxic drive' (hypoxia replacing hypercapnia as a stimulus to breath) is often blamed, resulting in an inappropriate reduction in supplemental oxygen even in the presence of hypoxaemia. Nonetheless, oxygen supplementation in patients with chronic hypercapnoeic respiratory failure can result in an increase in hypercapnia. The Haldane effect (haemoglobin binding to oxygen as hypoxaemia is treated results in displacement of CO$_2$ bound to haemoglobin, thus releasing CO$_2$ into plasma) and V/Q (ventilation–perfusion) mismatch due to oxygen induced reduction in pulmonary vasoconstriction are important

causes of hypercapnia which have been found in these patients. The significance of 'hypoxic drive' in COPD exacerbations is yet to be conclusively demonstrated. The most important cause from a clinical standpoint remains the inability to sustain such a high work of breathing.

- A common mistake is to interpret wheeze and evidence of airflow limitation as inadequate bronchodilator therapy, and beta-2 adrenergic agonist toxicity can contribute significantly to the patient's deterioration. Airflow limitation caused by acute mucosal inflammation, oedema and increased mucus production takes time to resolve, requires the inciting event to be removed and is expediated by corticosteroids.

- A course of corticosteroid, particularly if prolonged, places the patient at risk of developing opportunistic infection and adrenal suppression. TB is an important consideration. *Pneumocystis* infection can emerge even after the cessation of steroid treatment.

- The presence of chronic lung disease, immunosuppresive steroid therapy and previous courses of antibiotics and hospital admissions must be taken into consideration when deciding empirical antibiotic therapy for patients with suspected bacterial infective exacerbation of COPD.

Issues to Consider

- What are the normal physiological mechanisms behind respiratory drive?
- What forms of ventilatory assistance are useful in this situation, and how are they used? What are the indications for ventilatory assistance?

Further Information

http://www.goldcopd.org Global strategy for the diagnosis, management and prevention of

COPD, Global Initiative for Chronic Obstructive Lung Disease (GOLD) 2010. www.goldcopd.org.

http://www.thoracic.org/clinical/copd-guidelines/resources/copddoc.pdf American Thoracic Society/European Respiratory Society Task Force. Standards for the diagnosis and management of patients with COPD 2004.

A listless 45-year-old man

Cyril Sieberhagen and Jonathan Mitchell

A 45-year-old schoolteacher is referred by his GP with deranged liver function tests. He presents with a 1-year history of persistent lethargy. There seem to be no exacerbating or relieving factors. There are no other specific symptoms. Initial blood tests have revealed some abnormalities of his liver enzymes and he has been referred to the hepatology clinic for further investigation. He has never been jaundiced.

On further questioning he admits to having used intravenous heroin in his teens, but says he has been clean since the age of 25. He has never been on a methadone replacement programme.

On examination he appears thin, but looks generally well. There is no evidence of jaundice or lymphadenopathy and he is afebrile. There are several tattoos on his upper torso and you notice some old scars in his antecubital fossae. There are a few spider naevi present on his upper chest, but no other signs of chronic liver disease. Cardiovascular and respiratory examination is unremarkable. The abdomen is soft and non-tender with no evidence of hepatosplenomegaly and no ascites. He is not encephalopathic.

Q.1   What additional information would you like to obtain from the history?

You arrange some further blood tests. The results are as follows:

Investigation 54.1 Summary of results

White cell count	7.3×10^9/L
Haemoglobin	13.5 g/dL
Platelets	100×10^9/L
INR	1.3
Sodium	138 mmol/L
Potassium	4.3 mmol/L
Bicarbonate	24 mmol/L
Urea	4.6 mmol/L
Creatinine	67 mmol/L
Glucose	5.6 mmol/L
Cholesterol	3.1 mmol/L
Calcium	2.23 mmol/L
Phosphate	0.88 mmol/L
Total protein	65 g/L
Albumin	43 g/L
Globulin	22 g/L
ALP	172 U/L
Bilirubin	20 mmol/L
AST	148 U/L
ALT	136 U/L
GGT	132 U/L
Autoimmune profile	Negative
IgG	16.8
IgA	3.9
IgM	1.3
Thyroid function	Free T4: 18.1 TSH: 3.5

Q.2 What do these results suggest? What further tests would you like to do?

The following tests are now available:

Investigation 54.2 Summary of results

Hepatitis B surface antigen	Negative
Hepatitis C IgG	Positive
Hepatitis C PCR	Positive with a viral load of 1 324 000 IU/mL

You review him in the outpatient clinic to discuss the results with him.

Q.3 What are you going to tell him regarding his results?

Q.4 How would you further manage this gentleman?

This patient underwent an ultrasound scan which shows a slightly fatty looking liver and normal sized spleen. Doppler studies of his portal vein shows normal flow. He went on to have a liver biopsy which confirms moderate inflammation and established cirrhosis.

Q.5 What are the options for treatment for this patient, and what complications might he face with regard to treatment?

He is found to be genotype 1 and commences a course of interferon and ribavirin. After 3 months, unfortunately, the treatment is stopped as his viral load has failed to fall and the side-effects of the treatment have become intolerable.

Q.6 How will you now follow him up?

Six months later he attends his planned outpatient appointment and complains of feeling more unwell. He has become increasingly fatigued and has developed some swelling of his ankles. His partner thinks that his eyes look a little yellow.

On examination, he is mildly jaundiced. There is mild ankle oedema and some shifting dullness on abdominal examination. His weight has increased by 3 kg since his last clinic visit.

Blood tests are as follows:

Investigation 54.3 Summary of results

White cell count	2.9×10^9/L
Haemoglobin	10.3 g/dL
Platelets	67×10^9/L
INR	1.9
Albumin	28 g/L
Globulin	22 g/L
ALP	312 U/L
Bilirubin	87 µmol/L
AST	111 U/L
ALT	165 U/L
GGT	278 U/L
Alphafetoprotein 1885 kiu/L (0–5)	

Q.7 Comment on the blood results. What is likely to have happened? What investigation would you like to arrange?

The following investigation is performed:

373

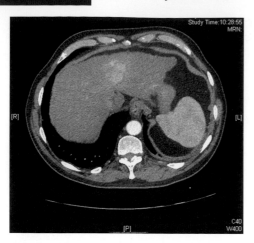

Study Time:10:28:55
MRN:

[R]

[L]

[P]

C40
W400

Figure 54.1 Courtesy of South West Liver Unit.

Q.8 What is this investigation? What does it show? What are his treatment options?

Answers

A.1 A complete history for risk factors for hepatitis should be taken. This includes enquiring about alcohol consumption, a family history of liver disease, blood transfusions (especially transfusions prior to September 1991), intravenous drug use and sharing of needles, a sexual history and significant foreign travel. It is also important to ask about close contacts with anyone with hepatitis.

Blood products used prior to 1991 were not always tested for hepatitis C, although the introduction of widespread treating varied from country to country.

A.2 The blood tests show a modest rise in his transaminases (ALT and AST) implying hepatic inflammation/mild hepatitis. His liver synthetic function (as demonstrated by normal albumin, normal clotting and a normal bilirubin) is well preserved at present. His platelet count is slightly low. This may reflect portal hypertension and hypersplenism. In this scenario, blood flow

through the portal venous system and therefore through the splenic vein is impaired. The spleen becomes engorged and has more opportunity to remove platelets from the circulation. This raises the possibility of an established cirrhosis.

In view of his history of intravenous drug use, viral hepatitis is high on the list of possibilities. Serology for viral hepatitis should be done. However, the net should be thrown wide and other forms of liver disease should be screened for. A ferritin and alpha-1 antitrypsin are important in ruling out inherited liver diseases.

A.3

- He has hepatitis C. It is likely that he contracted the virus through IV drug use in his teens and has been infected between 15 and 20 years. His viral load is high.
- Hepatitis C is a blood-borne virus that is spread through contact with infected blood. Only 15–20% of people infected

Answers *cont.*

with hepatitis C will clear the virus while 80–85% of infected people will develop chronic infection. In order to confirm chronic infection, a positive antibody test must be accompanied with a positive hepatitis C PCR.

- The main complication of chronic hepatitis C is the development of cirrhosis and the subsequent risk of developing hepatocellular carcinoma. Patients with hepatitis C often experience lethargy and the reason for this is not entirely clear. Commonly, people with hepatitis C infection are asymptomatic.

- There are also extra-hepatic complications of hepatitis C including: cryoglobulinaemia, leading to glomerulonephritis and a vasculitic skin rash.

- There are six genotypes of hepatitis C. There is treatment available for hepatitis C and this will depend on his genotype.

- It is important to cut down alcohol use in the context of hepatitis C as concomitant alcohol use may lead to acceleration of his liver disease.

- All patients with a diagnosis of hepatitis C should be screened for other blood-borne viruses including HIV.

A.4 He will need an ultrasound of his abdomen and Doppler studies of his portal vein to investigate the possibility of portal hypertension.

He also needs a blood test to check his genotype. This shows him to be genotype 1.

Liver biopsy can be an important way of assessing the degree of inflammation and fibrosis. The presence of cirrhosis reduces the chance of successful treatment.

However, recent advances in the use of non-invasive markers of fibrosis have reduced the number of liver biopsies performed. Consideration should be give to the use of these techniques including transient elastography or serum markers of fibrosis.

A.5 Hepatitis C is currently treated with a combination of interferon and ribavirin. There are two different preparations of interferon available: interferon alfa-2a and interferon alfa-2b. There is no current evidence to suggest that one product is significantly superior to the other.

Interferon works by enhancing the immune response to the hepatitis C virus rather than being directed specifically at the virus, while ribavirin is a non-specific antiviral agent that disrupts replication.

The duration of treatment is dependent on the genotype of hepatitis C. The current standard treatment is 48 weeks for genotypes 1, 4 and 5 and 24 weeks for genotypes 2 and 3. There is ongoing work being performed with regard to short course treatment in genotype 1, 2 and 3 patients.

Both interferon and ribavirin have significant side-effects that need to be discussed with the patient prior to starting them on treatment. These include:

Interferon

- Flu-like symptoms – this is a very common side-effect (up to 70% of patients).
- Decreased white cell count and neutropenia – this may require a dose reduction, withdrawing of the medication or support with granulocyte colony stimulating factor (G-CSF).
- Thrombocytopenia
- Depression – this may require treatment with an antidepressant.
- Irritability.
- Sleep disturbance.
- Anxiety.

The majority of these symptoms can be managed with good counselling prior to starting treatment, while the haematological side-effects may require dose adjustment or support with colony stimulating factors.

Ribavirin

- Haemolytic anaemia – this is caused by destruction of red blood cells.
- Cough, occasional shortness of breath, skin rash.
- Teratogenicity.

Significant anaemia may require a reduction of the ribavirin dose or support with erythropoietin (EPO). It is important to counsel the patient about the risks of birth defects prior to starting treatment and that any planned conception should be postponed until treatment has been completed.

The aim of treatment is to achieve a sustained viral response (SVR) – undetectable virus 6 months after completing treatment. The chance of achieving this differs depending on the genotype. Patients with genotype 1 have a 40–44% of achieving SVR, while patients with genotype 2 or 3 have an 80–85% of achieving SVR. Factors such as duration of infection, viral load, age and grade of inflammation and fibrosis also play an important role in determining the response to treatment. There are many new drugs currently in development and on the verge of commercial availability that may improve these outcomes. As yet these new drugs are expected to be used in combination with interferon and ribavirin but the landscape is rapidly evolving.

A.6   He has established cirrhosis and is therefore at increased risk of both hepatic decompensation and hepatocellular carcinoma (HCC). He should be reviewed regularly and entered into an HCC screening programme with 6-monthly ultrasound examinations and alphafetoprotein measurement.

Patients who have failed to clear the virus should always be considered for entry into clinical trials as soon as promising alternative therapies become available.

A.7   He now has evidence of significant synthetic dysfunction evidenced by a raised INR, depressed albumin and elevated bilirubin. He has a pancytopenia which is likely to be due to worsening hypersplenism and, by inference, increasing portal hypertension. This is further supported by the new development of fluid retention including possible ascites.

His alphafetoprotein is grossly elevated which, in the context of a patient with hepatitis C-related liver cirrhosis, is almost diagnostic of hepatocellular carcinoma.

He should have urgent cross-sectional imaging of his liver in the form of either a contrast enhanced CT or a contrast enhanced MRI.

A.8   This is a CT scan of the liver. You can tell that it is an arterial phase as bright contrast is seen within the aorta. A 4.5 cm enhancing lesion is seen in segment four of the liver. This is an arterialized hepatocellular carcinoma. The liver outline, in addition, appears irregular, consistent with the known cirrhosis.

In a patient with hepatitis C and HCC, the only curative option is liver transplantation. The tumour appears to be single and is less than 5 cm in diameter meaning he remains eligible. Surgical resection is not an option as his liver disease is advanced. Pending transplantation, his tumour could be treated with transarterial chemoembolization to allow 'bridging' to the curative procedure.

Revision Points

Hepatocellular Carcinoma

Epidemiology

Hepatocellular carcinoma (HCC) is the third most common cause of death in the world leading to more than 600 000 deaths annually. Highest rates are in Asia and are linked to a high prevalence of hepatitis B. However, rates are rising alarmingly in Western nations due to rising incidences of HCV, alcohol and NASH-related liver disease. More common in men.

Causes

Approximately 80% of cases occur in livers where established cirrhosis is already present. Chronic hepatitis B infection is the largest cause but HCC can occur in cirrhosis of any cause including alcohol and NASH. In viral hepatitis, HCC is possibly linked to incorporation of parts of the viral genome in host cells.

Diagnosis

Elevation of the serum marker alphafetoprotein (AFP) may be absent in up to 40% of cases in Western nations. Its use as a screening tool is limited, therefore. Standard screening of at-risk populations generally still consists, however, of 6-monthly ultrasound examinations with measurement of AFP. One or two cross-sectional imaging techniques are required to confirm the diagnosis. As HCC is generally a hypervascular tumour, multiphase CT is essential.

Symptoms

The majority of HCCs do not cause symptoms until they are at an advanced stage. Capsular involvement may cause pain and invasion of the portal vein may lead to new ascites or hepatic decompensation. ˙

Treatment

- Traditionally the outcome for most HCCs has been poor with curative resection of transplantation only suitable for 5% of patients. However, treatment options have changed dramatically over the last 10 years.
- Resection is still an option in patients with well-preserved liver function and without portal hypertension. Liver transplantation remains the gold standard but tumours must be small (<5 cm or no more than 3 lesions <3 cm in diameter) and the availability of donor organs is a major limiting factor.
- Small tumours can now be treated very successfully with ablative techniques such as radiofrequency ablation.
- Intermediate-sized tumours can be treated with transarterial chemoembolization (TACE) in which chemotherapeutic agents and embolic material are injected directly in to the tumour via its arterial supply. There are many techniques and the field is evolving rapidly.
- Systemic chemotherapy has traditionally had very poor results although there have been some promising data on the use of the multi-kinase inhibitor sorafenib.

Issues to Consider

- What are the implications of maternal hepatitis C infection in childbirth?
- What is NASH?
- Why has a vaccine still not been produced against hepatitis C?
- Why cannot patients with poor liver function have liver tumours resected surgically?

Further Information

www.hepctrust.co.uk *UK-based advocacy group for HCV patients.*

www.hepatitisaustralia.com *Excellent web resource for all types of hepatitis.*

A 74-year-old man with confusion and oliguria

Randall Faull

A 74-year-old man was brought into the emergency department confused and drowsy. According to his wife he had been unwell for approximately 1 week with a diarrhoeal illness, with nausea and anorexia. The changes to his mental state had appeared over the past 24 hours, and he had become bedridden. There was no history of chest pain.

Immediately prior to this acute illness he had been independent and well, although he had a past history of type II diabetes mellitus and ischaemic heart disease. He had been treated for hypertension for approximately 10 years. His current medications are combination perindopril/indapamide 5/1.25 mg one per day; gliclazide MR 30 mg twice daily; metformin 500 mg twice daily; aspirin 150 mg once daily; and celecoxib 200 mg once daily.

On examination, the man was drowsy but easily roused, and unable to give a clear history. His tongue was very obviously dry. Blood pressure was 100/55 mmHg lying, and he was unable to stand to check for a postural drop. Pulse rate was 90 and regular, although difficult to feel. Temperature was 36.5°C. There was no evidence of right or left heart failure, and his chest was clear to auscultation. Pedal pulses were not palpable, and he had a soft right carotid bruit. ECG is unchanged from previous.

An indwelling catheter was placed in his bladder, and it drained 50 mL of dark urine. Urinalysis showed protein + and blood +. A finger prick blood sugar level was 5.0 mmol/L. Urgent blood results included the following:

Investigation 55.1 Summary of results

Sodium	143 mmol/L	(N: 137–145)
Potassium	7.8 mmol/L	(N: 3.5–4.9)
Chloride	105 mmol/L	(N: 100–109)
Bicarbonate	8 mmol/L	(N: 22–32)
Urea	65 mmol/L	(N: 2.7–8.0)
Creatinine	850 µmol/L	(N: 50–120)
Phosphate	3.5 mmol/L	(N: 0.65–1.45)
Calcium	1.64 mmol/L	(N: 2.10–2.55)
Albumin	30 g/L	(N: 34–48)
Haemoglobin	145 g/L	(N: 135–175)

You insert an intravenous catheter and commence a 5% dextrose infusion at an initial rate of 1 litre per hour.

Q.1 What are the most likely causes and contributing factors to his renal impairment?

Q.2 What are the priorities in his management in the emergency department?

Q.3 How do you treat the hyperkalaemia? How do you manage the renal impairment?

Q.4 How do you decide whether he needs to be acutely dialysed?

Q.5 How do you distinguish acute from chronic renal failure? Is it important?

Q.6 What (if any) changes would you make to his medications (short-term and long-term)?

Q.7 How do you manage his recovery from the acute renal impairment?

Answers

A.1 It is likely that he has developed acute renal failure secondary to dehydration and intravascular hypovolaemia, with consequent reduction in renal blood flow. A key question is whether he has acute or chronic renal failure (or both). The clinical picture, rapid deterioration and dramatically deranged biochemistry (particularly the severe hyperkalaemia and acidosis) is highly suggestive of marked acute deterioration in renal function.

An additional important possibility to consider is that the patient is septic associated with infectious diarrhoea, which would further predispose him to acute renal failure. This can occur in severe infectious diarrhoeal illnesses such as *Salmonella*. He was afebrile when seen in the emergency department, but this does not completely preclude an infectious illness, and a precipitating infection should be sought carefully.

A contributing factor to the acute deterioration in his renal function may be the use of celecoxib. While this non-steroidal anti-inflammatory drug (NSAID) may have less gastrointestinal toxicity, it has the same adverse effects as other NSAIDs on renal function.

Similarly, while the angiotensin converting enzyme inhibitor perindopril he is taking would not be a causative agent in his acute renal deterioration, in the setting of intravascular depletion and hypotension it would exacerbate deterioration of renal function by further lowering the blood pressure and also interfering with autoregulation of glomerular blood flow. It should be stopped for the time being.

A.2 The priorities of treatment in the emergency department are the most immediately life-threatening abnormalities:
- Severe hyperkalaemia is the most obvious priority, because of the high risk of refractory cardiac arrhythmias and death.

Answers *cont.*

- He is hypotensive with evidence of poor peripheral perfusion, and so resuscitation with intravenous fluids is a high priority.
- There is also the possibility of contributory sepsis, and so intravenous broad-spectrum antibiotics should be considered.

The other biochemical abnormalities (low bicarbonate, high phosphate, low calcium), while impressive, are not immediately life threatening, and should correct with resolution of the severe renal impairment. The confusion and drowsiness are secondary to the acutely deranged biochemistry and should respond rapidly to appropriate treatment of the renal failure.

A.3 Severe hyperkalaemia is an emergency requiring rapid and aggressive treatment. While an electrocardiogram is a useful adjunct investigation and will show abnormalities such as peaked T waves and broadening of the QRS complex, at this potassium level it should not be used as a means of deciding whether to treat. Protocols for treatment of hyperkalaemia should be standard items in emergency departments, and consist of a combination of cardioprotective and potassium-lowering manoeuvres using calcium gluconate and dextrose-insulin. An example of such a protocol is shown in Box 55.1.

The approach to management of the renal impairment is to initially rapidly correct the underlying cause. In this case, infusion of intravenous fluids to correct the hypovolaemia/hypotension is necessary. Careful monitoring of the patient's fluid status, preferably by a combination of clinical assessment and invasive monitoring as available in a high-dependency unit. Accurate urine output measurements must be charted, and fluid input re-assessed regularly. A risk of rapid correction of intravascular depletion is fluid overload, particularly if the patient remains oliguric.

Fluid resuscitation may be all that is required to re-establish a good urine output

---

Box 55.1 Example of a protocol for treatment of hyperkalaemia

Treatment of Serum K⁺ Greater Than 6.5 mmol/L *OR* ECG Changes Present

- Give 10 mL calcium chloride 10% IV over 5 minutes (OR if calcium chloride not available, give 10 mL calcium gluconate 10% IV), then
- Via a separate line, or only after careful flushing of the same line, give 100 mL sodium bicarbonate 8.4% IV over 30 minutes, then
- Give 10 units neutral insulin (Actrapid or Humulin R) IV and 50 mL 50% glucose IV over 5 minutes.
- Give Resonium 30 g by mouth or 30 g PR as enema.
- Repeat full biochemistry (including BGL if insulin given) in 1 hour.
- You may need to repeat the above steps and correct causative factors, e.g. dehydration, over replacement of K⁺, use of K⁺ sparing diuretics, etc.
- In severe, intractable hyperkalaemia, haemodialysis may be required.

Additional Interventions to be Considered

- β-agonist therapy (e.g. salbutamol 20 mg in 4 mL administered by nebulizer) is recommended in some protocols for treatment of hyperkalaemia.
- Consider holding NSAIDs, ACE inhibitors or any other potassium potentiating medications.

Answers *cont.*

and recovery, although frequently if the condition has been present for any more than a few hours the patient will remain oliguric without improvement in biochemistry.

A.4 The absolute indications include;
- Severe pulmonary oedema in an oliguric/anuric patient.
- Severe intractable hyperkalaemia with imminent threat of life-threatening arrhythmias.
- Acute uraemic pericarditis manifested by typical pain and an audible pericardial rub. The latter is potentially life threatening because of the risk of intrapericardial haemorrhage and tamponade, and any acute dialysis must be conducted *without* anticoagulation.

Relative indications include lesser degrees of fluid overload and hyperkalaemia, severe acidosis and severe hyperphosphataemia, plus occasional situations where a dialyzable exogenous toxin complicates the clinical presentation.

The best treatment is rapid correction of the underlying cause of acute renal impairment, but dialysis is sometimes required as an interim measure.

In this patient, the most important indication for acute dialysis is the severe hyperkalaemia. While the acute treatment of hyperkalaemia is usually able to quite quickly (minutes to hours) lower potassium to relatively safe levels, it is not a sustainable option unless a good urine flow is established.

It is also reasonable to initiate acute dialysis for less 'compelling' reasons in patients with multiple acute medical problems, based on the assumptions that there is less acute reversibility to their underlying problems, and that correction of adverse biochemical abnormalities such as severe acidosis

is likely to improve their short-term outcome. A simple example of this is a hypotensive septic patient in an intensive care setting with progressive acute renal failure.

A.5 Determining whether the patient is suffering from acute or chronic renal failure (or acute on chronic renal failure) will fundamentally alter your approach to their treatment. Acute renal failure in isolation is potentially completely reversible with timely therapy, whereas the management of established chronic renal failure is very different and much more dictated by medium and long-term goals and outcomes. The biochemical abnormalities seen in this case will respond to reversal of acute renal failure, whereas if the underlying problem is chronic renal failure the most appropriate intervention is chronic dialysis. Patients with underlying chronic renal failure of any severity are also very prone to acute deterioration, even with relatively minor insults such as dehydration or introduction of an NSAID. This is a plausible scenario for this patient.

The most simple and reliable way to determine whether the patient has underlying chronic renal failure is by careful history and review of previous investigations. The latter includes finding reports of previous biochemistry. For example, knowing that a patient such as this has a usual serum creatinine of 300 µmol/L fundamentally alters your expectations about response to treatment and overall treatment goals. Not uncommonly also the patient will be aware of a history of renal impairment, and may even know results of previous blood tests. The history of diabetes and vascular disease is also a clues, at a minimum to categorize him as at risk of renal impairment.

Answers *cont.*

On the other hand, the normal haemoglobin level (albeit probably increased somewhat by intravascular hypovolaemia) argues against preceding underlying severe renal impairment, which would usually be accompanied by significant anaemia. A simple additional investigation is abdominal imaging (usually a renal tract ultrasound) to determine the size and appearance of the kidneys. Small, echogenic kidneys are diagnostic of underlying chronic renal failure, whereas acute renal failure alone usually has normal appearing kidneys.

A.6 Acutely all of his current medications should be stopped. He is hypotensive and so the combined ACE inhibitor/diuretic should not be given. The ACE inhibitor will also hinder recovery from the acute renal failure due to interference with glomerular blood flow autoregulation. The half life of the oral hypoglycaemic gliclazide will be prolonged in the setting of deteriorating renal function, increasing the risk of prolonged hypoglycaemia. Metformin serum levels also increase in renal impairment, which in turn increases the risk of lactic acidosis. His diabetes would probably be best managed in the short term with an intravenous insulin infusion and close monitoring of blood sugar levels. He will require a number of invasive investigations and treatments, and so it would be preferable to withhold the aspirin. Finally, the celocoxib is likely to have contributed to his acute renal deterioration, and should also be stopped.

Longer term medications will depend to a large extent on the level of renal function to which he recovers. He will need to resume antihypertensives, and an ACE inhibitor may be the best option again, particularly in view of his history of cardiac disease. In moderate to severe renal impairment hyperkalaemia can be a limiting side-effect of ACE inhibitors, so that will need to be monitored. Unless his underlying renal impairment is quite mild (e.g. GFR >45 mL/min), it will be best to avoid metformin use, and NSAIDs should be avoided if he has any significant degree of residual renal dysfunction.

A.7 It is likely that he will remain oliguric or anuric for a prolonged period (days to even weeks), failing to clear urea and creatinine and requiring regular dialysis. During this treatment phase his biochemistry must be monitored regularly, preferably at least daily, and the dialysis parameters adjusted to maintain safe levels of hydration and biochemical indices, in particular potassium. Fluid intake must be dictated by urine output, with account taken for insensible fluid losses. An accurate fluid balance chart, regular assessment of state of hydration, and daily accurate weighing of the patient, are all simple but vital tasks. At times there is an obligate excess fluid intake, for example for intravenous therapy or feeding (or nasogastric feeding). Attempts to increase the urine output with diuretics in this phase are unlikely to be fruitful, and additional fluid will need to be removed by regular dialysis.

The recovery phase from an episode of acute renal failure (acute tubular necrosis) is heralded by a steady increase in the urine output, followed some days later by stabilization and then fall in the serum creatinine.

Often urine output will dramatically increase to very large volumes; this is the dangerous 'polyuric phase' of recovery after acute renal failure, which requires even more careful monitoring of fluid status. Fluid intake must not be reduced, as a patient who is producing 500–1000 mL of urine per hour will quickly become profoundly hypovolaemic. Intravenous fluid, where

Answers *cont.*

volume is still dictated by the urine output (input = output + insensible losses, i.e. 'chase the urine'!) is essential. Ongoing daily weighing, assessment of state of hydration and an accurate fluid balance chart continue to be fundamental tasks.

Patients in the polyuric recovery phase waste salts, and supplementation of potassium is frequently necessary (whereas before you were trying to get rid of it).

Sodium and chloride can be adjusted in the intravenous fluids. The severe acidosis recovers as renal function improves, as do the derangements in phosphate and calcium levels. Occasionally supplemental calcium is needed, particularly if tetany is present. Oral phosphate binders may be useful during the established phase of acute renal failure, although only if the patient is taking adequate amounts of food.

Revision Points

Acute Renal Failure

Pre-renal – due to inadequate perfusion, with structurally intact nephrons:

- Hypotension.
- Hypovolaemia (dehydration, blood loss, burns).
- Heart failure (low cardiac output).
- Shock (septic, toxic, cardiogenic, other).
- Drugs (ACEI, NSAIDs, ARBs).

Intrinsic renal – structural and functional damage to nephrons:

- Vascular:
  - macrovascular: renal artery or vein obstruction
  - microvascular angiopathy: TTP/HUS, pre-eclampsia.
- Glomerular:
  - glomerulonephritis (immune complex (e.g. post-infectious), anti-basement

membrane antibodies (Goodpasture's), ANCA (Wegener's)).

- Tubular:
  - acute tubular necrosis (ischaemia or toxins)
  - drugs and crystals.
- Interstitial:
  - infections (pyelonephritis)
  - interstitial nephritis (drug or allergen)
  - amyloidosis (deposit in the tubules).

Post-renal – obstruction to passage of urine:

- Ureteric obstruction (kidney stones, retroperitoneal fibrosis).
- Bladder outlet obstruction (prostate cancer, neurogenic bladder).
- Renal injury/trauma.

Issues to Consider

- What are the most common causes of renal failure leading to dialysis?
- What forms of dialysis are available, and how are they chosen for individual patients?
- What are the indications for renal transplantation?
- What are the other complications of NSAID therapy?

Further Information

http://emedicine.medscape.com/ article/243492-overview *eMedicine acute renal failure.*

Pannu, N., Klarenbach, S., Wiebe, N., et al., 2008. Renal replacement therapy in patients with acute renal failure: a systematic review. Journal of the American Medical Association 299 (7), 793–805. *Free full text at: http:// jama.ama-assn.org/cgi/content/full/299/7/793.*

Index

Page numbers followed by 'f' indicate figures, 't' indicate tables, and 'b' indicate boxes.

A

Index

D

Index

Index